Food Safety in the Middle East

Food Safety in the Middle East

Edited by

Ioannis N. Savvaidis
Department of Environmental Health Sciences, College of Health Sciences, University of Sharjah, Sharjah, United Arab Emirates; Laboratory of Food Chemistry and Food Microbiology, Department of Chemistry, University of Ioannina, Ioannina, Greece

Tareq M. Osaili
Department of Clinical Nutrition and Dietetics, University of Sharjah, Sharjah, United Arab Emirates; Department of Nutrition and Food Technology, Jordan University of Science and Technology, Irbid, Jordan

ELSEVIER

ACADEMIC PRESS
An imprint of Elsevier

Academic Press is an imprint of Elsevier
125 London Wall, London EC2Y 5AS, United Kingdom
525 B Street, Suite 1650, San Diego, CA 92101, United States
50 Hampshire Street, 5th Floor, Cambridge, MA 02139, United States
The Boulevard, Langford Lane, Kidlington, Oxford OX5 1GB, United Kingdom

Notices
Knowledge and best practice in this field are constantly changing. As new research and experience broaden our understanding, changes in research methods, professional practices, or medical treatment may become necessary.

Practitioners and researchers must always rely on their own experience and knowledge in evaluating and using any information, methods, compounds, or experiments described herein. In using such information or methods they should be mindful of their own safety and the safety of others, including parties for whom they have a professional responsibility.

To the fullest extent of the law, neither the Publisher nor the authors, contributors, or editors, assume any liability for any injury and/or damage to persons or property as a matter of products liability, negligence or otherwise, or from any use or operation of any methods, products, instructions, or ideas contained in the material herein.

British Library Cataloguing-in-Publication Data
A catalogue record for this book is available from the British Library

Library of Congress Cataloging-in-Publication Data
A catalog record for this book is available from the Library of Congress

ISBN: 978-0-12-822417-5

For Information on all Academic Press publications
visit our website at https://www.elsevier.com/books-and-journals

Publisher: Charlotte Cockle
Acquisitions Editor: Nina Bandeira
Editorial Project Manager: Emerald Li
Production Project Manager: Bharatwaj Varatharajan
Cover Designer: Matthew Limbert

Typeset by MPS Limited, Chennai, India

Contents

List of contributors

Aisha Abushelaibi Higher Colleges of Technology, Abu Dhabi, United Arab Emirates

Anfal Al Katheeri Higher Colleges of Technology, Abu Dhabi, United Arab Emirates

Akram R. Alaboudi Department of Pathology and Public Health, Faculty of Veterinary Medicine, Jordan University of Science and Technology, Irbid, Jordan

Moza Abdullah Al-Busaidi Research and Innovation Sector, Ministry of Higher Education, Research and Innovation, Sultanate of Oman

Anas A. Al-Nabulsi Department of Nutrition and Food Technology, Jordan University of Science and Technology, Irbid, Jordan

Abdullah F. Alsayeqh Veterinary Medicine, College of Agriculture and Veterinary Medicine, Qassim University, Buraidah, Saudi Arabia

Wageh Sobhy Darwish Food Control Department, Faculty of Veterinary Medicine, Zagazig University, Zagazig, Egypt

Waleed Rizk El-Ghareeb Department of Public Health, College of Veterinary Medicine, King Faisal University, Al-Ahsa, Saudi Arabia

Dima Faour-Klingbeil DFK for Safe Food Environment, Food Safety and Regulatory Systems Compliance, Hannover, Germany; Centre for Rural Development, Humboldt University of Berlin, Germany

Ihab Habib Department of Veterinary Medicine, College of Agriculture and Veterinary Medicine, United Arab of Emirates University, Al Ain, United Arab Emirates; Department of Environmental Health, High Institute of Public Health, Alexandria University, Alexandria, Egypt; Centre for Biosecurity and One Health, School of Veterinary Medicine, Murdoch University, Perth, Australia

Kok-Song Lai Higher Colleges of Technology, Abu Dhabi, United Arab Emirates

Swee-Hua Erin Lim Higher Colleges of Technology, Abu Dhabi, United Arab Emirates

Mohamed Yousif Ibrahim Mohamed Department of Veterinary Medicine, College of Agriculture and Veterinary Medicine, United Arab of Emirates University, Al Ain, United Arab Emirates

Alaa Eldin M.A. Morshdy Food Control Department, Faculty of Veterinary Medicine, Zagazig University, Zagazig, Egypt

Amin N. Olaimat Department of Clinical Nutrition and Dietetics, Faculty of Applied Medical Sciences, The Hashemite University, Zarqa, Jordan

Tareq M. Osaili Department of Clinical Nutrition and Dietetics, University of Sharjah, Sharjah, United Arab Emirates; Department of Nutrition and Food Technology, Jordan University of Science and Technology, Irbid, Jordan

Ioannis N. Savvaidis Department of Environmental Health Sciences, College of Health Sciences, University of Sharjah, Sharjah, United Arab Emirates; Department of Chemistry, University of Ioannina, Ioannina, Greece

Ewen C.D. Todd Ewen Todd Consulting, LLC, Okemos, MI, United States

About the editors

Ioannis N. Savvaidis

Ioannis N. Savvaidis is a professsor in the Department of Environmental Health, College of Health Sciences, University of Sharjah, United Arab Emirates. He is a graduate of London University (United Kingdom) and a holder of PhD in Microbiology. He has been actively involved in teaching of various courses, related to Life and Health Sciences, including General Microbiology, Food Microbiology, Food Quality Management, Food Toxicology, and Food Preservation. His research interests include Novel Techniques of Food Preservation, Use of Natural Antimicrobials in Food Safety and Quality, The Microbial Ecology of Traditional Mediterranean and Middle Eastern Foods, and especially Food Safety issues regarding the growth, survival, and monitoring of foodborne pathogens in these Foods and Foods Products. He has been a visiting professor of the American University of Beirut and Qatar University.

Tareq M. Osaili

Tareq M. Osaili is a professor of Food Safety at Jordan University of Science and Technology, Jordan, and currently he is the Vice Dean of the College of Health Sciences at the University of Sharjah, United Arab Emirates. He finished his PhD in Food Science from the University of Arkansas, United States. In the past two decades, his research focused on detection and inactivation of pathogenic microorganisms in foods using innovative techniques and assessment of food safety knowledge, attitude, and practice of the communities. He has published more than 130 original research and review articles in peer-reviewed international journals and contributed in many book chapters. Prof. Osaili has been selected as an expert at the Joint FAO/WHO Expert Meetings on Microbiological Risk Assessment (JEMRA) for 5 years (2018–22).

Preface

The impact of foodborne disease has been discounted in many parts of the world, including the Middle East, based on the limited resources allocated to its control. However, in some ways this type of illness has a silent impact on the public which society considers as unfortunate but acceptable as a mild illness short-lived. I wrote in 2004 that at present, there is no clear connection between government policy and a reduction in foodborne illness. Although national disease statistics may show gradual declines over long periods for some pathogens associated with food, other problems, including new pathogens, tend to emerge. In some ways this has not changed for many Middle Eastern countries in the 21st century. The implementation of risk-based and preventive food safety systems is generally voluntary and still far from being addressed in regulating the safety of the locally sold foods, and whole-genome sequencing used in epidemiological investigations of foodborne outbreaks to identify and characterize pathogens is still not a standard tool or used in many countries, including the Middle East, due to limited skills or resources. One of the problems is that international food safety regulations and requirements continue to evolve to adapt to food safety challenges responding to the rapid changes along the global supply chain, and Middle Eastern countries need to be in the forefront of these rather than following in a reactionary way, especially in dealing with imports and exports. Although there is a continuing demand for traditional and unique Middle Eastern foods both in the Levant and Gulf countries, consumer perception within the Middle East is changing due to globalization along with business and marketing, and that presents new food safety challenges.

In the Middle East, the true incidence of foodborne infections is difficult to determine since there are limited systematic surveillance efforts to detect sporadic cases and outbreaks, and also to provide isolates that could be used for source attribution and risk assessment at national and regional levels. Unfortunately, most foodborne disease incidents are only covered in the press, if at all, with relatively few in scientific publications or epidemiological or medical reports to show what went wrong in the food production or preparation that led to the contamination. These press news items are typically limited in that they cover the initial complaints and government action against the commercial suppliers or food preparers but do not follow up to discover the etiological agents or the factors contributing to the outbreaks.

Generally, local and national governments tend to punish with fines and even imprisonments managers and staff in those establishments that are found to be responsible for foodborne illnesses even if the actual cause is not known. Although much of the book is devoted to pathogen-related illnesses, there are also issues with the overuse of pesticides and uncontrolled use of veterinary antimicrobial agents which are not well understood. The presence of heavy metals in wastewater and foods, and mold contamination of crops leading to production of mycotoxins, particularly aflatoxin, is of concern. In foodservice establishments the proportion of trained individuals is relatively low, except for those working in the hospitals. Studies on food safety knowledge, attitudes, and practices of food handlers in foodservice establishments in the Arab countries are growing slowly since the last decade. However, they are still a few in number. Although certification of foodservice and food processing employees is required in Arab-speaking countries everywhere where food is processed, prepared, and served commercially, food handlers are not in strong favor of monitoring and controlling the temperature of food, which was similarly reflected in their self-reported practices. Information on food handlers' knowledge and self-reported practices indicate that there are inadequacies in existing food safety training and underscore the need for continuous training and refresher courses that integrate learning on foodborne diseases and their causative agents and be able to identify food hazards to implement appropriate preventative and control measures.

This is not to say that some concerns are not being addressed. Awareness of the public should be that Arab citizens have the right to access safe food. Laws have been put in place or are being considered to give governments more powers to prevent and control foodborne illnesses. Improvements in conducting investigations of complaints of illness are also being established such as a National Rapid Alert System, enhanced laboratory capacity, and government and private contractors creating online and in-person courses to meet the necessary food safety standards. Many of these food control agencies now have credibility with the public. However, improved epidemiological surveillance systems are required as essential for enhancing national and regional prevention and control systems. This is especially important not only for residents of these countries but for making tourists safer, and less likelihood that imported and exported foods are contaminated. For processed foods, it is important that a multihurdle approach is used to prevent pathogen growth where added preservatives, inactivation treatments, and appropriate packaging to retain both freshness and safety of perishable food products. It is also critical that collaboration between Arab and international Food Safety regulators, as well as sustaining capacity building efforts, is enhanced.

Because it was predicted in 1997, unless the global accident rate is reduced, by the year 2015, an airliner will crash somewhere in the world almost weekly, a White House Commission on Aviation Safety and Security was created, and its principal focus was on reducing the rate of accidents by a factor of five within a decade with a modernization of safety and security systems. The implementation of such systems around the world did substantially reduce the risks of crashes. We need something similar for countries to take food safety seriously and reduce the number of illnesses, hospitalizations, and deaths as well as the years lost to disabilities brought on through chronic infections and poor quality of life resulting in early deaths as measured by Disability-Adjusted Life Years (DALYs). Let us remind ourselves of these large numbers. According to the WHO, 1 in 10 people who eat contaminated food fall ill. Each year worldwide, unsafe food causes 600 million cases of foodborne diseases and 420,000 deaths with 30% of foodborne deaths occur among children under 5 years of age. In contrast, in 2020, there were 137 civil aviation crash fatalities worldwide. A staggering 33 million years of healthy lives (DALYs) are lost due to eating unsafe food globally each year, and this number is likely an underestimation. The Eastern Mediterranean Region, which includes the Middle Eastern countries, has the third highest estimated burden of foodborne diseases per population, after the African and South-East Asia Regions. More than 100 million people living in the Eastern Mediterranean Region are estimated to become ill with a foodborne disease every year with 37,000 deaths; 32 million of those affected are children under 5 years. Both typhoid fever and hepatitis A are contracted from food contaminated by the feces of an infected person, and brucellosis is commonly caused by unpasteurized milk or cheese of infected goats or sheep. Half of the global cases of brucellosis are in people living in this region, with more than 195,000 people infected every year, causing fever, muscle pain or more severe arthritis, chronic fatigue, neurologic symptoms, and depression. In addition to disease incidence and deaths, the disease burden in terms of DALYs is very high with 33 million DALYs of which children under 5 years old bore 40% of this burden. Maybe a high-level commission is needed to address these shameful numbers, but however it is tackled Middle Eastern Arab nations need to vigorously pursue regional strategies to minimize the risks of foodborne disease to their populations and visitors alike, and this book should be a stimulus to those responsible to move in this direction.

This is the first comprehensive book on *Food Safety in the Middle East*. Its contents should appeal to any with an interest in food safety in the region, especially students, researchers, government officials, food processing consultants or technologists, and even concerned everyday consumers.

Ewen C.D. Todd
Ewen Todd Consulting LLC, Okemos, MI United States

Chapter 1

Traditional foods, food safety practices, and food culture in the Middle East

Ioannis N. Savvaidis[1,2], Anfal Al Katheeri[3], Swee-Hua Erin Lim[3], Kok-Song Lai[3] and Aisha Abushelaibi[3]
[1]Department of Environmental Health Sciences, College of Health Sciences, University of Sharjah, Sharjah, United Arab Emirates, [2]Department of Chemistry, University of Ioannina, Ioannina, Greece, [3]Higher Colleges of Technology, Abu Dhabi, United Arab Emirates

1.1 Introduction

The consumption of food constitutes a basic need in life as its consumption helps provide the organism with nutritional support. Food is a composite mixture of various ingredients that are consumed for nutrition, health, and well-being of humans. Food may consist of essential nutrients such as carbohydrates, proteins, fats, minerals, and vitamins. For humans, however, the process of achieving satiety is often shared with family, friends, and visitors, or to a lesser extent, strangers (Fox, 2003). Food defines history, culture, and tradition. In addition, food also plays a vital and important role in the promotion of health and disease prevention. Nutritionists have claimed that to survive, humans require four main types of food, which are vegetables, grains, dairy products, and meats (Fox, 2003). In addition, for reasons that initially started off as improving taste and promoting safety, the practice of cooking has now evolved to become a necessity, developing into symbolic representations of certain cultures and geographical regions. The practices of food intake are affected by factors such as genetic, social, psychological, and cultural (Castro, 2004).

Food habits between cultures have changed over time, providing variation ranging from traditional to modern; this evolution is not only attributed to migration but also attributed to urbanization. Furthermore, behavior toward food and eating, despite being conditioned during childhood, is closely related to tradition and culture. What is eaten and not eaten distinguishes the palate of various cultures; this is applied also to the method of preparation

Food Safety in the Middle East. DOI: https://doi.org/10.1016/B978-0-12-822417-5.00009-X

and special dishes. The passing of certain methods of food preparation or dishes from one generation to the next that is still in use today can be referred to as "traditional foods (TFs)." Moreover, TFs can also be defined as foods that have been through simple processing methods such as drying, cooking, and natural fermentation (Prakash, 2016). It is important to preserve the heritage of TFs as it will give people an identity.

The Middle-Eastern countries are in a region where tremendous valuable and diverse natural resources may be found. This attribute has significantly impacted the region through the import of foreign labor and modernizing of the region over time. Even though urbanization has made life easier, holding on to history and traditional culture remains as an important aspect of life in the people of the Middle-Eastern countries, despite the transition of people from rural areas to urban cities.

TFs and the Middle East are inextricably linked and there is common knowledge that food plays a huge role in the Middle East. Regions within the Middle East have their own unique dishes and special taste when authentic TFs are concerned. Culture preferences, affordability, and influences of education and media in addition to individuals needs are categorized according to the variety of food availability (Kuhnlein & Receveur, 1996). To understand certain people's choices toward food, their consumption, or their food culture, it is necessary to understand their religion and tradition (Nam, Jo, & Lee, 2010). Therefore in this chapter, various aspects of TFs in the Middle-Eastern countries, their nutritional values, preparation, and health aspects will be discussed. In addition, consumer perception and the relevance of TF consumption in the modern world along with future prospect and awareness efforts to sustain their presence in the current days going into the future will be discussed.

1.2 The Middle East—history of the Middle-Eastern foods

Middle East is a term describing a geographical area that extends from Egypt to Afghanistan, or the region in which Islam was developed. This book will only cover the Arabic-speaking Middle East countries, which include Egypt, Jordan, Palestine, Lebanon, Syria, Yemen, and the Arabian Gulf countries (Bahrain, Kuwait, Iraq, Oman, Qatar, Saudi Arabia, and the United Arab Emirates). These countries share similar social, political, economic, culture, religion, language, and ancestry. The main religion is Islam and the climate tends to be hot and dry with most parts receiving some rainfall, but usually amounts are small or irregular to sustain a continuous settled agriculture. Nowadays one could look at various aspects of the Middle East through examining other notions and values, apart from food, culinary habits, and so on. The landscape and country territories of the Middle East areas have undergone geographical changes in view of the continuing wars in the area and as a result of people having to dislocate, migrate, or escape to seek a better and safe future for their families. On the contrary, a number of Gulf countries have been changing, in terms of population diversity, as a result of the tourist boom, property development, infrastructure, and so on, attracting huge funds for investment in computer technologies, and this is due to both natural available oil/gas revenues in the area, as well on strategic plans of local governments to attract outside funds, so as to increase prosperity, health, and education in the area. It may also be therefore said that due to the influx of expats and of several communities into this area, we have seen changes in the TFs and in food culture. Such changes may have an impact on the existing food nutritional habits as well as on food quality and food safety standards and consequently may alter the food culture behavior of the various people ethnicity who constitute the Middle East.

The peak in Islamic Civilization (Kirk, 2016) contributed to development in culture, economy, and science. Islam was not the only religion practiced at that time; Christianity and Judaism were also present; these also influenced food preparation and dietary practices. Islam prohibits the consumption of pork and blood along with drinking alcohol (Tajkarimi, Ibrahim, & Fraser, 2013). Such prohibitions have contributed to a change in the eating style of Muslims as they create dishes with less fat contents, which conversely lowered the chance of developing noncommunicable chronic diseases that can be avoided.

The world's first written recipes were Middle Eastern, found on stone tablets dating from the 17th century BC. But the major Middle-Eastern medieval recipe collections were written in the palaces of Baghdad during Islam's golden age, between the 7th and 13th century, the very moment when Europe descended into the Dark Ages.

Arabic foods were transported by Turkish conquerors at Topkapi Palace and the Aya Sofya in Istanbul. From the 15th century onwards, the Ottomans carried the flame of Middle-Eastern TFs and cuisine that we also see also today in the Eastern Mediterranean culture (Greece, Cyprus etc.) as well as in the most of Central European countries, due to the emigrants, mostly during the last decades of the closing 20th century and after the devastating World Wars I and II.

Middle-Eastern food is moving beyond, simply being recognized for well-known dishes such as kebabs and Shawarmas, to embracing its modern positioning as a healthy, superfood with infused gastronomy designed to bring people together.

With the benefits of being wholesome, tasty, and healthy food, this cuisine combines the best of both worlds and a range of external environmental influences, as well as changes in consumer expectations from food and drink are skyrocketing Middle-Eastern food into mainstream culture. This may just be the beginning of the greatest shift in the food space, in which food from this region forms the basis for other cuisines to aspire to.

1.3 Traditional foods of the Middle East

1.3.1 General aspects

It's quite hard to put a clear-cut definition between traditional and non-TFs, especially with the great changes in the food culture in the Middle East and in the Gulf. In general, TFs are those foods that are commonly consumed in a country, through customs and traditions. They are highly accepted by the local communities and additionally people know how to prepare TFs, to be included in local dishes. TFs are often recognized by consumers with characteristics linked to regional identity and sensory quality, sold under different trademarks and, in general, consumers show a favorable attitude toward such products (Guerrero, 2001). Traditional means proven usage in the community market for a time period showing transmission between generations; this time period should be the one generally ascribed as one human generation, at least 25years (EU, 2006). Recently, a definition of TF has been developed through the work of the EuroFIR FP6 Network of Excellence. This is an elaborative definition, which includes statements about traditional ingredients, traditional composition, and traditional type of production and/or processing (EuroFIR, 2007; Trichopoulou, Soukara, & Vasilopoulou, 2007).

1.3.2 Types of Middle-Eastern foods

The Arab cuisine is identified as regional dishes covering the Arabian countries from the Maghreb to the Fertile Crescent and the Arabian Peninsula. Every region within the Middle East has its own unique type and way of eating TFs. In fact, rice is one of the essentials of food in the Gulf countries. Many recipes use rice as their main ingredient. Dishes such as Chicken Machboos (spiced chicken and rice), Kabsa (mixed rice with meat, vegetables and spices), Maqluba (rice, meat and vegetables), and Mandi (rice, meat, saffron) are dishes that are mainly consumed during lunchtime.

Parathas or chapatis is another TF eaten in the Gulf; mainly influenced by the Indian diet due to the immigrants from Indian subcontinent. Date bread is a common food consumed in Arabian Gulf along with thin pan bread. Millet bread, Sorghum bread, wheat bread, and flat bread are all types of foods that are consumed frequently in the Gulf region. Moreover, broad beans, chickpeas, and black-eye beans are common types of legumes that are consumed in the Middle East. Milk (cow, camel, goat, sheep) and milk products such as, labneh (kind of "Greek yogurt"), soft white cheese, butterfat milk (or laban as known in the area), ghee, and hard cheese are also considered TFs in the Middle East.

Meat, fish, and their products like goat meat, camel meat, fermented fish sauce like Mehiawah or Tareeh, and certain types of fish like hamour, sheri, tuna, barracuda, grouper, trevally, emperor, and pomfret (FAO, 2011) are main ingredients in preparing traditional meat or seafood dishes in the

Middle East. Sweets and confectioneries include corn flour sweet, nashab or darabeel (nut rolls), sesame sweet, and sweet samosa. Lastly, other products like Dakkous (hot tomato sauce), Hab (seeds), Baharat (mixed species), chickpea snack, and Arabic coffee (Musaiger & Miladi, 1993) are also considered TF. Other regions in the Middle East have distinguished food like Hummus, kibbeh, Mansaf, Masgoof, Shawarma, and Tahini (Amr & Yaseen, 1994; Ayaz, Sawaya, & Al-Sogair, 1986). All these foods described are considered TFs and served in both normal and special occasions.

1.3.3 Current trends

It is widely accepted that the Middle East area and especially the Gulf countries over the past 4–5 decades, mainly as a result of a massive influx of mostly Asian communities, including also other expats have witnessed changes, with regard to the local food cultural habits. However, at the same time, national dishes have regained their character and local consumers welcomed new food cultural influences, as an alternative, to their TFs. A transformation of what was perceived last century as staple foods of the Middle East (bread, rice, dates, meat, fish, or dairy based on camel milk, and so on) has been taking place and what is certain and widely admitted by food connoisseurs, that Middle-Eastern foods (mostly) have themselves emigrated to Europe and the United States. This has been due to the emigrants of the so-called "diaspora" (educated mostly Lebanese, Syrians, or other Arab-speaking countries) that sought jobs and a stable future for themselves or for their families fleeing to Western affluent countries. However, producers of local traditional Middle-Eastern types of foods have been confronted with new challenges to further improve the safety, healthiness, and convenience of their products, by means of different innovations, which will enable them to maintain and expand their foods to global markets.

1.3.4 Importance of traditional foods

Certain groups of people are associated with a certain type of TF. Food knowledge among a group of people living together is commonly passed from generation to another; this is one method to sustain their culture, a part of which is food. In fact, TF plays an important role not only in the physical nourishment but also in cultural attributes in most communities worldwide (Pufall et al., 2011) providing an identity to that people group. A concept by Hippocrates that has existed since ancient times has been stated as "food as medicine" (Ranfa, Maurizi, Romano, & Bodesmo, 2014). TFs that are nutrient enriched have a long history of supporting health and wellness. Dates, for example, is a nutrient-rich TF, widely consumed in the Gulf mostly but also in some of the MENA countries. Dates are considered as one of the essentials in every Gulf family's larder due to its essential sources of nutrients such as fiber, sugar, magnesium, calcium, potassium, and carbohydrates (Khan, 2018).

Nowadays, traditional knowledge and practices from various continents have been integrated with modern science, which then led to the formation of new food models. For example, combining Asian, Mediterranean, African, Central and Latin American, and other traditional and ethnic foods will produce a new type of "combinational food equation." This new type of food may also be nutrient rich and considered as a new traditional "fusion" food. Moreover, TFs and ingredients have the potential to boost the health, medicinal, and nutraceutical values (Prakash, 2016).

The importance of TF divulges an exploration of culture. Hence, what we consume, how we acquire it, who prepares it, and who eats first are the forms of communication, heritage, and culture. TFs help us to discover attitudes, practices, and rituals along with strengthening the bonds between individuals, communities, and countries (Boutaud, Becuţ, & Marinescu, 2016). Therefore continuing the practice of making and eating TF holds an enormous amount of ethnic history and roots, as it serves as an important reminder of tradition and identity of formation.

1.4 Food safety practices

Food safety practices in the Middle East, including the Gulf area, generally have not seem significant changes over the past half decade. However, these areas have welcomed new food practices, as culturally certain areas have been affected by the influx of various communities, mainly in certain Gulf countries (UAE, Qatar, etc.) and to a lesser extent in the upper Middle-Eastern area. It is well documented in the aforementioned countries, expatriates may in some cases amount up to 80%–86% of the total population, and food practices therefore have been changing over the past two to three decades (Gulf Migration, 2016).

TF practices are still native and followed by the local consumers, especially those areas that have remained avoid of emigrants, expatriates, tourists, business travelers, and so on. Due to the high temperatures that are characteristic especially in the Gulf area, including parts of the upper Middle East (July, August) during summer, fresh foods (mostly of animal origin) are prone to rapid spoilage, quality degradation, and most importantly hazards related to foodborne infectious diseases.

One of the most significant factors, affecting Food Safety practices, is the temperature of the environment, affecting the survival and growth of all types of bacteria, and usually those of concern to humans, such as *Listeria monocytogenes*, *Salmonella* spp., *Staphylococcus aureus*, and *Escherichia coli* O157:H7 if found in food products. Refrigeration is mostly available for most of the consumers living in rural areas and cooling (by means of refrigeration) of households (A/C), supermarkets (by means of refrigeration), food processing companies (by means of refrigeration), and transport of food items (by means of refrigeration) are all widely available. However, during summer months, even under controlled cooling conditions, fresh foods or food products bought from supermarkets or even from local markets (fish or meat) may become exposed to high ambient temperatures (and as these being considered highly perishable) may present a food safety risk to the consumers. Apart from the temperature factor of the environment, it is widely accepted that other food safety practices such as personal hygiene, safe food handling of food products at home, prepared cooking modes of foods, all contribute significantly to food safety practices.

As with other areas globally, food practices especially in the Middle East have relied upon TFs processing preparations, either at homes or restaurants/caterings levels. Unless effective measures and practices are applied, by the consumers either at home or at the caterings, or even at large social events (e.g., during Ramadan period), all types of food preparations (homemade, restaurants/and caterings) easily perishable, as well as nonperishable food products, are likely to be contaminated with microorganisms. In some cases, food-borne pathogenic bacteria may be contaminating food products, thus posing serious health risks to the consumers, especially children, pregnant women, the elderly, and the immunocompromised or those with chronic health-related diseases. It is thus absolutely crucial, and in order to minimize risks and hazards related to food safety practices, to follow strict hygienic conditions from farm (fields) and up to the (plate) "fork"—A food safety ritual or quote widely postulated by scientists and in order to avoid foodborne illnesses.

The main global challenges of the foodborne diseases can be summarized as: (1) the identification of emerging foodborne pathogens; (2) the increase in the proportion of the foodborne illnesses susceptible groups (e.g., children, elderly, and pregnant women, and people with immunocompromised diseases) in the developed countries; (3) the increase of food globalization via food trading, which spread the pathogens all over the world; (4) the increase of the tourism activity between countries, which may spread some new foodborne pathogens and put select people at risk; (5) the introduction of new pathogens into a new environment, which might affect the sensitivities of these pathogens to antibiotics; thereby, producing resistance to antibiotic; and (6) the increasing rate of consuming food outside the home, which enhances the risk related to poor handling practices of some food establishments (WHO, 2015).

Unsafe practices still exist among the people of the Middle East, especially in the Arabian Gulf region. Especially, in remote areas locals, farmers, and/or their families may consume their freshly available produce, such as raw milk that may be contaminated with pathogenic bacteria (e.g., *Brucella* spp). In one study, it was reported that raw camel milk samples sold in Saudi Arabia were commonly contaminated with *S. aureus* (70%) and *Salmonella*

(24%) (El-Ziney & Al-Turki, 2007). These results emphasize the unsafe food practice of the consumption of raw camel milk and possible foodborne diseases or outbreaks. Under hot climatic conditions, pathogenic bacteria contaminating food products multiply quickly and thus may reach high numbers, posing severe food safety risks and in some cases involving even human fatalities. The Gulf area over the past decade has seen the emergence of reoccurrence of an important microorganism (*Brucella* spp) that is responsible for milk-borne-related disease known as Brucellosis. The region witnessed approximately 100 cases of human Brucellosis per 100,000 persons/year. The highest incidence rates of Brucellosis have been reported to occur in Iraq, Saudi Arabia, and Jordan (Rubach, Halliday, Cleavel, & Crump, 2013).

Homemade preparations and practices are still part of daily activities in the Middle East and the Gulf areas, posing food safety risks such as improper cooking, unhygienic food handling, as well as high ambient temperature are all being factors contributing to both spoilage of food products (and also potentially unsafe for consumption) by the presence, survival, or growth of bacteria, potentially causing a foodborne infection. A study conducted in the Eastern Mediterranean region (Turkey, having similar food safety practices, as in the Middle East) concluded that that a high percentage (87%) homemade preparations were responsible for foodborne outbreaks, mainly due to improper hygienic practices, improper keeping storage temperatures during food processing, as well as inadequate heating before serving the food (Karabudak, Bas, & Kiziltan, 2008).

Another practice that may be posing a food safety risks in the Middle East area is the purchase of raw materials, sold unpackaged, and if available as bulk products in open fresh produce markets, may be of questionable quality. These products may be held at room or under environmental (in some cases during summer months) abuse temperature conditions, raising serious concerns about their microbiological safety. According to Ismail (2006) the quality of raw materials used for making traditional "Hawashy" or hummus was questionable as no heat treatment was used in the preparation of hummus (apart from boiling of the chick peas) thus raising concerns about the microbiological safety of the product. Hummus on most occasions is a product that is held at room temperature, and as result of the various types of bacteria introduced from raw materials or upon processing, or even cross-contamination, may be contaminated with both spoilage and foodborne-causing infections-bacteria, such as *Listeria* and *E. coli* spp. (Al-Nabulsi et al., 2013).

Scenes of food practices that are characteristic of the Middle East area, and to a lesser extent of the Gulf nowadays, may involve street food preparations to be sold right on that day, prepared by vendors on the streets and/or within small shops (e.g., "fateh" (a chickpeas with yogurt meal), ful medames (cooked beans), or mutabal (eggplant), hummus and felafel (chick peas/tahini) preparations, and so on). These foods prepared on certain big city streets, both highly trafficked (e.g., as in Beirut scenes of barbequing meat, or hand-pressed pomegranate fresh juice) and air-borne polluted, are likely to be frequently contaminated (and also from food handler's hands) with bacteria; therefore incidents of foodborne pathogens or even further occurring illnesses are likely. It is well established that, both *Listeria* spp., being abundant in the environment, and *S. aureus*, a commonly found microorganism on the hands or skin of humans, may contaminate foods, and if conditions allow the growth of these bacterial species in high numbers, incidents of foodborne infections are likely.

Numerous reports have revealed the risks associated with consuming contaminated street-vended foods that have high levels of coliform bacteria and pathogenic bacteria, such as *E. coli*, *Salmonella* spp., *S. aureus*, *Bacillus cereus*, *Clostridium perfringens*, and *Vibrio cholera* (Cho et al., 2011; El-Obeid, Aziz, Mousa, & Alzahiri, 2014; Hanashiro, Morita, Matt, Matt, & Torres, 2005). Ismail (2006) reported that street foods have been found to harbor certain foodborne pathogens and high bacterial counts in different countries in the Middle East region.

In the Gulf area, El-Obeid et al. (2014) conducted a study involving 56 samples purchased from 10 different street vendors. Samples were tested for microbial contaminants (*Salmonella* spp., *L. monocytogenes, E. coli*, and *E. coli* 0157:H7). Out of the 56 samples, only two samples "Biryani" and "Khabess" contained *E. coli*. However, these two samples tested negative for *E. coli* O157:H7. The microbial contamination of the Qatari traditional street-vended foods was low (3%). The authors concluded that the low (%) microbial population of the street-vented foods may be attributed to both the Food Safety training (required) program of food handlers in Qatar and the food inspection tests, conducted by the Food Health Inspectors on a regular basis. Food service employees can spread foodborne diseases by hand due to poor personal hygiene, unhygienic living conditions, and inadequate training. Food handlers may contaminate foods through contact with feces, urine or noses, ears, or skins.

Interestingly, it was also recently reported that sharing food practices during public gatherings, feasts, labor camps, schools, and military camps in the GCC region was a major pathway of exposure to foodborne pathogens, such as *Shigella* spp., *Salmonella* spp., *Campylobacter coli*, *C. jejuni*, hepatitis A virus, rotavirus, and parasites (Todd, 2017a).

What seems to emerge as a key and important issue, especially in rural and remote areas, is the increasing need to educate locals, farmers, or consumers on implementing efficient pasteurization processes, in order to protect themselves and also the public health of their community members. Changing consumer habits, such as effective cooking processing of food products (that are likely to bear foodborne pathogenic microorganisms), proper and hygienic handling of foods, as well as in relation to the keeping of food products, under controlled refrigerated conditions, are very important issues in the region and will contribute positively to food safety standards and practices of the Middle East and the Gulf areas.

1.5 Culinary food preparations

The nutrients found in TFs depend on the preparation process. Cooking methods in the Middle East vary from stir frying, boiling, grilling; Tannoor is a traditional oven that is made from clay, but nowadays it is made of stainless steel (Al-Khusaibi, 2019). These methods may increase or lessen the nutritional value of the dish. It is stated that stir frying has little to no impact toward increasing or decreasing the nutritional value in fired food (Fillion & Henry, 1998), unlike boiling where a lot of nutritional values are lost. Moreover, grilling limits nutrient degradation as food is cooked in very high heat through short amount of time. Most of the foods in the Middle East are prepared using the above methods. Although the preparation method of the TFs is similar, the initial steps before boiling or frying may be different. Some TFs require soaking or marinating some ingredients before cooking as this step is important in enhancing the flavors or making the texture of the dish softer. For instance, Harees is a dish that is often eaten in Gulf countries. The basic ingredient of the dish is wheat. Before preparation, the wheat must be soaked in water to soften the wheat before putting it on fire to cook. Hummus and falafel (main ingredient being chick peas) are also dishes that are soaked before starting the cooking method. Foods like Shawarma, Tikka, Machboos, and Biryani are dishes that involve marinating the meat in a mixture of spices before cooking as it will induce the flavors and tenderness of the meat. Table 1.1 lists various types of TF preparations, their preparation/cooking methods, and the countries or the Middle East and regions that are widely consumed.

1.6 Food culture

In Western Europe and also in the United States, consumers nowadays, as a result of either a new trend toward a new healthier lifestyle or perhaps a need to more "natural," without chemical additives (posing toxicity in some cases to humans), have been seeking new foods that could be nutritional and having also potential functional benefits. Over the past decades, individuals, either traveling to the Middle East and Gulf areas for recreation, business, or those expatriates returning home have been acting as the best ambassadors of the Middle-Eastern cuisine and Arabic foods—a healthy diet with functional natural ingredients. Greater awareness of food from this region among modern consumers has allowed Middle-Eastern cuisine to emerge in new forms, and traditional flavors and spices such as harissa, za'atar, zhug, sumac, kefir, labneh, and tahini are becoming an increasingly popular spices

TABLE 1.1 Methods of cooking and traditional food preparation in the Middle East.

Plant-based Arab food				
Method of cooking	**Dish**	**Preparation method**	**Countries**	**References**
Boiling	Lentil soup	• Lentil is rinsed and soaked in cool water • Lentil is boiled until cooked • Vegetables, chicken stock, and spices are added into boiled lentil	Middle East region	de Almeida Costa, da Silva Queiroz-Monici, Pissini Machado Reis, and de Oliveira (2006)
	Bulgur	• Bulgur is boiled in water, salt, and oil	Turkey	Caba, Boyacioglu, and Boyacioglu (2011)
	Hummus	• Chickpeas are rinsed and boiled • Food processor is used to blend chickpeas • Tahini, olive oil, lemon juice, garlic, salt, cumin are added to chickpeas mix	Middle East region	Tajkarimi et al. (2013)
	Tabouleh	• Bulgur is boiled in water, salt, and oil • Garlic, parsley, mint, tomato, lemon juice, olive oil, and salt are added	Middle East region	Al-Marzooqi, Burke, Al Ghazali, Duffy, and Yousuf (2015)
	Kushari	• Lentil, rice, pasta, and chickpeas are boiled separately • Onion rings are fried • Garlic, coriander, red pepper flakes, and salt are added to tomato sauce	Egypt	Grivetti (2002)

(*Continued*)

TABLE 1.1 (Continued)

Plant-based Arab food				
Method of cooking	**Dish**	**Preparation method**	**Countries**	**References**
	Makdous	• Eggplants are boiled, drained, and cut into half and flattened using heavy objects • Eggplants are exposed to sunlight until dried • Chopped red pepper and walnut are added inside eggplants • Eggplants are stored inside jars to be cured in olive oil	Syria	Porreca et al. (2020)
Frying	Fattoush	• Arabic bread is coped into squared and deep dried until golden for garnishing • Lettuce, tomato, cucumber, green peppers, radishes, green onions, and parsley are added in a large bowl • Olive oil, lemon juice, garlic, sumac, pomegranate molasses, mint, salt, and pepper are added into the vegetables	Middle East region, Lebanon, Turkey, Greece	Todd (2017b)

(*Continued*)

TABLE 1.1 (Continued)

Plant-based Arab food				
Method of cooking	Dish	Preparation method	Countries	References
	Falafel	• Chickpeas are soaked overnight • chickpeas and chopped onion, parsley, coriander, garlic are added to food processor • Falafel mixture is shaped into balls and deep fried until golden	Egypt and Middle East region	Ismail and Kucukoner (2017)

Meat and fish Arab food				
Method of cooking	Dish	Preparation methods	Countries	References
Boiling	Meat/chicken Hareese	• Chicken or meat is boiled until tender • Bones are completely removed from chicken or meat • Wheat berries, cinnamon, salt, pepper is added into chicken or meat and covered with stock	United Arab Emirates	Habib, Ali, Ibrahim, and Afifi (2011)
	Meat Salona	• Lamb is boiled and then drained • Onion, garlic, turmeric, cinnamon bark, salt, pepper, and spices are cooked with meat • Tomato, potato, carrots are added to simmer and served	Saudi Arabia, Arabic region	
Frying	Machboos	• Chicken is rinsed and rubbed with spices • Chicken is fried in ghee or samin until browned • Garlic, tomato, dried lemon, cinnamon, cardamom, and coriander and potato are added to fried chicken	Gulf region	Habib et al. (2011), Sawaya et al. (1998)

(Continued)

TABLE 1.1 (Continued)

Meat and fish Arab food				
Method of cooking	Dish	Preparation methods	Countries	References
		• Rice is added after the removal of chicken from the pot to be boiled • Onion is fried for garnishing		
	Kibbeh,	• Minced meat and onion are cooked • Small amount of cooked meat bulgur and spices are processed into food processor • Kibbeh mixture are shaped into golf balls and filled with minced meat. • Kibbeh is deep fried in oil	Mediterranean, Lebanon, and nearby countries	Hoteit et al. (2020)
Grilled	Kofta	• Ground beef, parsley, onion, cumin, cinnamon, coriander, salt, and pepper are added into food processor to be minced • Kofta is shaped into oblong and placed in grill to be cooked	Mediterranean, Lebanon, and nearby countries	Hoteit et al. (2020)
	Kebab	• Cubed shaped lambs are mixed with garlic, olive oil, lemon juice, salt, and pepper • Lambs are threaded into skewers • Lamb skewers are grilled to be cooked	Mediterranean, Lebanon, and nearby countries	Hoteit et al. (2020)

(Continued)

TABLE 1.1 (Continued)

Meat and fish Arab food				
Method of cooking	**Dish**	**Preparation methods**	**Countries**	**References**
	Tikka	• Cubed shaped chicken breast is mixed with yogurt, garlic, ginger, lemon juice, coriander, cumin, turmeric, paprika, salt, and pepper • Chicken cubes are threaded into skewers and grilled	Mediterranean, Lebanon, and nearby countries	Hoteit et al. (2020)
	Shawarma	• Chicken breasts are combined and marinated with garlic, coriander, cumin, pepper, paprika, salt, lemon juice, and olive oil • Grill the marinated chicken breast and serve with bread, yogurt	Mediterranean, Jordan	Ahmed, El-Hakem, and Ibrahim (2015), Tajkarimi et al. (2013)

Beverages				
Method of cooking	**Drink**	**Preparation method**	**Countries**	**References**
Boiling	Yansoon	• Yansoon seeds and water are boiled, strained, and served	Arab countries	Mohammad and Abu-Rumman (2018), Saeed et al. (2013)
	Gahwa	• Boiled water is added into a pot • Arabic coffee and cardamom are added and brought to boil at low heat	Arab countries, Saudi Arabia	Ismail (2013), Jalloun and Alhathlool (2020), Rasheed and Al-Sowielem (2003)

(*Continued*)

TABLE 1.1 (Continued)

Beverages				
Method of cooking	Drink	Preparation method	Countries	References
		• Saffron is added into the dallah • Arabic coffee is strained and served		
	Chai Karak	• Tea, water, cardamom, saffron, and sugar are added into saucepan and boiled • Evaporated milk is added, boiled, strained, and served	Arab Gulf states, United Arab Emirates	
	Haba Al hamra	• Milk, custard, and condensed milk are mixed and boiled • Soaked cress seeds, saffron, rose water, and cardamom are added into the mixture	Arab countries, Qatar	Kilshaw et al. (2016)
Soaking	Qamar al-Din	• Dried apricots are soaked in warm water until it is dissolved • Sugar is added to strained dried apricots and served cold	Arab countries, Iraq, Levant	Amr (2015)

(*Continued*)

TABLE 1.1 (Continued)

Beverages				
Method of cooking	**Drink**	**Preparation method**	**Countries**	**References**
	Zhourat	• Zhourat is soaked in hot water, strained, and served with honey	Middle East	Obón, Rivera, Alcaraz, and Attieh (2014)
	Jellab	• Jellab syrup, water, and rose water are added and served	Lebanon, Jordon, Palestine and Syria	Montagnese et al. (2019)
Sweets				
Method of preparation	**Dish**	**Preparation method**	**Countries**	**References**
Boiling	Halwa	• Sugar and water are mixed until dissolved on low heat • Tapioca flour and water are mixed and added into the sugar and water mixture • Nutmeg, cardamom, and saffron are added until halwa is formed • Roasted nuts and sesame seed are added as garnishing	Middle East and Gulf countries especially Oman	Ali, Al Zuhaibi, Waly, Devarajan, and Johnson (2015), Musaiger and Miladi (1993)
Frying	Luqmat or Leqemat	• Flour, sugar, powdered milk, cardamom, saffron yeast, water, oil, eggs, and yogurt are mixed into pancake batter consistency	United Arab Emirates	Habib et al. (2011)

(*Continued*)

TABLE 1.1 (Continued)

Sweets				
Method of preparation	Dish	Preparation method	Countries	References
		• A scoop is taken and slowly dropped into frying oil until browned • Luqmat is served with date syrup		
	Qatayef	• Flour, semolina, baking powder, yeast, and water are mixed • The batter is cooked into small circles • Cream is added in the middle and pinched from the sides • Qatayef is deep fried and garnished with pistachio	Middle East region, Saudi Arabia, Kuwait	Al-Amiri, Ahmed, and Al-Sharrah (2020)
Tanoor/oven	Kunafeh	• Kadayif noodles are spread in butter-coated pan • Cheese is added on top of the kadayif noodles • Kunafeh pan is inserted into the oven until cheese is melted • The pan is flipped, syrup is added before serve	Mediterranean	Montagnese et al. (2019)
	Um Ali	• Bread is cut into small pieces and spread in dish • Nuts are sprinkled on top of bread • Milk, condensed milk, and sugar are brought to boil then poured over bread • The dish is baked until browned before serve	Middle East and Gulf countries	

(Continued)

TABLE 1.1 (Continued)

Sweets				
Method of preparation	**Dish**	**Preparation method**	**Countries**	**References**
	Maamol	• Ghee, sugar, flour, rose water, and milk are added to make the dough • Dates are added into food processor to make dates filling • A piece of dough is flattened, and a date filling is added to make cookie ball • Maamol is baked and served	Arab countries, Saudi Arabia	ElQuliti & Khashoggi (2017)
	Basbousa	• Selmolina, sugar, baking powder, yogurt, and coconut flakes are mixed • Mixture is poured into baking pan and baked • Syrup is poured into the basbousa before serve	Turkey, Jordan, Egypt, Morocco, Arabic region	
Oven method	Halwa	• Sugar and water are mixed until dissolved on low heat • Tapioca flour and water are mixed and added into the sugar and water mixture • Nutmeg, cardamom, and saffron are added until halwa is formed • Roasted nuts and sesame seed are added as garnishing	Middle East and Gulf countries especially Oman	Ali et al. (2015), Musaiger and Miladi (1993)

in Western dishes. Consumers are increasingly seeking transparency and authenticity: Middle-Eastern cuisine—with its emphasis on simplicity and natural ingredients—has benefited as a result.

Middle-Eastern cuisine is increasingly influencing not just what but also how we eat. While its dishes and tastes are becoming more widespread in the Western world today, evidence suggests this is just the beginning. Western food culture has transformed in the last two decades—driven by factors including globalization, changing lifestyles, health, well-being, and sustainability. During this revolution, Middle-Eastern cuisine has grown its presence in nontraditional markets dramatically—bringing rich, authentic dishes considered both flavorsome and healthy to tables across the world.

1.6.1 Eating habits

Hospitality is of utmost importance in this part of the world, and there is strong emphasis on enjoying meals with family and friends. Middle-Eastern hospitality is unique and those offered food or invited by locals at home mostly, if not wishing to even sample or nibble the food, may be in for a pleasant surprise, as the locals may insist on trying their homemade preparations.

This traditional offering may be traced to even early inhabitants in the area, inviting one another of all together sitting around food meal preparations, after a day with scotching sun in the desert as it was with nomads or those sitting onboard of fishing vessels. However, even today in modern megacities, like Cairo, Dubai, Beirut, Jeddah or Damascus, the eating habits still retain the elementary culinary must foods, as previously mentioned, and consumers nowadays have valued the various benefits (freshness, nutritional, wholesomeness) of the Middle-Eastern foods.

1.6.2 Religious or fest meals

Arabic or Middle-Eastern foods may trace their origins from prehistoric times in Mesopotamia, around Iraqi and the upper Arabic region area, or even dating back to early nomads, caravans, locals before the arrival of Islam. Early communities, usually residing in small villages or passing through the desert (not constantly staying in one place) and those by the sea coast all relied on simple food items available readily, like camel milk, dates livestock-based products like yogurt, cheese, and fish/seafood. Apart from these basic staple foods, that sustained life in the area, it is important to note the role of beverages that played in these areas. It has been said that as early as prehistoric times, milk as a beverage was available usually as camel milk and or even before as goat milk playing a key role in maintaining life, sustaining therefore all living dependent forms such as humans, animals, even plant species, and so on. Especially according to the Islamic culture or even dating back to the Old Testament, the goat was a highly valued animal and slaughtered in religious fests (Eid-ul-Adha) and amazingly enough even in modern eras, locals of the area are still honoring this tradition, paying tribute to the religious norms. Even probably not well known to the average consumer is the fact that fermentation was accidentally discovered in the Middle-Eastern area, as milk stored in leather flask and under high ambient temperatures turned sour and turning into yoghurt.

Finally, it is important to highlight the fact that fermentation, a unique process sustaining life even in prehistoric or after the spread of Islam, or at the aftermath of the Ottoman empire (Lewis, 1980) had its origins in the Middle East. The important role of wine and of other products in the region ("arak") has been acknowledged by food historians, in a way sustaining early inhabitants in the regions, that traveled days through deserts and without access to fresh, safe, and hygienic water at its source. Wine or related beverages in a way played a kind of a food safety role, having no harmful surviving bacteria that would pose risks of food-borne related infections. This is probably not widely even today known and most importantly, the origin of the word "al-cohol" may have its roots to Arabic origin. The Middle East and the Gulf areas were home to important scientists, the so well-known "Al-Chemists" and paved a path to the Medieval Europe, by transferring existing knowledge and practical expertise on Chemistry, Mathematics, Geometry and Astrology, as well as Agriculture. The agricultural practices as applied by the Arabs were all developed in Spain (Andalusia, or Al-Andalus, a Muslim-ruled area of the Iberian Peninsula) with the spread of the Islam in Europe.

1.7 Nutritional and health aspects of traditional foods

Many foods, whether traditional or not, are important in the diet and can make a significant contribution in achieving basic nutritional requirements (Musaiger, Al-Mohizea, Al-Kanhal, & Jaidah, 1990). Due to a change in food habits in the Arab countries to more processed foods and convenient fast foods of late, consumption of TFs has been reduced. As people in the Middle East become more affluent and can afford food of other cultures, local TFs are being side lined and being replaced by novel processed foods. It is widely known that healthy food plays an important role in the prevention and treatment of undernutrition, overnutrition, diet-related, and nonrelated communicable diseases (NCDs) such as obesity, diabetes, cardiovascular diseases (CVDs) and some types of cancers. Data available on the nutritional and health aspects of Middle-Eastern cuisine (Montagnese et al., 2019) show that the Middle-Eastern diet is low in saturated fats, high in monounsaturated fats and omega-3 fatty acids. Another study found that Arab diet is nutritionally balanced as it contains a lot of fresh fruits and vegetables along with unprocessed grains (Salari, 2002). Nevertheless, the health risk of developing noncommunicable diseases nowadays is still relatively high due to the inactive lifestyles that people have developed.

Recently and over the last decade, the prevalence of NCDs such as obesity, diabetes, hypertension, blood lipids, and lipoproteins has been on the rise in the countries of the Middle East, even exceeding the percentage in developed countries. Eating healthy is a crucial factor in reducing the risk of developing nutrition-related diseases. Moreover, factors such as culture, ethnic heritage, personal preferences, habits, and other traditions may manipulate cultural diets (Bawadi & Al-Sahawneh, 2008). Additionally, new foods and ingredients have been introduced to the diet of the Arab countries. This results in a nutritional transition due to the replacement of traditional diets with diets higher in fats and processed foods (Mokhtar et al., 2001; Ng, Zaghloul, Ali, Harrison, & Popkin, 2011). The chance of consuming high amounts of processed food could play an important role in the development of CVDs. Physical activity may also be considered in preventing the progression of medical complication of diseases (Galal, 2003). Despite this fact, the incorporation of physical activity in the lifestyle of people within the Middle East region is relatively low. According to a survey done by WHO, between 21.6% and 86.8% of Middle-Eastern countries' population are physically inactive (Sibai et al., 2010). Although the above reasons may be an attribute to the health aspect of consuming TF, the perceptions that consumers developed toward consuming TF may also have an association with the change of eating style.

1.8 Consumer perception and pattern of traditional foods in the Middle-Eastern countries

Food culture arises from where people are originated; whether they still live there or not, their way of living has been shaped by various resources (Wahlqvist & Lee, 2007). Traditional cuisine is usually very popular among local people; however, the practice of consuming TF today has evolved due to changes in perception and lifestyle. The younger generation may have a belief that TF is not tasty nor popular, and that the Western diet is ideal; this perception inevitably contributes to their intake.

A study done at a UAE University showed that the majority of their participants agree that Emirati TFs are healthy (Dhaheri, Maawali, Laleye, & Washi, 2014). Furthermore, based on the questionnaire the younger generation misses having TF, which comprises mainly plant based, rich in grains, legumes, vegetables, fruits along with little animal products more regularly. TF is known for its long period of preparation as it enhances the flavors. Due to longer preparation time, people would rather buy TF from a restaurant than prepare it from home as it saves time. Moreover, cooking, cleaning, and raising children were the main roles for women in the past and they consumed a lot of time (Keddie, 2012). Due to modernization, women have had to go out and work; this trend has resulted in the reduction of the availability of TF.

Discovering new cuisines that were not present previously will replace the consumption of TF with other types of food. In fact, fast food is now easily accessible and available in most of the Middle East countries unlike TF, which may only be considered a delicacy and is only available in limited places. As a consequence, other cuisines are prized in the place of TF because of their exoticness and special taste, notwithstanding the price.

Globalization has caused the evolution of food consumption from TFs to Western foods. Consumers' method of purchasing power of food has changed, accompanied by the change in lifestyle, and with this change, increased nutrition-related disease (Musaiger, 2011). For instance, the prevalence of NCDs in the Middle East and North Africa has increased over the last two decades (Golzarand et al., 2012). A study related to food patterns by adults in the UAE in 1998 found that older people preferred to consume TF more compared to the younger generations; this could be because older people are more attached to the tradition and heritage (Musaiger & Abuirmeileh, 1998).

There are many factors that change consumer consumption pattern of TFs. One of these factors is income. The increase of income in some of the Middle-Eastern countries and specifically the Gulf countries has resulted in a significant change in dietary pattern. Oil export and revenues were the main reasons behind the marked rise in the consumption of meat, poultry, milk, and eggs between 1980s and 2005 (Musaiger, 2011). Another factor that aids in changing consumer patterns is urbanization. People in the Middle East and Gulf countries used to grow their own vegetables, fruits, spices, and herbs. However, as people shifted from rural areas to urbanized areas, their incomes increased and so they have sacrificed fresh fruits, vegetables, pulses, potatoes, and other roots to food that is rich with sugar, salt, and fats (Schmidhuber, 2005).

Improvement of food processing might be a reason toward changing consumer patterns. Advances in food processing made it possible for a variety of food to be available in the markets. People in the past used to own an animal that is able to provide milk and milk products and used to take time to prepare the product that they want, compared to directly just buying it off the shelf today. Although improvements in food processing speed up the process of availability of certain food, the processing of food also has a negative impact when consumed in the long term (Musaiger, 2011).

1.9 Future prospect and awareness efforts—maintaining the heritage

TFs are an essential part of the Middle East and Gulf countries region; even though the preparation methods are different, the basic recipes are the same. This is because of the strong bond between countries that the Middle East region has, which is made up of their culture, religion, agriculture crops, and climate. It is important to preserve heritage so that future generations will know what TFs are.

The aim of preserving heritage is not to hold on the same old habits that our fathers have had. Sheikh Zayed, the Founding Father of the UAE once mentioned "He who does not know his past cannot make the best of his present and future, for it is from the past we learn" (Hashemi, 2009).

The date palm is commonly found in the Middle East; this has been known since prophet Mohammed as he used dates for breaking his fast-during Ramadan, he considered dates to be a superfood containing all-essential nutrients which serve to line an empty gut before actual food is consumed. Millions of Muslims now follow his way to break their fast by dates providing evidence of the importance of food culture preservation (Petzen, 2020). The passing of food habits similar to the one from Prophet Mohammed emphasizes on the fact that cultural heritage is not manifestation of people; what matters is the wealth of knowledge and skills that are passed from our prophet through to the next generation.

1.9.1 Evolution and modernization of traditional food

Throughout years, industrial food processing has made food evolutionize through time. The United States Department of Agriculture has defined industrial food processing as any raw agriculture commodity that has been subjected to washing, cleaning, milling, cutting, chopping, heating, pasteurizing, blanching, and cooking along with the addition of other ingredients (Mayo Clinic Health System, 2017). The concept of food processing has played a central part in human evolution (Wollstonecroft, 2011). TF standards have been difficult to achieve because of a great deal of care before processing is required. As a result, people have switched from organic food to exported and processed food. The transition from conventional diets to refined foods may be attributed to an improvement in the supply and affordability of these processed items. Food processing has standardized TF by introducing a series of steps that may speed up the period of preparation but resulted in a good quality of food.

Food has not been the same as it used to be. In fact, manufactures, restaurants, and food businesses are working toward fulfilling consumer's needs, resulting in innovation of new products. Due to the expansion of food industry, companies are shifting from creating original TF to food with new flavors. Moreover, food packing may also be considered new in the Middle-Eastern countries and so businesses may have found an opportunity with the changes occurred within the area and begin to manufacture food that may seem to consumers convenient, ready to eat, and tasty. Oppose to our ancestors where they used the weather to preserve their food, hence within the presence of technology, new innovative ways of preserving have been introduced through packaging. These involved cans, trays, boxes, bags, wrappers, cartons, and aseptic packaging.

1.10 Current trends in the Middle East and Gulf countries—conclusions

Middle Eastern including Mediterranean cuisine is defined by the presence of fundamental elements, which play an important role in locals' beliefs and practices and in relation to their religion, language, and culture.

The "basic" food products of the Eastern Mediterranean, the Levantine cuisine are considered traditional and widely consumed even nowadays, rapidly penetrating other continents (Europe, America) including: Cereals (mostly wheat, barley), olive oil and olives, dried and fresh vegetables, fruits, honey, yogurt, cheese, meat, and fish, all being symbols of a simple and healthy life. Apart from the benefit of the Middle-Eastern foods in relation to nutrition, being healthier to humans, they also add to the improvement of taste. Open to the influences of foreign civilizations, the Middle-Eastern food products together with new ethnic products and ingredients, seasoning, and so on, have somehow undergone a transformation over the past decades owing to the food practices of the diverse communities that have emigrated to both Middle East and the Gulf areas. What remains of all that in today's Middle East? How are TFs eaten nowadays? In what way do modern cooking methods reflect the survival of a recipe from the past?

1.11 Conclusions

The famous dictum of the French gastronomist Jean Anthelme Brillat-Savarin, at the beginning of the 19th century, "Tell me what you eat, and I will tell you who you are" has been profoundly shaken in this era of globalization. Enticing diners with its fusion of Mediterranean and Middle-Eastern influences, it taps into an appetite for bold ingredients, soulful flavors, and a more social way of eating—with a focus on sharing plates or shamelessly messy but undeniably satisfying, street food. It's a trend we're seeing so far and could be attributed to several global food trends—including the growth in the vegan/vegetarian movements converging to create a perfect storm—due to the unique strengths of Middle-Eastern cuisine. It is widely accepted that the global food and beverage industry have been undergoing changes as new culinary trends continuously emerge in United States, Europe, and also including the Middle East and the Gulf regions. When it comes to Arabic cuisine, the general consensus is that the region has not widely undergone major changes in relation to the TFs consumed in the Middle-Eastern cuisine. These areas as previously mentioned, especially the Gulf countries, and major cities such as Doha, Dubai, Abu Dhabi, Riyad, Kuwait, and Bahrain, have all seen new culinary trends with food cultural landscapes emerging from diverse cuisines, including Italian, Mexican, Japanese, Indian, Chinese, and so on. Levantine cuisine is sweeping the globe, combining its fusion of Mediterranean and Middle-Eastern influences, with for bold healthy ingredients, soulful flavors and suggesting a more social way of eating—with a focus on sharing plates or shamelessly messy, but undeniably satisfying, street food.

Similarities of TF in the Middle Eastern and Gulf region are testament of the interspersing of culture and people. Sharing traditions and culture within this region needs to be continued so that the next generation is able to participate in the making and consuming of these foods. This ensures the food heritage remains unique to this region, in addition to serving as a reminder to them of their roots. Local governments need to take an active and major role in sustaining the consumption of TF more frequently, beyond specific occasions. This will not only protect TFs in the Gulf and Middle East but also preserve food cultures in years to come, strengthening a more wholesome social establishment within countries.

Concluding, the rest of the world is finally catching up on the delights of Middle-Eastern cuisine and it's going to be a wonderful to see how it grows and evolves on a global scale.

References

Ahmed, A. M., El-Hakem, N. A. B., & Ibrahim, G. A. (2015). Chemical and microbial assessment of beef and chicken shawarma sandwiches in Ismailia governorate and its impact on consumer health. *Egyptian Journal of Environmental Chemistry and Health*, *1*, 686–693.

Al-Amiri, H. A., Ahmed, N., & Al-Sharrah, T. (2020). Fatty acid profiles, cholesterol composition, and nutritional quality indices of 37 commonly consumed local foods in Kuwait in relation to cardiovascular health. *MedRxiv*. Available from https://doi.org/10.1101/2020.11.18.20233999.

Ali, A., Al Zuhaibi, K., Waly, M., Devarajan, S., & Johnson, E. (2015). Growth performance, fasting plasma glucose lipid profile of Sprague-Dawley rats fed different levels of Omani halwa. *Pakistan Journal of Nutrition*, *14*(8), 503–510.

Al-Khusaibi, M. (2019). Arab traditional foods: Preparation, processing and nutrition. In M. Al-Khusaibi, N. Al-Habsi, & M. Shafiur Rahman (Eds.), *Traditional foods: History, preparation, processing and safety* (pp. 9–35). Springer International Publishing. Available from https://doi.org/10.1007/978-3-030-24620-4_2.

Al-Marzooqi, H. M., Burke, S. J., Al Ghazali, M. R., Duffy, E., & Yousuf, M. H. S. A. (2015). The development of a food atlas of portion sizes for the United Arab Emirates. *Journal of Food Composition and Analysis*, *43*, 140–148. Available from https://doi.org/10.1016/j.jfca.2015.05.008.

Al-Nabulsi, A. A., Osaili, T. M., Shaker, R. R., Olaimat, A. N., Attlee, A., Murad, A., ... Holley, R. A. (2013). Survival of E. coli O157:H7 and Listeria innocua in tahina (sesame paste). *Journal of Food, Agriculture and Environment*, *11*, 303–306.

Amr, A. S. (2015). Traditional ethnic foods: Examples of Arab's response to the harsh environment of the Levant and Iraq. *Journal of Saudi Society for Food and Nutrition*, *10*(1–2), 1–18.

Amr, A. S., & Yaseen, E. I. (1994). Thermal processing requirements of canned chickpea dip. *International Journal of Food Science & Technology*, *29*(4), 441–448. Available from https://doi.org/10.1111/j.1365-2621.1994.tb02085.x.

Ayaz, M., Sawaya, W. N., & Al-Sogair, A. (1986). Microbiological quality of tehineh manufactured in Saudi Arabia. *Journal of Food Protection*, *49*(7), 504–506. Available from https://doi.org/10.4315/0362-028X-49.7.504.

Bawadi, H. A., & Al-Sahawneh, S. A. (2008). Developing a meal-planning exchange list for traditional dishes in Jordan. *Journal of the American Dietetic Association*, *108*(5), 840–846. Available from https://doi.org/10.1016/j.jada.2008.02.016.

Boutaud, J., Becuţ, A., & Marinescu, A. (2016). Food and culture. Cultural patterns and practices related to food in everyday life. *International Review of Social Research*, *6*, 1–3. Available from https://doi.org/10.1515/irsr-2016-0001.

Caba, Z., Boyacioglu, M. H., & Boyacioglu, D. (2011). Bioactive healthy components of bulgur. *International Journal of Food Sciences and Nutrition*, *63*, 250–256. Available from https://doi.org/10.3109/09637486.2011.639748.

Castro, J. M. D. (2004). The time of day of food intake influences overall intake in humans. *The Journal of Nutrition*, *134*(1), 104–111. Available from https://doi.org/10.1093/jn/134.1.104.

Cho, J. I., Cheung, C. Y., Lee, S. M., Ko, S. I., Kim, K. H., & Hwang, I. S. (2011). Assessment of microbial contamination levels of street-vended foods in Korea. *Journal of Food Safety*, *31*, 41–47.

de Almeida Costa, G. E., da Silva Queiroz-Monici, K., Pissini Machado Reis, S. M., & de Oliveira, A. C. (2006). Chemical composition, dietary fibre and resistant starch contents of raw and cooked pea, common bean, chickpea and lentil legumes. *Food Chemistry*, *94*(3), 327–330.

Dhaheri, A., Maawali, A., Laleye, L., & Washi, S. (2014). Nutritional knowledge of Emirati traditional foods and body image perceptions among UAE University students. *Emirates Journal of Food and Agriculture*, *26*(10), 853. Available from https://doi.org/10.9755/ejfa.v26i10.18801.

El-Obeid, T., Aziz, H. A., Mousa, R., & Alzahiri, A. (2014). Survey on the microbial quality of traditional foods sold by street vendors in Qatar. *Austin Journal of Nutrition and Metabolism*, *1*, 1–4.

ElQuliti, S. A. H., & Khashoggi, G. A. (2017). A feasibility study for snacks manufacturing/retailing investment project. *American Scientific Research Journal for Engineering, Technology, and Sciences (ASRJETS)*, *31*(1), 1–23.

El-Ziney, M. G., & Al-Turki, A. (2007). Microbiological quality and safety assessment of camel milk (*Camelus dromedaries*) in Saudi Arabia (Qassim region). *Applied Ecology and Environmental Research*, *5*, 115–122.

EU. (2006). Council Regulation (EC) No509/2006 of 20 March 2006 on agricultural products and foodstuffs as traditional specialties guaranteed. *Official Journal of the European Union*, *L 93*, 1–11.

EuroFIR. (2007). FOOD-CT-2005–513944, EU 6th framework food quality and safety programme. Available from http://www.eurofir.net. Accessed June 2007.

FAO. (2011). Markets in the Middle East: Market, trade and consumption. *GLOBEFISH, Food and Agriculture Organization of the United Nations*. Available from http://www.fao.org/in-action/globefish/fishery-information/resource-detail/en/c/338542/.

Fillion, L., & Henry, C. J. K. (1998). Nutrient losses and gains during frying: A review. *International Journal of Food Sciences and Nutrition*, *49*(2), 157–168. Available from https://doi.org/10.3109/09637489809089395.

Fox, R. (2003). *Food and eating: An anthropological perspective*. Available from http://46.17.89.115/publik/foxfood.pdf.

Galal, O. (2003). Nutrition-related health patterns in the Middle East. Available from https://web.a.ebscohost.com/abstract?direct = true&profile = ehost&scope = site&authtype = crawler&jrnl = 09647058&AN = 12412481&h = 3RlkkVMseFYl2%2bdOmcbevZ1Z5c4fwY%2bBMVQFAw3-Um1KPkG8%2bxfzrV2fcxEo2UGacmvFn7%2fdKLqbrbr1HJxogYg%3d%3d&crl = c&resultNs = AdminWebAuth&resultLocal = ErrCrlNotAuth&crlhashurl = login.aspx%3fdirect%3dtrue%26pro-file%3dehost%26scope%3dsite%26authtype%3dcrawler%26jrnl%3d09647058%26AN%3d1-2412481.

Golzarand, M., Mirmiran, P., Jessri, M., Toolabi, K., Mojarrad, M., & Azizi, F. (2012). Dietary trends in the Middle East and North Africa: An ecological study (1961 to 2007). *Public Health Nutrition*, *15*, 1835–1844. Available from https://doi.org/10.1017/S1368980011003673.

Grivetti, L. E. (2002). Street foods: Edited by A.P. Simopoulos and Ramesh V. Bhat, 2000, 186 pages, hardcover, $198.25. Karger, Basel, Switzerland. *The American Journal of Clinical Nutrition*, *75*(2), 337–338. Available from https://doi.org/10.1093/ajcn/75.2.337.

Guerrero, L. (2001). Marketing PDO (products with denominations of origin) and PGI (products with geographical identities). In L. Frewer, E. Risvik, & H. Shifferstein (Eds.), *Food, people and society. An European perspective of consumers' food choices* (pp. 281–296). Berlin: Springer Verlag.

Gulf Migration (2016). GCC: Total population and percentage of nationals and foreign nationals in GCC countries (national statistics, 2010–2016) (with numbers). Available from https://gulfmigration.org/gcc-total-population-percentage-nationals-foreign-nationals-gcc-countries-national-statistics-2010-2016-numbers/.

Habib, H., Ali, H., Ibrahim, W., & Afifi, H. (2011). Nutritional value of 10 traditional dishes of the United Arab Emirates. *Ecology of Food and Nutrition*, *50*, 526–538. Available from https://doi.org/10.1080/03670244.2011.620880.

Hanashiro, A., Morita, M., Matt, G., Matt, M., & Torres, E. (2005). Microbiological quality of selected street foods from a restricted area of São Paulo city, Brazil. *Food Control*, *16*, 439–444.

Hashemi, B. A. (2009). On the legacy of Sheikh Zayed Bin Sultan. *The National*. Available from https://www.thenationalnews.com/lifestyle/on-the-legacy-of-sheikh-zayed-bin-sultan-1.516604.

Hoteit, M., Zoghbi, E., Al Iskandarani, M., Rady, A., Shankiti, I., Matta, J., & Al-ãJawaldeh, A. (2020). Nutritional value of the Middle Eastern diet: Analysis of total sugar, salt, and iron in Lebanese traditional dishes. *F1000Research*, *9*, 1254.

Ismail, M. (2013). Different doses of Arabic coffee improve serum lipid profile, uric acid and liver enzymes of experimental rats. *Food and Public Health*, *3*(4), 228–233. Available from https://doi.org/10.5923/j.fph.20130304.07.

Ismail, M., & Kucukoner, E. (2017). Falafel: A meal with full nutrition. *Food and Nutrition Sciences*, *8*(11), 1022–1027. Available from https://doi.org/10.4236/fns.2017.811074.

Ismail, S. A. (2006). Microbiological quality of Hawashy consumed in Ismailia, Egypt. *Journal of Food Safety*, *26*, 251–263.

Jalloun, R. A., & Alhathlool, M. H. (2020). Arabic coffee consumption and the risk of obesity among Saudi's female population. *Journal of the Saudi Society for Food and Nutrition (JSSFN)*, *13*, 59–67.

Karabudak, E., Bas, M., & Kiziltan, G. (2008). Food safety in the home consumption of meat in Turkey. *Food Control*, *19*, 320–327.

Keddie, N. R. (2012). *Women in the Middle East: Past and present*. Princeton University Press.

Khan, G. A. (2018, May 13). Dates: A Middle Eastern delicacy. *Arab News*. Available from https://www.arabnews.com/node/1301551/saudi-arabia.

Kilshaw, S., Miller, D., Tamimi, H., El-Taher, F., Mohsen, M., Omar, N., ... Sole, K. (2016). Calm vessels: Cultural expectations of pregnant women in Qatar. *Anthropology of the Middle East, 11*. Available from https://doi.org/10.3167/ame.2016.110204.

Kirk, G. E. (2016). *A short history of the Middle East: From the rise of Islam to modern times*. Routledge.

Kuhnlein, H. V., & Receveur, O. (1996). Dietary change and traditional food systems of indigenous peoples. *Annual Review of Nutrition, 16*, 417–442. Available from https://doi.org/10.1146/annurev.nu.16.070196.002221.

Lewis, B. (1980). The Ottoman Empire and its aftermath. *Journal of Contemporary History, 15*, 27–36.

Mayo Clinic Health System. (2017). Processed foods: What you should know. *Mayo Clinic Health System*. Available from https://www.mayoclinichealthsystem.org/hometown-health/speaking-of-health/processed-foods-what-you-should-know.

Mohammad, A., & Abu-Rumman, A. (2018). Analysis of Pimpinella anisum (Yansoon) seeds using gas chromatography mass spectrometry. *International Journal of Chemical Studies, 6*, 3033–3037.

Mokhtar, N., Elati, J., Chabir, R., Bour, A., Elkari, K., Schlossman, N. P., ... Aguenaou, H. (2001). Diet culture and obesity in Northern Africa. *The Journal of Nutrition, 131*(3), 887S–892S. Available from https://doi.org/10.1093/jn/131.3.887S.

Montagnese, C., Santarpia, L., Iavarone, F., Strangio, F., Sangiovanni, B., Buonifacio, M., ... Pasanisi, F. (2019). Food-based dietary guidelines around the world: Eastern Mediterranean and Middle Eastern countries. *Nutrients, 11*(6), 1325. Available from https://doi.org/10.3390/nu11061325.

Musaiger, A. O. (2011). *Food consumption patterns in the Eastern Mediterranean region*. Arab Center for Nutrition. Available from https://www.cabdirect.org/cabdirect/abstract/20113393009.

Musaiger, A. O., & Abuirmeileh, N. M. (1998). Food consumption patterns of adults in the United Arab Emirates. *Journal of the Royal Society for the Promotion of Health, 118*(3), 146–150. Available from https://doi.org/10.1177/146642409811800304.

Musaiger, A. O., Al-Mohizea, I. S., Al-Kanhal, M. A., & Jaidah, J. H. (1990). Chemical and amino acid composition of four traditional foods consumed in the Arab Gulf states. *Food Chemistry, 36*(3), 181–189. Available from https://doi.org/10.1016/0308-8146(90)90053-7.

Musaiger, A. O., & Miladi, S. (1993). *Traditional foods in the Arab Gulf*. FAO.

Nam, K.-C., Jo, C., & Lee, M. (2010). Meat products and consumption culture in the East. *Meat Science, 86*(1), 95–102. Available from https://doi.org/10.1016/j.meatsci.2010.04.026.

Ng, S. W., Zaghloul, S., Ali, H. I., Harrison, G., & Popkin, B. M. (2011). The prevalence and trends of overweight, obesity and nutrition-related non-communicable diseases in the Arabian Gulf States. *Obesity Reviews, 12*(1), 1–13. Available from https://doi.org/10.1111/j.1467-789X.2010.00750.x.

Obón, C., Rivera, D., Alcaraz, F., & Attieh, L. (2014). Beverage and culture. "Zhourat," a multivariate analysis of the globalization of a herbal tea from the Middle East. *Appetite, 79*, 1–10. Available from https://doi.org/10.1016/j.appet.2014.03.024.

Petzen, B. (2020). Middle Eastern food: Six lenses. *The Geography Teacher, 17*(3), 94–103. Available from https://doi.org/10.1080/19338341.2020.1796746.

Porreca, F. I., Unsain, R. A. F., Carriero, M. R., Sato, P. D. M., Ulian, M. D., & Scagliusi, F. B. (2020). Dialogues and tensions in the eating habits of Syrian refugees living in São Paulo, Brazil. *Ecology of Food and Nutrition*, *59*(2), 175–194. Available from https://doi.org/10.1080/03670244.2019.1681419.

Prakash, V. (2016). Chapter 1—Introduction: The importance of traditional and ethnic food in the context of food safety, harmonization, and regulations. In V. Prakash, O. Martín-Belloso, L. Keener, S. Astley, S. Braun, H. McMahon, & H. Lelieveld (Eds.), *Regulating safety of traditional and ethnic foods* (pp. 1–6). Academic Press.

Pufall, E., Jones, A., Mcewen, S., Lyall, C., Peregrine, A., & Edge, V. (2011). Perception of the importance of traditional country foods to the physical, mental, and spiritual health of labrador inuit. *ARCTIC*, *64*. Available from https://doi.org/10.14430/arctic4103.

Ranfa, A., Maurizi, A., Romano, B., & Bodesmo, M. (2014). The importance of traditional uses and nutraceutical aspects of some edible wild plants in human nutrition: The case of Umbria (central Italy). *Plant Biosystems*, *148*(2), 297–306. Available from https://doi.org/10.1080/11263504.2013.770805.

Rasheed, P., & Al-Sowielem, L. S. (2003). Prevalence and predictors of premenstrual syndrome among college–aged women in Saudi Arabia. *Annals of Saudi Medicine*, *23*(6), 381–387. Available from https://doi.org/10.5144/0256-4947.2003.381.

Rubach, M., Halliday, J., Cleavel, S., & Crump, J. (2013). Brucellosis in low-income and middle-income countries. *Current Opinion in Infectious Diseases*, *26*(5), 404–412.

Saeed, I. A., Ali, L., Jabeen, A., Khasawneh, M., Rizvi, T. A., & Ashraf, S. S. (2013). Estrogenic activities of ten medicinal herbs from the Middle East. *Journal of Chromatographic Science*, *51*(1), 33–39. Available from https://doi.org/10.1093/chromsci/bms101.

Salari, S. (2002). Invisible in aging research: Arab Americans, Middle Eastern immigrants, and Muslims in the United States. *The Gerontologist*, *42*(5), 580–588. Available from https://doi.org/10.1093/geront/42.5.580.

Sawaya, W. N., Al-Awadhi, F., Aziz, A., Al-Rashdan, A., Mahjoub, B. T., & Al-Amiri, H. (1998). Nutritional profile of Kuwaiti composite dishes: Minerals and vitamins. *Journal of Food Composition and Analysis*, *11*(1), 70–88. Available from https://doi.org/10.1006/jfca.1997.0558.

Schmidhuber, J. (2005). The growing global obesity problem: Some policy options to address it. In *Paper presented at the 97th seminar of the European Association of Agricultural Economists*. University of Reading, England, April 21–22, 2005.

Sibai, A., Nasreddine, L., Mokdad, A., Adra, N., Tabet, M., & Hwalla, N. (2010). Nutrition transition and cardiovascular disease risk factors in Middle East and North African countries: Reviewing the evidence. *Annals of Nutrition & Metabolism*, *57*, 193–203. Available from https://doi.org/10.1159/000321527.

Tajkarimi, M., Ibrahim, S. A., & Fraser, A. M. (2013). Food safety challenges associated with traditional foods in Arabic speaking countries of the Middle East. *Trends in Food Science & Technology*, *29*(2), 116–123. Available from https://doi.org/10.1016/j.tifs.2012.10.002.

Todd, E. C. D. (2017a). Foodborne disease and food control in the Gulf States. *Food Control*, *73*, 341–366.

Todd, E. C. D. (2017b). Foodborne disease in the Middle East. In S. Murad, E. Baydoun, N. Daghir, & A. Badran (Eds.), *Water, energy & food sustainability in the Middle East: The sustainability triangle* (pp. 389–440). Springer International Publishing. Available from https://doi.org/10.1007/978-3-319-48920-9_17.

Trichopoulou, A., Soukara, S., & Vasilopoulou, E. (2007). Traditional foods: A science and society perspective. *Trends in Food Science and Technology*, *18*(8), 420–427.

Wahlqvist, M. L., & Lee, M.-S. (2007). Regional food culture and development. *Asia Pacific Journal of Clinical Nutrition*, *16*(Suppl. 1), 2–7.

WHO (World Health Organization). (2015). WHO initiative to estimate the global burden of foodborne diseases: Fourth formal meeting of the Foodborne Disease Burden Epidemiology Reference Group (FERG): Sharing new results, making future plans, and preparing ground for the countries. Available from http://apps.who.int/iris/bitstream/handle/10665/159844/9789241507950_eng.pdf?seq uence = 1. Accessed December 15, 2018.

Wollstonecroft, M. (2011). Investigating the role of food processing in human evolution: A niche construction approach. *Archaeological and Anthropological Sciences*, *3*, 141–150. Available from https://doi.org/10.1007/s12520-011-0062-3.

Chapter 2

Overview on food safety in the Middle East

Ewen C.D. Todd
Ewen Todd Consulting, LLC, Okemos, MI, United States

2.1 Introduction

2.1.1 Background on Arab countries

The Arabic-speaking Middle East countries can be separated into two main geographic regions, the Eastern Mediterranean countries (Egypt, Jordan, Lebanon, Palestine, Syria) and the Arabian Gulf countries [Bahrain, Kuwait, Iraq, Oman, Qatar, Saudi Arabia, and the United Arab Emirates (UAE)]; Yemen has a coast bordering both the Red Sea and the Arabian Sea. All of these countries have major water shortages and have traditionally relied on scarce seasonal rains and more recently on deep wells to tap into aquifer ground water and the establishment of high-energy desalination plants. Overuse of deep wells has resulted in brackish water, especially near the coasts, increasingly unsuitable for drinking or irrigation. The high Lebanon and anti-Lebanon mountain ranges give moisture to Lebanon and Syria, and rivers allow drinking water and irrigation in Iraq (Tigris and Euphrates) and Egypt (Nile) with the River Jordan and its Yarmouk tributary supplying limited water for irrigation to Jordan and the Palestinian West Bank. Unfortunately, typically the quality of surface water for potable consumption is poor. However, for all of these countries available water is a shrinking commodity especially with global warming. Some communities are forced to use water that may be polluted with agricultural chemicals and sewage effluent. Thus food safety may be compromised from food contaminated with pathogens from the environment and opportunities for their growth under high ambient temperatures. Another factor affecting health are past and current civil wars and invasions affecting mainly, Iraq, Syria, and Yemen, where public health systems are adversely affected, displaced persons and refugees are crowded into camps, and foreign troops are present in contained army bases. Under these conditions, foodborne illness reporting was very limited.

Food Safety in the Middle East. DOI: https://doi.org/10.1016/B978-0-12-822417-5.00008-8

This chapter gives examples of foodborne outbreaks in each of these countries but is not meant to be comprehensive. Of the seven countries bordering on the Arabian Gulf, six of these belong to the Gulf Cooperation Council (GCC): Bahrain, Kuwait, Oman, Qatar, Saudi Arabia, UAE. The GCC is a regional political organization comprising the energy-rich Gulf monarchies, with Iraq one time as an associate member. Yemen, which borders both Saudi Arabia and Oman, was in negotiations for GCC membership, but the current civil war has stalled that. For the purposes of this chapter they are considered together. Some of outbreak information have been previously reported in Todd (2017a, 2017b).

2.2 Foodborne disease incidents in Arab Middle East countries in the Eastern Mediterranean

2.2.1 Egypt

Egypt has the highest population of a Middle East country with over 102 million inhabitants and Cairo as its very large capital city (7.7 million) (https://www.worldometers.info/world-population/egypt-population/). Foodborne disease illnesses in institutions are more likely to be reported more often than small incidents in other settings. In October 2008, over 1400 children in primary, middle, and secondary schools in Darin village, in the Nile delta province of Mansoura, were hospitalized after claiming to eat tainted school biscuits, which were later found to be "bacteriologically sound," but a toxin was suspected (LaBudde, 1998). Most of the students were discharged, but five remained in intensive care units. The distributor was detained by police on the order of the provincial governor. This was apparently only one of the several episodes of apparent poisonings in schools at that time. Food poisoning affecting 161 students occurred on April 29, 2013, at Al-Azhar, Cairo's centuries old seat of Sunni learning, and Egypt's top Islamic university, less than a month after a mass poisoning incident at the same university left more than 500 students hospitalized (Masriya, 2013). Investigations were initiated within the university and by the Ministry of Health, and apparently "bad tuna" had been served at the campus cafeteria. There were no deaths. If tuna was the vehicle of the outbreak, scombroid poisoning was the likely cause of the illnesses. The allergic-like symptoms generally begin 15–60 min after ingestion and usually resolve in a few hours. Scombroid fish poisoning occurs after fish, most frequently tuna, with high levels of accumulated histamine or other biogenic amines is eaten. The outbreaks saw the sentencing of the dorm's director, the university's kitchen manager, and eight chefs to 5 years in prison.

It is not just local families or students who may be affected by foodborne illness but visitors. Tourism has been the major economy in Egypt for many years, but it can be threatened not only by the risk of terrorism but also by foodborne illness (Costa, 2008). Tourists might not stop coming to Egypt because of a few reports of diarrhea; however, widespread reporting of severe cases, and lawsuits, will make tour operators much more selective in their destinations of choice, and they can bring pressure on the Egyptian hospitality industry to improve its hygienic standards. Multiple reports of illness have been reported from Nile River cruises and resort town on the coast. From September to November, 2008, 34 cases of hepatitis A imported from Egypt were reported to the German public health authorities (Bernard & Frank, 2009). Investigations pointed to a continuing common source of infection, most likely linked to Nile river cruises. In addition, eight French cases who had been traveling on a Nile cruise and one on a Red Sea diving safari were documented (Couturier et al., 2009). One specific cruise ship was mentioned by 6 of 10 Belgian cases (Robesyn, Micalessi, Quoilin, Naranjo, & Thomas, 2011). Those who took a Nile cruise had typically done this in combination with a hotel stay. At least three different ships and three different hotel accommodations were mentioned in the travel histories of the French cases. The patients affected had not been vaccinated, which emphasized the need for more effective travel advice before trips to hepatitis-A-endemic countries (Sane et al., 2015). Possible sources of infection might have been contaminated food obtained from a common food catering company consumed onboard, contaminated tap water supplies for the ships' bunkers, or a common exposure on shore (e.g., a restaurant where tourist groups from various ships were taken during day trips). As all of these ships continuously traveled up and down a short stretch of the river (Aswan to Luxor and back) with standard stops along the way, the cases possibly shared an exposure on land. Both the long incubation period of hepatitis A (15–50 days) and long delays in collecting information on the individual cases precluded any rapid intervention on location. No specific food source was identified but could have been juices as recognized in an earlier major outbreak. In 2004 tourists returning from Egypt included 351 hepatitis-A-case patients from nine European countries who were infected with a single hepatitis A virus (HAV) strain (genotype 1b) (Frank et al., 2007). The case-control study identified orange juice most likely contaminated during the manufacturing process, for example, by an infected worker with inadequate hand hygiene or by contact of fruit or machinery with sewage-contaminated water. Citrus fruit and citrus juices have occasionally been implicated as vehicles of HAV and *Salmonella* infections, with contamination typically occurring during production or preparation just before consumption. As HAV is resistant to acid, it likely can survive for prolonged periods in orange juice.

2.2.2 Jordan

In September 1989, a 183-case outbreak of salmonellosis occurred in a university hospital in Amman after employees, patients, and visitors ate in the cafeteria (Khuri-Bulos, Khalaf, Shehabi, & Shami, 1994). The incubation period ranged from 16 to 72 h. Symptoms included diarrhea (88%), fever (71%), abdominal pain (74%), dehydration (34%), and bloody stool (5%). Eighty-four were hospitalized. Cultures of eight food items were negative, but stool culture on 90 of 180 patients and 11 of 61 kitchen employees yielded *Salmonella* Enteritidis (SE) group D1. A cohort study revealed a food-specific attack rate of 72% for the steak and potato meal and 18% for the rice and meat meal. Stratified analysis of the steak and potato meal revealed that the potatoes were implicated most strongly. Cultures were obtained from all kitchen employees, who showed no symptoms of illness, but 11 of 61 grew SE group D1. One asymptomatic, culture-positive employee had prepared the mashed potatoes on September 23, 16 h before the first case presented at the hospital emergency with severe gastroenteritis symptoms. All of the food workers had negative stool cultures 3 months earlier. The potatoes were mashed by machine but peeled after boiling and mixed with milk by hand, using a ladle and no gloves. Two different batches, the first of which was served exclusively to hospitalized patients and the second to a few remaining patients and employees, were prepared and served within 30–60 min of preparation. From the epidemiological data, it can be assumed that the infected handle fecally contaminated only the second batch of potatoes, thus sparing most of the highly susceptible inpatients from exposure. Further, while potatoes clearly were implicated, individuals who ate steak only had an elevated risk of being attacked. This probably was due to surface contamination of foods being served on the same plate. Kitchen employees harboring *Salmonella* were excluded from work until they had three negative stool cultures taken 1 week apart; it took 6 weeks for them to return to work. Stool surveillance that was routinely carried out in the hospital was ineffective in detecting infected employees to prevent this outbreak and the investigators recommended that employees adhere to proper hygienic practices including thorough washing of hands, especially when preparing food.

In late summer, 2006, over 1000 persons suffered from salmonellosis after eating chicken shawarma at a well-known franchise operation in Zarqa (Khalaf, 2006). Many of those ill were briefly hospitalized. It was suggested that the source of the *Salmonella* could have been the mayonnaise, likely made with unpasteurized eggs, used in the shawarma preparation and left at ambient temperatures, which was typical at the time being in vats uncooled on the counter. This would allow the growth of any *Salmonella* present. However, the falafel and undercooked chicken could also have been sources. The restaurant owner was fined 135 dinars ($190), which was hardly a punitive amount. Each municipality in Jordan monitors its restaurants as well as oversight by the Ministry of Health, and it was speculated that inspectors in Zarqa might have been less stringent in their review of food safety practices than in Amman.

In August 2007 nearly 250 persons were treated for gastroenteritis from *Salmonella* after eating contaminated chicken shawarmas (sandwiches) from a restaurant in the Baqaa Palestinian camp northwest of Amman, prompting the authorities to ban the operations of 600 fast food outlets until "the proper mechanisms are set up to ensure that this does not occur again" (Sreeraman, 2007). The chicken had been "poorly cooked" and the owner of the shop was arrested. There were similar incidents involving shawarma chicken the previous year. The health and water ministers had just resigned following a large waterborne outbreak with hundreds of cases suffering from diarrhea and fever. This Baqaa camp, established in 1968, has 100,000 Palestinian refugees who face high poverty and high unemployment rates. Authorities began a campaign following the outbreak to clamp down on fast food restaurants not adhering to health and safety regulations, causing estimated costs of between 100,000 and 250,000 Jordanian dinars (approximately USD141,000–353,000) a day to the industry (Rahimi, 2007). A month earlier in July, two ministers resigned over a water contamination scandal that saw more than 1000 Jordanians needing hospital treatment. A third outbreak occurred in October 2007, with about 300 persons ill after eating hummus at a restaurant in Jerash; 90 of them suffering from diarrhea and fever were taken to Jerash and Amman hospitals (Anonymous, 2007). The restaurant was closed pending an investigation that was considering both salmonellosis and cholera. In July 2012, 16 people were admitted to hospitals in Zarqa (east of Amman) suffering from similar symptoms after apparently eating poisoned food in Awajan district (Anonymous, 2012). As typical in press reporting of outbreaks, nothing is usually released on the causes of the illnesses, and in this outbreak, the patients recovered uneventfully. However, the media became more interested in the following incident where fatalities occurred.

In 2014 a Jordanian family was vacationing at the Dead Sea, and they ate burgers at their resort. They ordered food from a restaurant near the resort's pool and ate some of it there before taking the rest to their hotel room (Azzeh, 2014a). Severe symptoms of vomiting, fatigue, and abdominal pain occurred shortly afterwards, and the resort's nurse was called to check on their situation. The family was then taken to a local hospital where the resident doctor maintained that they had food poisoning and referred them to a hospital in Amman for gastric lavage, as it could not be performed at his hospital, and gave each of them an injection to relieve the symptoms until they reached Amman. Unfortunately, the 3-year-old son died on the way. In Amman, the mother and daughter were admitted to intensive care and the mother died 2 days later. The father and daughter made a gradual recovery. It was speculated that remaining 7–8 h outside the hospital without receiving the necessary treatment might be the reason why the condition of the family worsened and the boy died. Although several forensic doctors said that food poisoning was the cause of the deaths, the Health Ministry formed a committee comprising doctors from public and university hospitals to identify the exact cause of death. The restaurant where the family ate dinner was temporarily closed down. In December, the Amman prosecutor general charged the administration of the Holiday Inn Resort Dead Sea of causing the death of the mother and her child because it was determined that the resort did not follow standard health procedures when preparing the food, based on answers given by hotel employees and experts giving testimonies in toxicology and forensic medicine (Husseini, 2014). Tests carried out by the Jordan Food and Drug Administration on samples of the leftover food ordered by the family from the hotel's pool restaurant and taken to their room revealed high levels of the *Bacillus cereus*. However, tests showed that food from the hotel's kitchens conformed to health standards. This case was widely reported and discussed, and the family threatened to sue those responsible for "seriously harmful" rumors accusing the husband and father of the victims of being responsible for their deaths (Azzeh, 2014b). From the information available, it would seem that *B. cereus* was responsible for the illnesses and deaths. Although deaths from preformed cereulide enterotoxin are rare, Bottone (2012) documents four fatal cases in children or young adults.

A man and child died, and 826 people were hospitalized after suffering from a foodborne illness after eating at a restaurant outside Amman at a Palestinian refugee camp in July 2020 (Anonymous, 2020a). The restaurant had been offering half-price shawarmas, the rotisserie meat snack. Health officials found that the meat had not been refrigerated in what were heat-wave temperatures. Three people, including the restaurant owner, were detained. Laboratory tests have confirmed the presence of two types of bacteria in the shawarma meals, including the *Enterococcus faecalis* and *Campylobacter*. Jordan had been experiencing high temperatures in at the time, with Amman exceeding 40°C. According to a Ministry of Health spokesperson, the restaurant was allowed to reopen on condition of rectifying its hygiene situation but "there was no full compliance," and a second outbreak was followed days later by another mass poisoning at a similar outlet in the same camp (Anonymous, 2020b). One thousand people were hospitalized in the two incidents, which exposed a lack of enforcement of food safety rules, especially in impoverished areas. Poorer areas were seeing brisk demand over the Eid Al Adha holiday as families saved money to eat cheap meals outside. The source of the food poisoning was traced to contaminated stock from a distribution center. The authorities confiscated five tonnes of meat and half a tonne of potatoes from the facility. The ministry closed 20 restaurants in the Baqaa area, as well as one in Amman "as a precautionary measure." However, the investigation has yet to publicly reveal full details of the outbreak including incubation period, symptoms, experiences, and the pathogen(s) found in the ill persons; *Enterobacter faecalis* is considered a fecal contaminant but not a typical human pathogen. *Campylobacter* is certainly found in raw chicken and could have recontaminated cooked chicken, but although it could survive, it would not multiply rapidly in cooked chicken or kitchen environments (Park, Ro, Jo, Park, & Yoon, 2014). Nevertheless, low levels of *Campylobacter* spp. can cause human infections.

2.2.3 Lebanon

Although Lebanon does not have an historic foodborne disease surveillance system, a number of studies over the years have indicated some of the epidemiological disease issues that have affected residents in the country in the past and continuing into today. Several outbreaks were documented many decades ago. In the 1940s, according to Berberian (1946) cheese poisoning was by far the commonest form of food poisoning in Syria and Lebanon. It was usually contracted from green cheese, made from unpasteurized goat's or sheep's milk and only occasionally from cow's milk. The cheeses were produced locally in small quantities by farmers, villagers, and dairymen; they have a central hole in which salt is placed. From the symptoms of nausea, vomiting, diarrhea, prostration, and muscular cramps, 1–2 h up to 6 h after consumption, the author concluded that the agent was *Staphylococcus aureus*, which was found in cheese samples from four outbreaks at levels between 2.7 and 10.6 million/g of cheese. Salt added during production may inhibit some pathogens but not *S. aureus*.

A well-investigated outbreak occurred after a catered lunch meal was served at a bank cafeteria in May 2004; 32 employees suffered from diarrhea, fever, and abdominal pains 5.5–22.5 h (mean, 10.3 h) after eating chicken noodles au gratin (Hanna, Adib, & Daoud, 2009). A few cases had systemic infections. SE was confirmed in stool and blood cultures within 48–72 h after hospital admission of the first cases, and also in leftovers of the suspect food. The dish had been served at the bank in the past with no apparent health problems. Preparation normally starts in the evening prior to the day the dish is served. However, in this instance, some of the constituents had been prepared 3 days ahead, because the dish was to be served on a Monday, immediately after the week-end closure. No *Salmonella* was found in rectal and nasal mucosal swabs taken from all 18 kitchen workers, or in the tanker water supply (although it had high fecal coliform counts), but SE was found in a frozen batch of the same raw chicken breast consignment that had been used for the chicken noodles. The batch of chicken came from a large producer of poultry and eggs in Lebanon, who was advised of its potential involvement in a major foodborne outbreak. However, the investigators were refused access to the poultry-producing facility. It is highly likely that contaminated chicken carcasses had been, and would continue to be, shipped to many parts of Lebanon. That the same SE strain occurred in the patients, the raw chicken, and the leftover food was confirmed through random amplified polymorphic DNA-PCR. It would appear the 3-day delay in the chicken noodle preparation was significant in allowing the *Salmonella* present in the ingredients not only to survive but also to probably grow;

undercooking, cross-contamination, inadequate storage, and reheating all may have played a role in the outbreak but no more information was available to determine which. The bank management decided to sue the caterer and because they were aware of apparently inefficient way that public authorities were conducting the investigation, they took the initiative to call upon an independent investigative team to obtain solid evidence to win any court action. The caterers, concerned that they would be the only party blamed for the *Salmonella* outbreak, had succeeded in concealing some raw and cooked items from the destructive path of the public health authorities. These items were central to establishing contamination upstream from the caterer's kitchen. No action seems to have been taken against the poultry producer who was the source of the SE, a pathogen that is invasive of flocks and difficult to eradicate. The authors complained about the obsolete Lebanese laws dating back to the 1930s that still govern what should be done following a report of "food poisoning." Public health officers are mandated to stop the spread by destroying allegedly contaminated food items and closing down incriminated facilities. The result of this activity is generally agreeable to the public but does not help determine the cause to develop appropriate prevention and control strategies (Hanna et al., 2009). Also, because no investigation was done, many nonimplicated foods and ingredients would be discarded.

Vibrio parahaemolyticus has been found in Lebanese seafood (1.8%) and a number of *V. parahaemolyticus* isolates were recovered from hospitalized patients from July to October, 2017 (Fattel, Panossian, Salloum, Abboud, & Tokajian, 2019). These were characterized through whole genome sequencing and molecular typing as belonging to clone ST3 and had the presence of orf8, linking the isolates to the well-known pandemic O3:K6 serotype. All of the isolates had the tdh +, trh −, group-specific PCR + genotype, which is a characteristic of the O3:K6 pandemic clone. These came from patients suffering from gastroenteritis between the ages of 33 and 80, living in Matn, who recalled eating seafood. The lack of epidemiological data, as is the case in this study, was noted as a limitation in outbreak investigations. They recommended that more studies are needed to build a genome-based comparison between clinical and environmental isolates to determine the origin and source of contamination. A rare case of non-O1, non-O139 *Vibrio cholerae* occurred in Beirut in 2015, and the authors believed that a possible source was the consumption of contaminated water in the larger Beirut area (Zmeter, Tabaja, Sharara, & Kanj, 2018). In 2015 the main dumpsite serving the Beirut and Mount Lebanon areas closed and, consequently, rubbish piled up in the streets. Protests broke out due to the failure of municipalities to provide a proper solution, people were burning and dumping wastes along seashores and hillsides. Although the authors could not specifically identify a source of the *Vibrio*, they considered that the contamination of water sources from the trash, especially after heavy rains, led to the spread of infectious pathogens, including *V. cholerae*, in the population. However, a lack of effective nationwide surveillance mechanism results in underreporting of infectious diseases, and the true rates of these diseases are often underestimated.

2.2.4 Palestine

Although foodborne illness is rarely reported for Palestinians, residents are exposed to pathogens on a regular basis. The study of Adwan, Alqarem, and Adwan (2015) indicates that fresh meat sold to the public can be heavily contaminated microbiologically (up to 10^7 total aerobic count CFU^{-1}), and the prevalence of *S. aureus*, *Salmonella*, and *Escherichia coli* in meats was 30%, 25%, and 95%, respectively. Among the tested *S. aureus* strains, 75% were enterotoxigenic. The results also showed that 89.5% of the *E. coli* found in the meat samples were enterohemorrhagic *E. coli* (EHEC), enteropathogenic *E. coli* (EPEC), enteroaggregative *E. coli* (EAEC), enterotoxigenic *E. coli* (ETEC), or diffuse adherent *E. coli* pathotypes. Elmanama, Arafa, and Abu-Owda (2017) found that the bacteriological quality of fresh vegetables salad sold in the local school canteens and restaurants in Gaza Strip, Palestine, was poor with samples having high total and coliform counts, and containing *E. coli* (53.5%), *E. coli* O157:H7 (1%), *S. aureus* (21.5%), *B. cereus* (14%), *Listeria* spp. (7.5%), *Listeria monocytogenes* (2%), *Salmonella* spp. (5%), and *Shigella* spp. (1%). The bacterial contamination could have arisen from washing vegetables with contaminated water or handling of vegetables by infected workers, since contaminated irrigated water and organic manure are widely used by Gaza farmers for soil fertilization.

Poisonings and rumors of deliberate poisonings are more likely to be in the news than foodborne illness incidents. The most famous was that of Yassar Arafat in October, 2004, when 4 h after eating dinner, he began to experience severe nausea, vomiting, and abdominal pain followed by watery diarrhea (Dickey, 2013). He died a month later and polonium was found in his clothing and later in his exhumed body. He was originally diagnosed having gastroenteritis, but he was likely deliberately poisoned by an undetermined agent in a political assassination.

2.2.5 Syria

As expected with on-going civil war and invasions by foreign forces, little is published on foodborne disease outbreaks or on the risks of contracting a foodborne illness. However, a study by Nashef (2018) of 277 Syrian refugee mothers of school-aged children in the Bekaa region of Lebanon may indicate what conditions would occur in Syria. The study showed that these mothers reported experiencing severe household food insecurity, low socioeconomic conditions, living in overcrowded spaces, high unemployment rate, low educational levels, and limited food safety knowledge. In fact, the situation in Syria would have been worse for them to have sought refugee status in another country. Only the most newsworthy of incidents involving food is being covered by the press. For instance, in November 2014, defected Syrian army soldiers posing as cooks infiltrated an Islamic State of Iraq and Syria (ISIS) camp and poisoned meals killing at least a dozen Islamic State militants and having 15 others transferred to nearby field hospitals after they ate a contaminated lunch at the Fath El-Sahel camp, where 1200 of them were based (Gee, 2014). The "cooks" immediately fled, along with their families, with the help of fellow revolutionaries. No details of the symptoms or the poison is given though it appears to have had a rapid onset, probably caused by a relatively tasteless chemical added to one or more foods in lethal doses.

2.3 Foodborne disease incidents in Middle East countries bordering the Arabian Gulf and the Arabian Sea

2.3.1 Bahrain

At least 750 people were treated after the island's biggest mass poisoning case ever caused by contaminated egg-and-mayonnaise sandwiches served at a wedding party in a Sitra village in early July 2002 (Correspondent. 2002). Most of the people were discharged following treatment, but a 23-year-old Bahraini man died 6 days after he was treated for food poisoning. He was a diabetic and had to be taken repeatedly to the hospital since the incident. His condition was made worse because of his sickle cell anemia condition. According to news sources, he might have lived if he had not been refused to be admitted to the hospital with a fever but hospital staff were unable to save him when he returned later the same day when the fever was worse. In April 2003 an outbreak of acute gastroenteritis affected 37 crew members of a British Royal Navy ship deployed in the Northern Arabian Gulf (Gallimore et al., 2005). Of 13 samples examined from the cases, five different viruses were identified including, three norovirus genotypes, a sapovirus, and a rotavirus. Fecal contamination of the salad at source was the most probable explanation for the diversity of viruses detected and characterized. The supplies had been sourced from Bahrain but had originated in another country in the Middle East. The contamination of the salad could have been untreated sewage sludge, which is used to fertilize food crops in some of the food source countries. Those sourcing food crops, particularly those that are eaten raw, should be aware of the agricultural practices in the region. Most outbreaks are given limited coverage through the media as illustrated in the following examples. Food samples taken from a restaurant tested positive for *Salmonella* following an investigation into an outbreak of a mass food poisoning in 2014 (AHN, 2014). The food control inspectors shut down the main restaurant, which was suspected of causing the food poisoning outbreak, as well as two affiliated branches, which remained closed until health requirements were met. The food stocks suspected of being contaminated with *Salmonella* were destroyed, and staff suspended from work, administered proper medication and given health tips to avert any future incidence of food poisoning. The inspectors found serious irregularities in storing food at the temporary restaurant branch located at the Autumn Fair, sufficient to allow the *Salmonella* to reproduce. Consumers were advised to strictly abide by health requirements in cooking and storing food, stressing the need to choose well-cooked food and observe personal hygiene, particularly hand washing before eating. Unfortunately, no details of the outbreak are given in this report. In 2019 it was reported that food served at a religious ceremony caused 27 persons including a young boy to be ill with abdominal pain, vomiting, diarrhea, and headache (Anonymous, 2019). Those affected were hospitalized but no details on the agent or cause were available.

2.3.2 Iraq

In recent years with the rise of the Islamic State of Iraq and the Levant, also known as the ISIS, fluid borders between Iraq and Syria with refugees and internally displaced persons (IDPs), presence of foreign troops, and a disrupted health system, it is not surprising that there are relatively few published outbreaks occurring in Iraq. This was compounded with healthcare staff trying to contain a major cholera outbreak and treat cases (Jameel et al., 2016). Apparently in 2015 45 fighters died after ingesting an iftar meal commemorating the conclusion of Ramadan in Mosul (Schachtel, 2015). It remains unclear whether the fighters died of food poisoning or intentional poisoning, similar to an attack in November when Free Syrian Army men who posed as cooks reportedly poisoned ISIS fighters' meals, killing a dozen. In another iftar event, on June 12, 2017, Iraq CDC informed about a food poisoning outbreak among 825 IDPs in Al-Khazir camp, Northern Iraq, after consuming an iftar breakfast provided by a nongovernment organization (NGO) (Kadhim et al., 2018; Sangar, 2017). The iftar was composed of rice, white bean broth, chicken, yogurt, date, and bread. The cases developed nausea/vomiting or diarrhea or abdominal pain. A retrospective cohort study was initiated. The large number of ordered meals from a NGO single restaurant led to suboptimal food preparation and storage, where the food was cooked in the early morning, at 9:00 a.m., and then transferred to the camp at 1:00 p.m. The food was distributed far later, between 4:00 and 5:00 p.m. The etiological agent was not identified. As a result, rigorous implementation of food handing instructions and health education of the food handlers at refugee camps was encouraged.

Before the disruption by ISIS, outbreaks were sometimes reported in the literature, as in the following *Clostridium perfringens* outbreak (Al-Mola & Al-Rawi, 2013). From a foodborne outbreak of undetermined origin in

Mosul, Iraq, stool specimens collected from those ill were positive for *cpe* gene, coding for the enterotoxin (CPE), the causative factor of *C. perfringens* food poisoning, whether *C. perfringens* counts were high or not ($<$ or $>10^3$ CFU g^{-1}). The authors point out that isolation of the causative agent from stool samples by direct plating is challenging, particularity if several days have passed since the onset of the illness, and the detection of the *cpe* gene directly from human stool samples is a rapid method for the identification of enterotoxigenic *C. perfringens* strains.

A very complete investigation was carried out by Asaad et al. (2014) with two likely pathogens responsible for many attending a restaurant in Tikrit City in June 2013. A total of 203 persons who attended the restaurant and 11 food handlers sought medical care for diarrhea (92.5%), nausea (87.5%), and vomiting (84.5%), and 82 (38.3%) were admitted to hospitals. The incubation period was 1–19 h after food consumption in the restaurant, with > two-thirds of cases ill within 8 h of eating. Apart of one death, all other patients recovered uneventfully. Of the stool specimens submitted, 32% were positive for *Salmonella* Typhimurium, and 30% of samples of leftover food and raw ingredients were positive for *S. aureus*, and 10% for coliform bacteria. Blood, urine, stool, and under the fingernail swabs were negative for all 13 food handlers. An environmental assessment conducted by health inspection team revealed that gloves were not used, and temperatures of cooked and cooled foods were not checked. Also, hands, cooking utensils, vegetables, and other food stuffs were inadequately washed. The overall personal hygiene of food handlers was unsatisfactory: only 1 worker of the 13 interviewed had a valid health card and none had attended food safety education and training session held by Health Inspection Section. More importantly, three workers had a history of diarrhea 2–3 days before the outbreak and had direct contact with the served foods. Laboratory analysis showed that hummus, chicken shawarma, fried lamb, raw meat kofta (lamb and chicken), and olive salad contained *S. aureus*. Although no tests for *S. aureus* enterotoxin were done or levels of the pathogen were determined, and no *S. typhimurium* serotyping and phage-typing results were available, the authors considered that the short incubation period, abrupt appearance of the signs and symptoms, and the microbiological results for cases' stool samples and leftover food items pointed to both *S. aureus* and *S.* Typhimurium as the etiological agents in this outbreak. The incubation period is more consistent with an intoxication rather than an infection, but the same *Salmonella* serovar was isolated from the ill patients. Although no pathogens could be found on the food handlers, their unhygienic practices were likely the source of contamination during the food preparation. Because of the limited capacity of the investigation team in this outbreak, the authors recommended strengthening the role of health inspection through regular examination and training of food handlers, monitoring restaurant environment and food processing, enhancing timely investigations of outbreaks, and raising the capacity of local public health laboratory.

2.3.3 Kuwait

Restaurants in various forms are very popular in Kuwait, and the number is increasing year by year. In 2016 it was estimated that there were more than 5000 restaurants in Kuwait, visited by over 650,000 people each day (Al-Kandari, Al-abdeen, & Jiwan, 2019). With this number, it is not surprising that there are reports of illnesses from restaurants in the press. In a general review of foodborne illness in Kuwait, Fattahova (2014) reported that food poisoning cases are frequent and increase during the summer due to high temperatures and consumption of fast food, with the most common symptoms of food poisoning being vomiting or diarrhea and sometimes fever; some of these could cause physiological or neurological disorders. However, the number of food poisoning cases is not accurate as many cases are not reported and are treated at home without medical aid. If they are ill enough, they are advised to go directly to the hospital rather than the polyclinic, because the polyclinic is usually overburdened with other cases. Emergency departments see many cases of suspect food poisoning, especially children. Some apparent food poisoning cases turn out to be really suicide attempts through excess drug consumption, which can appear to be linked to food. Also, some apparently food poisoning cases may be criminal in nature because an individual wants to blame an eating establishment for injuries unrelated to any food they ate there. The article continues by stating that the medical history of the patient is crucial. The information the patients provide matters, such as if they are sure of suspicious food they ate from a restaurant for instance, which indicates food poisoning. But if they say they didn't eat outside, and no other family member is experiencing any complications, then there is a criminal suspicion. However, there has to be more than a complainant's statement to incriminate a food source, especially a restaurant. In the following examples, many people were ill, indicating that a foodborne outbreak had occurred, but the agents were not determined. Three incidents that were reported by the press in 2018 give examples of the limited investigations that are publicly available.

In July, 2018, five American soldiers fell ill with *Salmonella* and more than 40 were suspected of being infected in Camp Arifjan in Kuwait, after an outbreak was attributed to food vendors (Myers, 2018). Although the source of the pathogen was not discovered, the command ordered all dining and medical facilities to be inspected and personnel given refresher training for public sanitation requirements and food handling and preparation procedures. Also, in July, the Kuwait News Agency reported on a mass food poisoning where 287 had fallen ill after eating from a falafel restaurant in Hawally area in Kuwait (Anonymous, 2018a). Most were hospitalized but released soon afterwards, and the restaurant was closed. The fact that no other details were given and the name of the restaurant was not released frustrated many in online discussions of this incident in the blog

Twofortyeightam (Mark, 2020). This occurred soon after video footage of the restaurant inspection went viral on social media. One of the coowners sent an audio message and pointed the finger at one of his shadow partners. However, the medical reports showed that all the food items that were served at the restaurant were contaminated but particularly for the mayonnaise through incompetent hygiene and food storage. In November 2018, public hospitals in Kuwait received around 130 foreign workers executing a government project with suspected food poisoning. No further details were announced on the incident (Anonymous, 2018b; 2018c). As in many GCC countries, foreign workers make up much of the work force, sometimes under less than ideal public health conditions.

2.3.4 Oman

A well-investigated outbreak in a hospital occurred in 2008, with 58 persons suffering from diarrhea (Al-Abri et al., 2010). All affected had eaten meals served by the hospital kitchen the previous day. A toxin-producing *B. cereus* strain was isolated from feces of patients and food handlers, and of food samples from the kitchen, where many violations of basic food hygiene standards were observed, despite a recent external quality assurance inspection. In January 2013, a food poisoning outbreak affected 300 employees of Oman's state-owned Petroleum Development Oman (PDO) at the Qarn Alam Camp (Vaidya, 2013). These had reported to the camp's clinic, mostly with a mild to moderate infection resulting in vomiting and diarrhea. Some were hospitalized. Both the company and Ministry of Health officials were working to identify the cause of the incident, but no other information was available. The PDO is the Sultanate's major exploration and production company, accounting for more than 70% of the country's crude-oil production and nearly all of its natural gas supply. In late August 2015 20 Omanis fell ill after consuming contaminated food at a restaurant in Saham province, and some were hospitalized (Rejimon, 2015). Although food samples were taken, the results are not known. The restaurant initially remained open but later Omani authorities closed the restaurant, jailed the staff, and fined them, but specific reasons were not given. Despite continuous crackdowns by the Omani authorities to ensure food safety and public hygiene, food poisoning cases are not uncommon. In August 2014 40 nationals fell sick after reportedly consuming contaminated food at a restaurant in Ibri province. A follow-up investigation showed that a massive quantity of foodstuffs found to be contaminated, improperly labeled, and not fit for consumption was confiscated early in 2015. Because of ongoing reports of unhygienic conditions for food, the 2014 the Consumer Protection Act administered by the Public Authority for Consumer Protection (PACP) has already begun to crack down on those restaurants that flout the rules with powers to impose larger fines and jail terms. For instance, a product will be termed adulterated if foreign substances are found in it that may change its composition and affect its durability (Anonymous, 2017). Malpractices include (1) if the product is past its expiration date; (2) any changes to the natural character of the product; and (3) if the labels are presented with details that are misleading and marked inappropriately.

2.3.5 Qatar

To improve standards of hygiene in restaurants, Qatar's Supreme Council of Health (SCH) has increased the number of inspections on food outlets and has launched a hotline for residents to report complaints on food poisoning (Walker, 2014). The council is responsible for monitoring food establishments and implementing Qatar's food laws along with the Ministry of Municipality and Urban Planning (MMUP). The SCH embarked on an intensive inspection campaign, collecting food samples from all restaurants and food outlets in the country including suppliers. According to the protocol, after a hotline call is received and a report is filed, a team from the SCH would visit the affected people, then inspect the related food outlet and collect samples for laboratory examination. An example of such a "crackdown" was in response to the illness of a family of four which suffered food poisoning after eating chicken, rice, and salad at a popular Turkish restaurant, which was closed down because a medical report prepared by the SCH's environmental health section confirmed that the outlet served contaminated food and violated health regulations. Tests conducted in the Central Food Laboratory at SCH found three types of bacteria that cause diseases in food served by the restaurant. Medical tests on the victims also showed that they were infected by the same bacteria, unfortunately unnamed, as well as one of the restaurant workers. Another popular Turkish restaurant was closed for 2 months after it was found that several customers were treated in the hospital for food poisoning symptoms including intense nausea, vomiting, and diarrhea. As part of the SCH's campaign, experts would undertake community awareness drives and organize seminars and training sessions about food contamination to improve understanding among owners and workers in food establishments. Other closures occurred because of serving food with moldy ingredients, rotten vegetables in the kitchen, insects in pasta, and generally violating the provisions of the food law. As a result of the law, the MMUP increased the number of spot-checks and naming and shaming erring establishments in Arabic on its website. A follow-up to one of these closed Doha Turkish restaurants was a trial when five staff were each been handed fines, jail sentences, and deportation orders after they were found guilty of causing food poisoning to approximately 20 customers ill with vomiting, nausea, and diarrhea (Santacruz, 2015). The restaurant was accused of serving spoiled and unsafe food in October 2014. An affected pregnant woman gave birth to her baby 2 months prematurely. The manager of the restaurant was fined

$2750 and sentenced to spend 3 months in jail, while three other staff members were each fined $1900 and sentenced to 1 month in jail. During an inspection, it was found that another staff member did not hold the necessary health certificate and was subsequently fined $2200 and also sentenced to 1 month in jail. As well as the staff members being sentenced to jail and fined, the Court of Environmental Misdemeanors also found that the restaurant itself was guilty of causing the food poisoning outbreak and issued the restaurant with $8800 in fines and ordered it closed for a further 3 months. These draconian measures may or may not discourage other establishments from serving food that puts the Qatar public at risk. But they were felt necessary because of the complaints made by the public, and in 2017 an amendment was made to the Food Control Law to provide for closing of shops, which shall be indicated with a sign and on the website and local newspapers at the expense of the violator (FAOLEX Database, 2020). Although little has been published in scientific journals or even in the national press about foodborne illness outbreaks, food handlers in Qatar have the potential to spread pathogens when they prepare and serve food through their unhygienic habits. Asim et al. (2019) found that the majority of managers and food handlers in Doha in the facilities studied were trained in food safety management systems. However, applying their knowledge into practice was not observed during the walk-through audits in 53 food service establishments. Caterers, in particular, did not keep employee hygiene records and the majority had no washroom facilities on site. In addition, during the walk-through audit, it was observed that several employees were working in the kitchen with their normal daily clothes without wearing aprons, gloves, and hair nets. These observations indicate an immediate need to educate employees, especially when they may be carrying and excreting organism such as parasites (Abu-Madi et al., 2011) and antibiotic-resistant *E. coli* (Eltai et al., 2018). In addition, there is a high antibiotic-resistant *E. coli* prevalence in chicken meat sold at retail in Qatar and resistant isolates were significantly higher among isolates from local chilled than from imported chilled and frozen chicken samples (Eltai et al., 2020).

2.3.6 Saudi Arabia

In the Kingdom of Saudi Arabia (KSA), a national policy for reporting, notifying, and recording incidents of bacterial food poisoning was established in 1984 (Aljoudi, Al-Mazam, & Choudhry, 2010). Since then *Salmonella* food poisoning outbreaks have been reported from different regions of KSA, exhibiting seasonal and regional variations, with chicken, meat, and rice being commonly incriminated food items, and have been frequently reported in the *Saudi Epidemiological Bulletin*. SE is the most frequent *Salmonella* serotype isolated from foodborne disease outbreaks in recent decades. According to ProMED (http://www.promedmail.org) editorials, restaurants and communal feasts and institutional feeding (such as in school cafeterias, hospitals, nursing homes, prisons), where large quantities of food are prepared several hours before serving, are the most common settings in which foodborne illness incidents occur. For instance, in 2005 a hospital in the Jizan Region received 19 suspected food poisoning cases that were ill after taking meals from a restaurant, including a woman who suffered from severe diarrhea, abdominal pain, vomiting, and dizziness (Fagbo, 2005). The restaurant was closed down and three of its workers were detained pending the results of laboratory tests. The report of an investigative committee could not find a specific cause but noted that the restaurant had earlier been responsible for some hygienic violations. In January, 2008, 92 patients sought medical care at hospitals and primary healthcare centers in Najran city (Southern Province), complaining of gastrointestinal symptoms: diarrhea, fever, vomiting, nausea, and abdominal pain, after eating from a newly opened restaurant. SE was isolated from patient but not food handler stools (Alfara & Al Mazroua, 2008). Although food items showed no growth for any pathogens, mayonnaise was prepared at the restaurant from blending egg yolk, oil, and garlic, and stored at ambient temperatures. At the end of each day, unused mayonnaise was kept for use on the following day, when it was sometimes mixed with a new batch of mayonnaise.

In 2006, 31 foodborne illness outbreaks, accounting for 251 cases, were reported in Qassim (Al-Goblan & Jahan, 2010). Located at the heart of the country, and almost in the center of the Arabian Peninsula, Qassim province has a population of 1.4 million and is the richest region in the country with a large agricultural economy. The highest proportion (64.5%) of the 31 outbreaks was reported during summer months of June to August. Men constituted 66.9% of the cases, and 68.1% were adults. *Salmonella* species was the commonest etiological agent, followed by *S. aureus*. In previous studies in Saudi Arabia, *Salmonella* had been important etiological agents. The majority (68.9%) in the Qassim study of the cases were ill after consuming commercially prepared foods. Consumption of contaminated meat, such as chicken with rice or shawarma sandwiches of chicken or mutton caused about two-thirds of the cases (67.7%). Al-Amoud and Al-Mazrooa (2000) described in more detail one shawarma outbreak in Riyadh involving eight persons suffering from SE where mayonnaise using raw eggs was the implicated ingredient. Other implicated foods in Qassim outbreaks included laban, camel milk, appetizer, mixed and green salads, as well as rice, potato chips and French fries, unspecified snacks, mayonnaise, popcorn, and chocolate.

Bakri et al. (2017) lists 14 outbreaks in Saudi Arabia from 2006 to 2011. An incident of food poisoning occurred in Taif city in 2006 when 39 of 64 members of families of four brothers living in four separate but adjacent houses suffered from vomiting, diarrhea (two with bloody diarrhea), abdominal pain, and fever (Abu Bakr, del, AlMazroua, & Al Hamdan, 2006). The mean incubation period was 10 h (median 2, range 2–24 h). Both blood and stool specimens were negative for the 20 patients who had been hospitalized. The only common food consumed was raw milk from which *E. coli* was subsequently isolated. The fact that the disease was severe for many of the patients with one death, and one of them had symptoms compatible with hemolytic uremic syndrome indicates the causative organism was a pathogenic *E. coli* strain. Several SE group D outbreaks occurred in 2007 and 2008. In May 2007 55 persons suffered from gastroenteritis and were hospitalized after having eaten meals at a restaurant in Bisha city (AlHonazil, Chaudhry, & Al-Enezy, 2008). Russian salad was the only meal item implicated, and SE was isolated from stool specimens or rectal swabs taken from 51 of those ill. The Russian salad had been prepared as follows: mayonnaise was made at the restaurant by blending egg yolk with oil and vinegar and mixed into carrots and cabbage. The salad was then placed in plastic containers to remain at room temperature for over 3 h. Any leftover Russian salad was used the following day. Although not determined, the most likely source of the SE would be the unpasteurized egg yolks. The same year, an SE outbreak of foodborne disease occurred in Riyadh.

In 2008, an outbreak in Najran city affected 92 people, who complained about gastroenteritis. Mayonnaise was prepared at the restaurant from blending egg yolk, oil, and garlic (Alfara & Al Mazroua, 2008). This was done by restaurant staff two to three times a week. During the day, most of the prepared mayonnaise was distributed in small containers to be served with the broasted chicken meal and kept not far from the oven. At the end of each day, unused mayonnaise was reused the following day, when it was sometimes mixed with a new batch of mayonnaise. Again, SE group D was the etiological agent. In fact, SE was the causative agents in four more outbreaks in 2009 and 2010 at Al-Hofuf, Khaiber, Riyadh, and Al-Ahsa (Bakri et al., 2017). At the Al-Hofuf outbreak, chicken shawarma from a restaurant was the vehicle. In the Khaiber valley outbreak, 55 cases of gastroenteritis were reported after the victims had a meal in a restaurant. In an outbreak at a college restaurant in Riyadh, 200 students suffered after eating Umm Ali (sweet pastry dessert) (AlGhamdi, Al-Sekaiti, & Al-Mazroa, 2010). Raw eggs were the most likely source of infection, while time—temperature abuse during preparation and storage of Umm Ali sweet was the most important contributing factor. In the fourth SE outbreak, 33 cases were reported ill in Al-Ahsa in which the patients had developed gastroenteritis, which associated due to SE group D. Al-Alwy, Al-Mazroa, and Naguib (2009) reported on an outbreak with a coinfection where 21 of 35 members of an extended family suffered from gastroenteritis and fever after being eating at a reception dinner prepared at the home of one of them on February 25, 2009, in Ahad Rafidah. The incubation period ranged from 36 to 63 h (mean 50, median 48 h). Out of the 24 stool samples collected from cases, five (20.8%) were positive for *Salmonella*, four (16. 4%) were positive for *Entamoeba histolytica*, and four (16. 4%) were positive for both. One food handler was positive for the *Entamoeba*. Meat and rice were the most likely vehicles.

In 2011, a group of 39 construction workers at the new Ha'il University buildings suffering from abdominal pain and severe diarrhea had eaten a green salad as a common source food (Maslamani, Al Mazroa, & Nooh, 2011). *S. aureus* was isolated from the salad and nasal swabs of two food handlers, and from undernail swab of one of the handlers. The time interval between food consumption and appearance of first symptom varied among the victims (30 min to 12 h), with a median of 6.5 h. Since one of these food handlers was working in preparing the green salad, he was considered the primary source for this outbreak. The food handlers and construction workers were friends and colleagues, living and eating together, and none of the food handlers had a health certificate to handle the food.

2.3.7 United Arab Emirates

Within the UAE, the Dubai Municipality reports foodborne disease statistics on an annual basis. In 2011 1663 cases were recorded; this gives 88 per 100,000, much lower than in Western countries (Saljila, 2011). Even lower numbers were given for 2014 (550) and for 2018 (800), which translate into 29 and 42 per 100,000, respectively (Al Ramahi, 2018; Masudi, 2014). However, the Municipality admits there are many more cases, since only half were confirmed. Although more than 200 cases were found to be caused by *Salmonella* infections, the cause of the remaining cases could not be verified. Officials shut down 180 restaurants over safety concerns; two reasons given were the summer's high temperatures and the improper refrigeration of foods. Sporadic cases were likely those at residences where there were improper food practices including cross contamination and undercooking.

In 2015, 25 students of the Emirates National School in Sharjah fell ill at their homes with abdominal cramps, nausea and vomiting, diarrhea, fever, and dehydration after they ate food at school at a food charity bazaar organized by the school (Afkarali, 2015). The students brought food from their homes to sell to each other and raise money for the charity. The foods exchanged included Arabic food, salads, cupcake, and sweets, but it was not possible to determine which food item was responsible for causing their illnesses, which started during the night for some. Based on the symptoms, the relatively short incubation period, and their rapid recovery, the students probably ingested staphylococcal enterotoxin, originating from poor food handling practices in one or more of the homes. Temperature abuse would allow *S. aureus* to grow followed by the production of enterotoxin in the food. For 25 students to be ill required at least 25 food items to be sold and eaten. Food prepared at home contributing to staphylococcal food poisonings is frequent in Middle Eastern countries (El Sheikha, 2015). Because the students ate the food during the afternoon of the exchange, there could have been opportunities for *S. aureus* growth and toxin production, and the teacher supervision for safe food handling did not seem to be evident, which is consistent with the publication of Abushelaibi, Jobe, Al Dhanhani, Al Mansoori, and Al Shamsi (2016) in a study of eight schools in Al Ain city, where inappropriate "behavior may expose students to bacterial food poisoning such as Salmonella and Staphylococcus." This included eating their meals in the playground.

In one particular outbreak in 2019 the Municipality closed a Jumeirah restaurant after 15 people were infected with *Salmonella* (Staff, 2019). The outbreak was likely caused by a hollandaise sauce that was prepared with raw eggs the use of which in ready-to-eat foods has been banned since 2012. The chef and person-in-charge of food safety have been held, and the restaurant rating was downgraded.

Asian and African employees working for a Sharjah-based building material company suffered from vomiting, fever, fatigue, and diarrhea starting 1 h after having eaten at an anniversary lunch organized by the company management (Afkar, 2019). One of the employees stated that he started to feel ill and took a pain killer for relief, but after 2 h his condition worsened and he soon found out that all his colleagues were also suffering from the same issue. Thirteen of the 18 ill were admitted to a local hospital and blood specimens were taken, but they recovered quickly. The meal consisted of rice, chicken, and fish, with watermelon and other foods for dessert. The restaurant manager stated that on the same day of the incident, 250 people had eaten meals from the restaurant without any complaint. Nevertheless, Sharjah Municipality temporary closed the restaurant and fined the owner. An undeclared "poisoning bacteria" was found in blood samples. Based on the symptoms, rapid onset and recovery, the only possibility is for a preformed toxin to have caused their illnesses. The *B. cereus* emetic toxin has caused similar symptoms from fried rice and staphylococcal enterotoxins have been associated with chicken products (CCFI (Committee on Control of Foodborne Illness) & International Association for Food Protection, 2011). It is not clear what was found in the blood, but it is unlikely to have been associated with this outbreak given the 1-h incubation period.

2.3.8 Yemen

Yemen is suffering from an extended civil war which began in 2015 between the Abdrabbuh Mansur Hadi-led Yemeni government and the Houthi armed movement, along with their supporters and allies. This has resulted in famine conditions and allowed a large cholera outbreak to develop. According to Friedrich (2019) and Weill, Domman, and Njamkepo (2019), Yemen is currently experiencing the largest cholera epidemic in recent history. The first cases were declared in September 2016, and over 1.1 million cases and 2300 deaths have since been reported. Even before the war, only a tiny proportion of Yemeni families was connected to the municipal supply; 13 million Yemenis—50% of the population—struggle daily to find or buy enough clean water to drink or grow food. Various estimates predict that the capital Sana'a could run out of water within a decade. As a result, 14.7 million Yemenis currently depend on humanitarian aid (Whitehead, 2015). Malnutrition and diarrhea kill 14,000 Yemeni children under five each year, and food aid can sometimes cause serious illnesses, as occurred in the following incident. In 2014 20 children arrived at al-Dali hospital in critical condition, and two died; the cause of death was beans provided by the World Food Program (WFP) (Alkhazzan, 2014). Medical sources indicated that most cases affected children between 5 and 15, and consisted of fever, blood in urine, severe diarrhea, as well as anemia; the two children who died had severe anemia and acute renal failure. More than 50 cases of the disease appeared not only in al-Dali, but in al-Azariq, also probably linked to the beans. The WFP had begun distributing more than 18,000 food baskets certified by the Yemen Bureau of Standards, to aid those displaced by violence in al-Dali whose residents have been caught in the crossfire between government troops and the rebels. This outbreak affecting children seems most likely to have been favism which is a hemolytic response to the consumption of fava (broad type) beans in some people who have hereditary Mediterranean type glucose-6-phosphate dehydrogenase (G6PD) deficiency. The peak seasonal incidence of favism in the Mediterranean where broad beans can be either eaten raw (as fresh in salads) or cooked (April and May) coincides with harvesting of the broad beans (Kattamis, Kyriazakou, & Chaidas, 1969), which is the time frame for this outbreak.

Epidemiological studies were conducted, and some foodborne disease outbreaks were reported before the civil war began and likely continued but are uninvestigated. For instance, Taha, Alghalibi, and Saeed Saleh (2013) determined the incidence of *Salmonella* infection in 250 enteric fever and 210 food poisoning cases attending Thamar general hospital and Dar Alshafaa medical clinic in 2008 through analyzing blood, urine, and stool specimens. Of the patients with enteric fever and food poisoning, 16.4% and 15.2%, respectively, were infected with different strains of *Salmonella*: the serovars isolated were: *Salmonella* typhi (45.6%), SE (24.4%), *Salmonella* paratyphi B (14.4%), *S. typhimurium* (13.3%), and *S. paratyphi* A (2.2%). However, only SE was isolated from both groups. For enteric fever, four serotypes were isolated, the most common being *S. typhi* (70.7%) followed by *S. paratyphi* (25.8%). The authors thought that *S. typhi* was spread predominantly within the household, for example, person-to-person transmission and poor hand-washing hygiene, whereas *S.* paratyphi and other serovars were mainly transmitted outside the home, for example, consumption of foods from street vendors. In Yemen, as well as in other GCC countries, there are many popular dishes that are eaten by hand (without a spoon) and shared between family members. Both SE (62.5%) and *S.* Typhimurium (37.5%) were isolated from patients with foodborne illnesses. In general, the standard of hygiene, quality control, and monitoring procedures for food preparation and storage in Thamar city was seen as low. Another source of pathogens including *Salmonella* is paper note currency. Notes of all the denominations were obtained from different occupational groups, mainly bus drivers, street hawkers, vegetable vendors, restaurants, butchers, and fish sellers in Taiz city, Yemen (Hanash, Al-baker, Al-harazi, Alkadasi, & Zaid, 2015). The following pathogens and indicator microorganisms were found: *E. coli* (50.3%), *S. aureus* (14.0%), *Klebsiella* spp. (4.4%), *Proteus* spp. (4.39%), *Salmonella* (1.3%), *Shigella* spp. (1.0%), and alpha hemolytic *Streptococcus* (0.1%). The authors considered currency notes could play a significant role in the transmission of potentially harmful microorganisms, and those handling food and money should avoid opportunities for cross-contamination.

2.4 Unique challenges to prevent and control foodborne illnesses from occurring in Arab countries

2.4.1 Mass gatherings

Mass gatherings are defined as of 1000 individuals upwards in a specific location for a designated period (WHO, 2009). Such occurrences put a strain on the local resources, such as food, drinks, accommodation, and healthcare, and can pose a health risk to the population. In 2009, Lebanon hosted the 6th Francophone Games. Pandemic A(H1N1)2009 virus presented a significant health threat at the time. A surveillance strategy was implemented for the timely detection and management of epidemiological events and outbreaks, in particular for A(H1N1)2009 virus cases (Haddad, Ammar, Khoury, Cox, & Ghosn, 2017). Data were collected and managed daily and feedback was generated through daily bulletins. A total of 299 medical consultations were reported, 29% of which related to infectious diseases. There were 10 cases reported as acute respiratory infections; all tested negative for A(H1N1)2009 virus within 24 h. Twenty-three cases of gastroenteritis were reported, in which 11 stool cultures were negative. While pandemic A(H1N1)2009 did not interfere with the Games, it was essential to strengthen surveillance and to have timely epidemiological information. This was achieved through preparedness, a multidisciplinary approach, timely management, and coordination. This type of surveillance is appropriate for future pandemics, such as for the COVID-19 coronavirus and its successors. Muslims are obligated to participate in the Hajj at least once in a lifetime if circumstances allow. This annual event to Mecca (Makaa) is the largest mass gathering in the world (upwards of 5 million pilgrims) and is considered a major public health concern for infectious diseases, including those borne by food and water. Saudi Arabia has extensive experience of providing healthcare at mass gatherings acquired through decades of managing millions of pilgrims at the Hajj (Memish et al., 2014). However, foodborne illnesses do occur as in 2003, when a large number of Iranian Hajjis presented to several hospitals in Al Madinah complaining of vomiting, nausea, abdominal pain, and diarrhea after eating food prepared in the kitchen of their caterer. A total of 414 persons was interviewed, 207 cases and 207 controls (AlMaghderi & Al-Mazroa, 2003). Four food items were eaten: rice, chicken along with bread and yoghurt obtained from a local supplier. *S. aureus* was believed to have been the etiological agent. In 2006 during the annual Hajj pilgrimage, a group of Saudi soldiers was diagnosed for having gastroenteritis following a rice lunch contaminated with *B. cereus* and *C. perfringens* (Bakri et al., 2017). But it is not only in Saudi Arabia that mass gatherings occur. For instance, during the 4-day Eid Al Adha holiday, when Aqaba is the site of one of the largest mass gatherings in Jordan, public health concerns during this holiday include foodborne and waterborne diseases (Abdullah et al., 2013). Millions of pilgrims attend Arbaeenia mass gathering in Iraq each year. Thousands of individuals work voluntarily at temporary rest areas (locally called Mawakib), distributed in most of Iraq governorates, to provide food and other services to the attendees (Lami et al., 2019). The potential for improper handling of food at Mawakib increases the risk of waterborne and foodborne diseases. There are also traditional Shi'a pilgrimages, such as the anniversary of death of Imam Moussa al-Kadhim in various locations in Iraq and Syria with 5–6 million pilgrims, and also the arts festival in Bosra, Syria, started in 1985, with 1.2–2.5 million attendees over 10 days (Ainsour & Fleischauer, 2013).

Mousavi and Jafari (2016) followed up on Iranian pilgrims to holy sites in Iraq who fell sufficiently ill to go to clinics in Najaf, Karbala, Baghdad, and Kazmain. Although the main complaint among pilgrims was acute respiratory tract infection, the authors considered that the high prevalence of gastroenteritis (7%) indicated that foodborne disease incidents probably occurred during their pilgrimage travels, and food preparation should be more closely monitored, and they should be advised to observe good personal hygiene principles. A more systematic review of Hajj pilgrims showed that gastrointestinal diseases, food-poisoning, and diarrhea were major concerns (Hoang et al., 2020). Pilgrims from Marseille, France, participating in the Hajj in 2016–18 underwent successive systematic rectal swabbing before and after their travel. Carriage of the main enteric pathogens was assessed by real-time PCR in the 376 persons studied. During the Hajj, 18.6% presented at least one gastrointestinal symptom, 13.8% had diarrhea, and 36.4% had acquired at least one enteric pathogen. EPEC and EAEC were the pathogens most frequently acquired by pilgrims (17.6% and 14.4%, respectively). A few also suffered from EHEC. Interestingly, pilgrims who suffered from diarrhea were more likely to wash their hands more often and be obese or overweight. Acquisition of pathogenic *E. coli* and other enteric bacteria in pilgrims can result in gastrointestinal distress often called Traveler's Diarrhea arising from the consumption of contaminated food and drink. Poor food safety and personal hygiene are the main risk factors for contracting foodborne and waterborne illnesses. For those pilgrims who have risks of underlying diseases, vaccination and medical examination before leaving for any mass gathering and using basic hygienic practices during the events would improve the likelihood that they would enjoy a healthy pilgrimage. Gautret, Benkouiten, Sridhar, Al-Tawfiq, and Memish (2015) also recommend regular use of alcohol-based hand rubs for pilgrims, as they require less time than traditional hand washing, act more rapidly, and contribute to sustained improvement in compliance associated with decreased infection rates. These would work to decontaminate hands and surfaces for *E. coli* and other pathogenic bacteria but would be less effective against parasites, norovirus, and HAV. Electronic syndromic surveillance is one way to enhance surveillance for mass gatherings (Fleischauer & Gaines, 2017). Despite its limitations and operational costs, syndromic surveillance may provide useful information to local health departments during a mass gathering. However, a preexisting infrastructure to support electronic data transfer, a capacity to quickly receive and interpret data, a thorough understanding of how to interpret and share these data with external stakeholders, and a plan to sustain any new surveillance enhancements are necessary before electronic syndromic surveillance can be used effectively during mass gatherings.

2.4.2 Migrant workers

Energy-rich Gulf states rely heavily on foreign workers across all sectors of the economy, from professionals to skilled workers and manual labor. Expatriates constitute almost 90% of the population in the UAE, two-thirds in Kuwait, half in Oman and Bahrain, and one-third in Saudi Arabia. The major group of migrant workers is from Asian countries, including India, Pakistan, Bangladesh, and the Philippines. In 2007 during Hajj season, a study was conducted in Mecca among food handlers, and samples of 504 participants from around the world were examined for parasitic intestinal infection using different stool examination techniques. Almost one-thirds (31.9%) were found to carry intestinal parasites including *Entamoeba coli* and *E. histolytica*, *Giardia lamblia*, and *Ascaris lumbricoides* (Bakri et al., 2017). Albreiki, Al-Ali, and Rayan (2004) found that 328 of 17,918 foreign workers in Al-Qatif area in the Eastern Province of Saudi Arabia who had previously been diagnosed as free of infection were asymptomatic carriers of *Salmonella*. The highest frequency was found among workers from Egypt (13.1%), while Filipinos and Indians were the lowest carriers (1.2%). In 2015–16, Humphrey et al. (2016) found that pathogens were detected in 57% of 75 male workers coming to the Qatar Red Crescent Worker's Health Center with the most frequent being *Salmonella* (27%), EPEC (21%), EAEC (15%), and ETEC (12%). Codetection of multiple pathogens was identified in 54% of positive stool specimens.

These kinds of data show that foreign workers in the retail food industry have the potential to cause foodborne disease outbreaks. Historically, this seems to have been the case. Between 1982 and 1986, of the 90 incidents, 1531 cases of foodborne diseases were reported in Saudi Arabia, whereas Saudis were involved in small incidents in which the food was probably mishandled at private homes, expatriates constituted the majority of cases of in relatively large foodborne outbreaks in which the food was probably mishandled in their camps (Alkanahl & Gasim, 1993). Dairy foods, meat, and chicken were the foods most frequently reported in association with foodborne diseases (36%, 30%, and 22% of incidents, respectively). *S. aureus* was the agent or the suspect agent of more incidents than *Salmonella* spp. Insufficient cooking and improper storage were the main factors suspected of contributing to incidents (17.8% and 13.3%, respectively). As noted by Al-Abri et al. (2010), many catering facilities in the region are manned by expatriate workers, typically from the Indian Sub-continent, and occupational health screening for such staff usually focuses on excluding the carriage of pathogenic parasites, which are of questionable importance. The need for continued education of such staff about food hygiene and for the enforcement of relevant regulations has been emphasized recently in the region.

2.4.3 Poison control centers

Poisons control centers are sources of expertise on the diagnosis and management of poisoning. Most centers provide emergency advice to the general public as well as to health professionals (WHO, 2019). These provide immediate, free, and expert treatment advice and assistance over the telephone in case of exposure to poisonous or hazardous substances. They also answer questions about potential poisons in addition to providing treatment management advice about household products, medicines, pesticides, plants, bites and stings, food poisoning, and fumes (AAPCC, 2020). The first poisons information center started in 1949 in the Netherlands. In the following decades, there was an expansion in the number of poisons centers in industrialized countries in the Americas, Europe, and Australasia. This was driven by the rapid increase in the development of new drugs and chemical products after the Second World War, and an associated increase in the incidence of poisoning. Since most health professionals were unfamiliar with the management of poisoning the need arose for a source of readily accessible, expert advice. In addition to providing emergency advice on the management of poisoning cases, poisons centers compile data on toxic exposures and on toxic substances. They have important roles in chemical safety and public health, which include characterizing the epidemiology of poisoning to prioritize preventive efforts; advising on the management of the health impacts of chemical incidents; surveillance of chemical exposures; and acting as sentinels to detect chemical release. Over the last decades there has been limited progress in establishing poisons centers, and as of February 2019, only 47%

of Member States had a such a center, with the most notable gaps being in the African, Eastern Mediterranean, and Western Pacific regions. However, Egypt, Palestine, and Saudi Arabia have established poison control centers. The Poison Control Centre of Ain Shams University in Egypt was established in 1981, being one of the earliest poisoning treatment facilities to be established in the Middle East. It has its own inpatient department, ICU and Analytical Toxicology unit (Halawa, Nageeb, & Guindi, 2013). It serves between 20,000 and 25,000 cases a year. In 2012, although the percentage of food poisoning was relatively high (14%), the authors admit that it does not reflect the real magnitude of the problem of foodborne disease in Egypt, since the vast majority of the food poisoning cases referred to the center were clinically of toxigenic type, such as scombroid, ciguatera, and botulism cases. The Palestinian Poison Control and Drug Information Center (PCDIC) was established at the An-Najah National University in 2006 to provide up-to-date information on medications and to help in the early diagnosis and management of poisoning cases including unintentional poisoning and suicidal poisoning, such as improper use of medications and pesticides (Sawalha, 2008). Calls are initiated before any treatment can be provided, and advice provided by the PCDIC was based on the nature of the call. The PCDIC has conducted both academic and nonacademic activities. The center introduced the concept of poison prevention weeks in Palestine and has conducted two so far. The PCDIC has published several articles in the fields of toxicology, rational drug use, complementary and herbal therapy, pharmacoepidemiology, and self-medication. Documentation of all enquiries is mandatory for analysis, evaluation, comparative purposes, and quality assurance. More information campaigns are needed to encourage people to use the services provided by the PCDIC. In Saudi Arabia, King Fahad Medical City (KFMC) poison control department was one of the very first poison control service in Saudi Arabia (KFMC, 2020). The initiative to establish the department started as a quality project proposal in 2012 to deal with all cases of poisoning and toxicology consultations in KFMC. The department is staffed by poison information specialists, clinical toxicologists, and backup medical toxicologists to answer inquiries about exposures to chemical agents, including household products, pharmaceuticals, natural toxins, pesticides, and industrial chemicals, and whether a particular exposure is toxic or not. Most of the advice given is for toxic substances other than considered for food poisoning cases, such as medicines, carbon monoxide, button batteries, cleaning products, nail polish remover, gasoline, kerosene, lamp oil, motor oil, lighter fluid, furniture polish, and paint thinner, pesticides, toxic plants, and toxic alcohols. This department cannot be considered a national center since currently it assists only the healthcare sector of KFMC with a long-term goal of serving the population of Riyadh. Yemen has no poison center but has the highest mortality rate for unintentional poisonings in Middle East Arab countries of 4 per 100,000 population according to WHO (2019).

2.4.4 Armed forces

Several Middle East countries have seen civil unrest for many years and been invaded by foreign troops, and sectarian wars have disrupted public health facilities. The impact of ISIS and conditions in refugee camps has been previously briefly discussed from brief media sources. Reports of gastrointestinal illnesses in "boots on the ground" have sometimes been published in scientific journals. For instance, when British troops invaded Iraq on March 21, 2003, they lived in minimal hygienic facilities for several weeks. During the first week of the conflict, they ate individual ration packs only, but centralized catering and locally produced fresh rations (including salads and fruit) were introduced during the second week (Bailey et al., 2005). Gastroenteritis was identified as the major cause of illness in hospital cases during this operation and probably diminished the operational effectiveness of those units affected. Admission rates were initially high because of exhaustion, dehydration, and poor living conditions during the first month of the conflict. A norovirus strain was identified from stool specimens, but the strain did not group within any of the 15 previously identified norovirus genotypes but was similar to novel strains identified in US military personnel during this same period. The authors believed that introducing fresh rations during a military operation, before adequate health and infection control measures were fully implemented, was inadvisable. In contrast, Royal Marines based elsewhere were not supplied with fresh rations during this period, and no outbreaks of gastroenteritis were reported.

Hundreds of thousands of American service members have been deployed to Afghanistan and Iraq since 2001. In the initial phases of operations in both Afghanistan and Iraq, large outbreaks of severe gastroenteritis secondary to norovirus and *Shigella* infections were reported in both British and American personnel (Aronson, Sanders, & Moran, 2006). Subsequently large outbreaks were less frequently reported, but diarrhea remained a common problem. More personnel deployed to Iraq than to Afghanistan experienced at least one episode of diarrhea; symptoms were of greater severity and a longer duration of illness. Diarrhea was associated with time spent off military compounds and eating local food. In Iraq, field laboratory testing found that ETEC and EAEC were the more frequently found pathogens than norovirus, *Shigella*, and parasites.

Even peace-keeping forces have been implicated with gastroenteritis and food poisoning as in the United Nations Interim Force in Lebanon (UNIFIL), which has been deployed in the country since 1978 and comprises both naval and armed forces. A study of medical records of 2054 patients of various nationalities treated in the UNIFIL Hospital from 1993 to 2000 showed there was a high incidence of infectious and digestive tract diseases resulted from disregard of basic sanitary principles that ought to be followed within areas of unfamiliar climatic and sanitary conditions. The most common reason for hospitalizations was salmonellosis, staphylococcal food poisoning, and viral hepatitis A and B. The highest proportion of contagious diseases was observed in 1996—when an epidemic of salmonellosis broke out in the Irish contingent, and in 1998 when an outbreak of staphylococcal food poisoning occurred in the Polish contingent (Buczyński, Korzeniewski, & Dziedziczak-Buczyńska, 2003; Korzeniewski, 2009).

2.5 Conclusion

As can be seen from the above review of foodborne disease in Arab Middle East countries, most incidents have been reported in the press with relatively few in scientific publications or epidemiological or medical reports. Press news items are typically limited in that they cover the initial complaints and government action against the commercial suppliers or food preparers but do not follow up to discover the etiological agents or the factors contributing to the outbreaks. Those cases with serious conditions and deaths are more likely to be reported, and they usually are public events such as wedding receptions, religious meals, or restaurants. Thus, even if incidents at homes may be frequent, they are rarely reported unless deaths occur. Generally, local and national governments tend to punish those establishments that are found to be responsible for foodborne illnesses even if the actual cause is not known; a microbiological agent or toxin has not been identified or the conditions that led to the illnesses. Such punishments can be fines, temporary closures. or even prison sentences.

Laws have been put in place to give governments more powers to carry out such penalties. Examples are the 2014 Omani Consumer Protection Act administered by the PACP (Anonymous, 2017), the Egyptian Law N1/2017 to establish the National Food Safety Authority (Abdel-Haleem & Ibrahim, 2017), and the Food Control Law of Qatar (FAOLEX Database, 2020; Walker, 2014). As a further example of more detail, the UAE Federal Law No. 10 of 2015 on Food Safety imposes standards and regulations for maintaining the safety and quality of food and ensuring the protection of public health and consumers (UAE, 2020). The law imposes strict penalties on those found to be endangering food safety across the UAE. Through its National Food Safety Committee, the Ministry of Climate Change & Environment works with its partners on implementing the law on safety of food and its executive regulations, which includes strict controls and standards to ensure food safety throughout the food chain. The law authorizes imposing fines of up to AED 100,000 (about US$27,230). The emirates of Abu Dhabi, Dubai, and Sharjah have policies that ensure that food is fit for human consumption including conducting the necessary research and studies on safe food and issue rules, regulations, and standards on food items sold or offered for human consumption. The Saudi Food and Drug Authority was established by royal decree in 2002 and has oversight of the Saudi food supply at the national level (SFDA, 2020). The Jordanian Food and Drug

Administration under the Ministry of Health became permanent law in 2008, with one of its responsibilities to ensure the safety of food stuffs, their quality, and their fitness for human consumption (JFDA, 2008). It is governed by a board of Directors with among other responsibilities to develop the general policy relating to food, drug, and their control; approve the required plans and programs; and follow their implementation. Improvements in conducting investigations of complaints of illness are also being established such as the National Rapid Alert System for Food, which was launched in 2017 to ensure proper implementation of response measures when serious food risks are detected (UAE, 2020). The system identifies the mechanisms of managing food risk alerts as well as banning and lifting of bans on adulterated and misbranded food. Despite these efforts, Faour-Klingbeil and Todd (2019) have reviewed the need for implementing national control systems in all MENA countries. However, these national agencies are not likely to address the prevention and control of local foodborne disease outbreaks. This is more the authority of municipalities such as Dubai, which has a Food Code, based on codes in western countries, to provide a set of model requirements to help food establishments achieve a higher degree of compliance with the food regulations, and attain a higher standard of food safety through adoption of good practices (Government, 2013). Recently, better pathogen detection systems involving pulsed-field gel electrophoresis (PFGE) have been employed in most Middle East countries. PulseNet Middle East is coordinated by both the Central Public Health Laboratory in Muscat, Oman, and the WHO Office for National Epidemic Preparedness and Response in Lyon, France (https://pulsenetinternational.org/networks/middleeast/). Reports on PFGE use are occasionally published, as in Fadlallah et al. (2019).

Certification of foodservice and food processing employees is required in Arab countries as occurs everywhere where food is processed, prepared, and served commercially, and private contractors create online and in-person courses to meet the necessary standards, for example, Boecker (https://www.boecker.com/food-safety-training/) and Laimoon (https://courses.laimoon.com/course/food-safety-manager-certificate). Such training has to be renewed on a periodic basis for managers and employees.

Overall, foodborne disease in Middle East countries is underreported, and improved epidemiological surveillance systems are required as essential for enhancing national and regional prevention and control systems. This is especially important not only for residents of these countries but also for making tourists safer and less likelihood that imported and exported food is contaminated. Climate change with hotter summers and less available potable and irrigation water will exacerbate the risks of pathogen growth and toxin production. Civil wars, sectarian strife, failed economies are factors over the years that have limited effective public health infrastructure to prevent and control foodborne illnesses in the Middle East, and these conditions still occur in some countries.

References

AAPCC (American Association of Poison Control Centers). (2020). Available from https://aapcc.org/. Accessed December 5, 2020.

Abdel-Haleem, A., & Ibrahim, N. (2017). Food regulations and enforcement in Egypt. *Reference Module in Food Sciences*, 1–6. Available from https://doi.org/10.1016/B978-0-08-100596-5.21188-8.

Abdullah, S., Sharkas, G., Sabri, N., Iblan, I., Abdallat, M., Jriesat, S., … Al-Nsour, M. (2013). Mass gathering in Aqaba, Jordan, during Eid Al Adha, 2010. *Eastern Mediterranean Health Journal*, *19*(Suppl. 2), S29–S33.

Abu Bakr, A., del, AlMazroua, M., & Al Hamdan, N. (2006). Foodborne outbreak among 4 families in Taif city, Saudi Arabia, July 2006. *Saudi Epidemiology Bulletin*, *13*(4), 28–31.

Abu-Madi, M. A., Behnke, J. M., Ismail, A., Al-Olaqi, N., Al-Zaher, K., & El-Ibrahim, R. (2011). Comparison of intestinal parasitic infection in newly arrived and resident workers in Qatar. *Parasites & Vectors*, *4*, 211.

Abushelaibi, A., Jobe, B., Al Dhanhani, F., Al Mansoori, S., & Al Shamsi, F. (2016). An overview of food safety knowledge and practices in selected schools in the city of Al Ain, United Arab Emirates. *African Journal of Microbiology Research*, *10*(15), 511–520, Accessed September 11, 2020.

Adwan, G. M., Alqarem, B. R., & Adwan, K. M. (2015). Prevalence of foodborne pathogens in meat samples in Palestine. *International Food Research Journal*, *22*(5), 1806–1812.

Afkar, A. (2019, October 2). UAE restaurant shut down after 18 workers suffer from food poisoning. *Khaleej Times*. Available from: https://www.khaleejtimes.com/news/uae-health/popular-uae-restaurant-shut-down-after-18-workers-suffer-from-food-poisoning. Accessed August 24, 2020.

Afkarali, A. (2015, December 18). 25 pupils suffer food poisoning in Sharjah. *Khaleej Times*. Available from https://www.khaleejtimes.com/nation/general/25-pupils-suffer-food-poisoning-in-sharjah. Accessed August 24, 2020.

AHN. (2014, February 2). Health Ministry announces initial food poisoning results. *Bahrain News Agency*. Available from http://www.bna.bh/portal/en/news/600495. Accessed September 7, 2020.

Ainsour, M., & Fleischauer, A. (2013). Public health considerations for mass gatherings in the Middle East and North Africa (MENA) region. *East Mediterranean Health Journal.*, *19* (Suppl. 2), S42–S47.

Al-Abri, S., Al-Jardani, A., Al-Hosni, M., Padmamohan, K., Al-Busaidi, S., & Beeching, N. J. (2010). A hospital acquired outbreak of Bacillus cereus gastroenteritis in a tertiary care hospital in Oman. Abstracts, 7th International Conference of the Hospital Infection Society, 10–13 October 2010, Liverpool, UK. *Journal of Hospital Infection*, *76*(S1), S65–S66.

Al-Alwy, M. M., Al-Mazroa, M. A., & Naguib, M. (2009). Foodborne outbreak in Ahad Rafidah, Saudi Arabia, February 2009. *Saudi Epidemiology Bulletin*, *16*(2), 13.

Al-Amoud, M., & Al-Mazrooa, M. (2000). Salmonella enteritidis outbreak, Riyadh, 1999. *Saudi Epidemiology Bulletin*, *7*, 24. Available from: https://www.fetp.edu.sa/view_bulletin_issue.php?bulletin_id = 26. Accessed September 8, 2020.

Albreiki, H. M., Al-Ali, A. K., & Rayan, A. J. (2004). Salmonella carriers among expatriate workers in Al-Qatif area. *Saudi Journal of Gastroenterology*, *10*(3), 140–143.

Alfara, N., & Al Mazroua, M. (2008). Food borne outbreak in Najran City, Saudi Arabia, January 2008. *Saudi Epidemiological Bulletin*, *15*(1), 5–6. Available from http://fetp.edu.sa/downloads/articles/y2008/A2008-V15-1-00207.pdf. Accessed September 8, 2020.

AlGhamdi, A. S., Al-Sekaiti, M. H., & Al-Mazroa, M. (2010). Foodborne Salmonella outbreak in a college, Riyadh, Saudi Arabia, October 2009 (1430 H). *Saudi Epidemiology Bulletin*, *17*(2), 14–15.

Al-Goblan, A. S., & Jahan, S. (2010). Surveillance for foodborne illness outbreaks in Qassim, Saudi Arabia, 2006. *Foodborne Pathogens and Disease*, *7*(12), 1559–1562.

AlHonazil, I. A., Chaudhry, A. J., & Al-Enezy, F. M. (2008). Food borne outbreak in Bisha City, Saudi Arabia, May 2007. *Saudi Epidemiology Bulletin*, *15*(2), 13.

Aljoudi, A. S., Al-Mazam, A., & Choudhry, A. J. (2010). Outbreak of food borne Salmonella among guests of a wedding ceremony: The role of cultural factors. *Journal of Family & Community Medicine*, *17*, 29–34.

Alkanahl, H. A., & Gasim, Z. (1993). Foodborne disease incidents in the eastern province of Saudi Arabia—A five-year summary, 1982–1986. *Journal of Food Protection*, *56*(1), 84–87.

Al-Kandari, D., Al-abdeen, J., & Jiwan, S. (2019). Food safety knowledge, attitudes and practices of food handlers in restaurants in Kuwait. *Food Control*, *103*, 103–110.

Alkhazzan, W. A. (2014). Deadly disease in Al-Dali governorate appears on eating beans. *Qary Net*. Available from http://qary.net/news-763918. Accessed January 3, 2016.

AlMaghderi, Y. S., & Al-Mazroa, M. A. (2003). Staphylococcus aureus food poisoning outbreak in AI-Madinah AI-Monawarah. *Saudi Epidemiological Bulletin*, *10*(2), 9, 10, 13. Available from https://www.fetp.edu.sa/view_bulletin_issue.php?bulletin_id = 36. Accessed September 14, 2020.

Al-Mola, A., & Al-Rawi, A. (2013). Detection of Cpegene in stool samples of food poisoning patients in Mosul/Iraq. *Science Journal of University of Zakho*, *1*(2), 414–419. Retrieved from https://sjuoz.uoz.edu.krd/index.php/sjuoz/article/view/143. Accessed August 4, 2020.

Al Ramahi, N. (2018, September 3). Dubai health authorities report 800 cases of food poisoning this year. *N UAE*. Available from https://www.thenational.ae/uae/health/dubai-health-authorities-report-800-cases-of-food-poisoning-this-year-1.766542. Accessed August 24, 2020.

Anonymous. (2007). Foodborne illness, hummus – Jordan: (Jerash), 2007-10-29 21:00:09 ProMed, PRO/AH/EDR. Archive Number: 20071029.3510. Accessed October 18, 2020.

Anonymous. (2012, January 2). 16 people food-poisoned in Zarqa. *Ammon News*. Available from http://en.ammonnews.net/article.aspx?articleNO = 15172#.VqUwlPkrKM8. Accessed September 5, 2020.

Anonymous. (2017, December 3). Oman consumer protection issues new regulations. *Oman Observer*. Available from https://www.omanobserver.om/oman-consumer-protection-issues-new-regulations/. Accessed September 8, 2020.

Anonymous. (2018a, July 9). Kuwait: Around 290 people poisoned from restaurant food. Available from https://www.gulf-insider.com/kuwait-287-people-poisoned-restaurant-food/. Accessed August 13, 2020.

Anonymous. (2018b, November 11). 130 foreign workers affected by food poisoning. *Arab Times*. Available from https://www.arabtimesonline.com/news/130-foreign-workers-affected-by-food-poisoning/. Accessed August 13, 2020.

Anonymous. (2018c, November 11). 130 foreign workers affected by food poisoning. *Arab Times*. Available from https://www.arabtimesonline.com/news/130-foreign-workers-affected-by-food-poisoning/. Accessed October 18, 2020.

Anonymous. (2019, September 11). Bahrain: Food from religious ceremony leaves 27 with 'food poisoning'. Available from https://www.gulf-insider.com/bahrain-food-from-religious-ceremony-leaves-27-with-food-poisoning/. Accessed September 7, 2020.

Anonymous. (2020a, July 20). Jordan 'rotten meat': Child dies and 800 poisoned near Amman. *BBC News*. Available from https://www.bbc.com/news/world-middle-east-53593948. Accessed September 4, 2020.

Anonymous. (2020b). Second mass poisoning in Jordan prompts food inspections. *The National*. Available from https://www.thenationalnews.com. Accessed December 5, 2020.

Aronson, N. E., Sanders, J. W., & Moran, K. A. (2006). In Harm's way: Infections in deployed American military forces. *Clinical Infectious Diseases, 43*(8), 1045–1051. Available from https://doi.org/10.1086/507539.

Asaad, A. M., Al Lami, F. B., Abdullatif, A., Kareem, A., Mahdi., & Mahmood, S. (2014). Food poisoning outbreak in Tikrit City, Iraq, 2013: *Staphylococcus aureus* and *Salmonella typhimurium* were the incriminated pathogens. *Iraqi Academic Scientific Journal, 13*(2), 169–175, ISSN: 16088360.

Asim, H. S., Elnemr, I., Goktepe, I., Feng, H., Park, H. K., Alzeyara, S., ... Kushad, M. (2019). Assessing safe food handling knowledge and practices of food service managers in Doha, Qatar. *Food Science and Technology International, 25*(5), 440–448. Available from https://doi.org/10.1177/1082013219830843.

Azzeh, P. L. (2014a, October 16). Mother dies 'of food poisoning'; daughter, husband in 'good condition'. *The Jordan Times*. Available from http://www.jordantimes.com/news/local/mother-dies-food-poisoning%E2%80%99-daughter-husband-good-condition%E2%80%99. Accessed September 4, 2020

Azzeh, P. L. (2014b, December 23). Family of Holiday Inn food poisoning victims to sue 'rumour-mongers'. *The Jordan Times*. Available from http://www.jordantimes.com/news/local/family-holiday-inn-food-poisoning-victims-sue-rumour-mongers%E2%80%99. Accessed September 5, 2020.

Bailey, M. S., Boos, C. J., Vautier, G., Green, A. D., Appleton, H., Gallimore, C. I., ... Beeching, N. J. (2005). Gastroenteritis outbreak in British troops, Iraq. *Emerging Infectious Diseases, 11*(10), 1625–1628. Available from https://doi.org/10.3201/eid1110.050298.

Bakri, M., AL Amin, F., Saleh, A. F., Saeed, A. T., Nabag, M., Haroon, M., & Mohamed, K. (2017). Food hygiene in past ten years in Saudi Arabia. *EC Microbiology, 7*(1), 04–13.

Berberian, D. A. (1946). Cheese poisoning in Syria and the Lebanon. *Journal of the Palestine Arab Medical Association, 1*(2), 30–37.

Bernard, H., & Frank, C. (2009). Cluster of hepatitis A cases among travellers returning from Egypt, Germany, September through November 2008. *Euro Surveillance: Bulletin Europeen sur les Maladies Transmissibles = European Communicable Disease Bulletin, 14*(3), 19096.

Bottone, E. J. (2012). Reply to "Can *Bacillus cereus* food poisoning cause sudden death?". *Journal of Clinical Microbiology, 50*(11), 3817.

Buczyński, A., Korzeniewski, K., & Dziedziczak-Buczyńska, M. (2003). Infectious diseases among military personnel in the catchment area of the United Nations Interim Force in Lebanon hospital, from 1993 to 2000. *Przeglad Epidemiologiczny, 58*(2), 313–323.

CCFI (Committee on Control of Foodborne Illness) & International Association for Food Protection. (2011). *Procedures to investigate foodborne illness* (6th ed.). New York: Springer.

Correspondent. (2002, July 7). Bahrain food poisoning victim dies. *Gulf News*. Available from https://gulfnews.com/uae/bahrain-food-poisoning-victim-dies-1.392986. Accessed September 7, 2020.

Costa, R. (2008). Food-borne illness and its effect on tourism in Egypt. *Food Safety and Environmental Health Blog*. Available from https://www.safefoodsblog.com/2008/11/international-food-safety/foodborne-illness-and-its-effect-on-tourism-in-egypt/. Accessed September 4, 2020.

Couturier, E., Roque-Afonso, A. M., Letort, M. J., Dussaix, E., Vaillant, V., & de Valk, H. (2009). Cluster of cases of hepatitis A with a travel history to Egypt, September-November 2008, France. *Euro Surveillance: Bulletin Europeen sur les Maladies Transmissibles = European Communicable Disease Bulletin, 14*(3), 19094. Available from https://doi.org/10.2807/ese.14.03.19094-en.

Dickey, C. (2013). Arafat's polonium poisoning mystery resurfaces. Available from https://www.thedailybeast.com/arafats-polonium-poisoning-mystery-resurfaces?ref = scroll. Accessed August 12, 2020.

Elmanama, A. A., Arafa, H. Z., & Abu-Owda, S. M. (2017). Bacteriological quality of fresh vegetables salad sold in schools canteens and restaurants in Gaza Strip-Palestine. *IUG Journal of Natural Studies, 25*(1), 1–12.

El Sheikha, A. F. (2015). Food safety issues in Saudi Arabia. *Nutrition and Food Technology, 1* (1), 1–4. Available from https://doi.org/10.16966/nftoa.103.

Eltai, N. O., Yassine, H. M., Al Thani, A. A., Abu Madi, M. A., Ismail, A., Ibrahim, E., & Alali, W. Q. (2018). Prevalence of antibiotic resistant Escherichia coli isolates from fecal samples of food handlers in Qatar. *Antimicrobial Resistance & Infection Control, 7*, 78. Available from https://doi.org/10.1186/s13756-018-0369-2.

Eltai, N. O., Yassine, H. M., El-Obeid, T., Al-Hadidi, S. H., Al Thani, A. A., & Alali, W. Q. (2020). Prevalence of antibiotic-resistant Escherichia coli isolates from local and imported retail chicken carcasses. *Journal of Food Protection, 83*(12), 2200–2208.

Fadlallah, S., Shehab, M., Cheaito, K., Haidar-Ahmad, N., El Hafi, B., Saleh, M., & Matar, G. M. (2019). PulseNet Lebanon: An overview of its activities, outbreak investigations, and challenges. *Foodborne Pathogens and Disease, 16*(7), 498–503. Available from https://doi.org/10.1089/fpd.2018.2581.

Fagbo, S. (2005, February 4). Food poisoning - Saudi Arabia (Jizan): Request for information. Archive Number: 20050204.0380. ProMED. Available from: http://promedmail.org/post/20050204.0380. Accessed September 8, 2020.

FAOLEX Database. (2020). Law No. 20 of 2017 amending some provisions of the Law No. 8 of 1990 on the organisation of food control. Available from http://www.fao.org/faolex/results/details/en/c/LEX-FAOC175438. Accessed September 13, 2020.

Faour-Klingbeil, D., & Todd, E. C. D. (2019). Prevention and control of foodborne diseases in Middle-East North African countries: Review of National Control Systems. *International Journal of Environmental Research and Public Health, 17*(1), 70. Available from https://doi.org/10.3390/ijerph17010070.

Fattahova, N. (2014, November 5). Food poisoning cases on the rise in Kuwait. *Kuwait Times*. Available from http://news.kuwaittimes.net/pdf/2014/nov/05/p05.pdf. Accessed September 8, 2020.

Fattel, L., Panossian, B., Salloum, T., Abboud, E., & Tokajian, S. (2019). Genomic features of Vibrio parahaemolyticus from Lebanon and comparison to globally diverse strains by whole-genome sequencing. *Foodborne Pathogens and Disease, 16*(11), 778–787. Available from https://doi.org/10.1089/fpd.2018.2618.

Fleischauer, A. T., & Gaines, J. (2017). Enhancing surveillance for mass gatherings: The role of syndromic surveillance. *Public Health Reports, 132*(Suppl. 1), 95S–98S. Available from https://doi.org/10.1177/0033354917706343.

Frank, C., Walter, J., Muehlen, M., Jansen, A., van Treeck, U., Hauri, A. M., ... Stark, K. (2007). Major outbreak of hepatitis A associated with orange juice among tourists, Egypt, 2004. *Emerging Infectious Diseases, 13*(1), 156–158. Available from https://doi.org/10.3201/eid1301.060487. Available from: http://wwwnc.cdc.gov/eid/article/13/1/06-0487. Accessed October 18, 2020.

Friedrich, M. (2019). Yemen's deadly cholera epidemic. *Journal of American Medical Association*, *321*(7), 637. Available from https://doi.org/10.1001/jama.2019.0151.

Gallimore, C., Pipkin, C., Shrimpton, H., Green, A., Pickford, Y., Mccartney, C., & Gray, J. (2005). Detection of multiple enteric virus strains within a foodborne outbreak of gastroenteritis: An indication of the source of contamination. *Epidemiology and Infection*, *133*(1), 41–47. Available from https://doi.org/10.1017/S0950268804003218.

Gautret, P., Benkouiten, S., Sridhar, S., Al-Tawfiq, J. A., & Memish, Z. A. (2015). Diarrhea at the Hajj and Umrah. *Travel Medicine and Infectious Disease*, *13*(2), 159–166.

Gee, C. (2014, November 8). A dozen ISIS fighters killed after chefs infiltrate camp and POISON terrorists' lunch. *Daily Mirror*. Available from https://www.mirror.co.uk/news/world-news/dozen-isis-fighters-killed-after-4590573. Accessed September 5, 2020.

Government. (2013). *Food code, Food Control Department, Municipality of Dubai*. Available from http://www.al-halabi.com/Portals/0/PDF/Food_Code_English_1.pdf.

Haddad, N., Ammar, W., Khoury, A., Cox, A., & Ghosn, N. (2017). Lebanon's experience in surveillance of communicable diseases during a mass gathering: Sixth Francophone Games, 2009. *Eastern Mediterranean Health Journal*, *23*(2), 118–124.

Halawa, H., Nageeb, S., & Guindi, E. (2013). Annual report of the Poison Control Centre, Ain Shams University Hospitals, Cairo, Egypt, 2012. *Ain Shams Journal of Forensic Medicine and Clinical Toxicology*, *21*(2), 27–34. Available from https://doi.org/10.21608/ajfm.2013.19165, ISSN 1687-1030.

Hanash, S., Al-baker, S. M., Al-harazi, T., Alkadasi, M., & Zaid, A. A. (2015). Prevalence of pathogenic bacteria from contaminated Yemeni currency notes in Taiz City. *Asian Journal of Research in Pharmaceutical Science*, *5*(1), 8–11.

Hanna, N. M., Adib, S. M., & Daoud, Z. (2009). Food-borne salmonella outbreak at a bank cafeteria: An investigation in an Arab country in transition. *La Revue de Santé de la Méditerranée orientale*, *15*(2), 470–474. Available from https://doi.org/10.4315/0362-028X-56.1.84.

Hoang, V. T., Dao, T. L., Ly, T. D. A., Sow, D., Belhouchat, K., Chaht, K. L., & Gautret, P. (2020). Gastrointestinal symptoms and the acquisition of enteric pathogens in Hajj pilgrims: A 3-year prospective cohort study. *European Journal of Clinical Microbiology & Infectious Diseases*, *40*(2), 315–323. Available from https://doi.org/10.1007/s10096-020-04018-z.

Humphrey, J. M., Ranbhise, S., Ibrahim, E., Al-Romaihi, H. E., Farag, E., Abu-Raddad, L. J., & Glesby, M. J. (2016). Multiplex PCR for detection of gastrointestinal pathogens in migrant workers in Qatar. *American Journal of Tropical Medicine and Hygiene*, *95*(6), 1330–1337. Available from https://doi.org/10.4269/ajtmh.16-0464.

Husseini, R. (2014, December 9). Holiday Inn Dead Sea resort management referred to court over October food poisoning deaths. *The Jordan Times*. Available from http://www.jordan-times.com/news/local/holiday-inn-dead-sea-resort-management-referred-court-over-october-food-poisoning-deaths. Accessed September 5, 2020.

Jameel, S., Shafek, M., Abdulmohsen, A., Mohamed, N., Naji, S., & Mohammed, T. (2016). The Isolation of Vibrio cholera and other enteric bacteria with molecular characterization of Vibrio cholera during the outbreak of Baghdad/Iraq in 2015. *Advances in Microbiology*, *6*, 699–715. Available from https://doi.org/10.4236/aim.2016.69069.

JFDA (Jordanian Food and Drug Administration). (2008). Law No. 41 of 2008, Jordan Food and Drug Administration Law. Available from Law No. 41 of 2008.pdf (jfda.jo). Accessed December 6, 2020.

Kadhim, K. P., Fathallah, K., Jaafar, A., Hamad, A., Saadoon, S., Awad, Z., & Lami, F. A. (2018). Food poisoning outbreak in Al-Khazir U2 camp of internally displaced persons - Iraq, Summer 2017.: EMPHNET sixth regional conference. *Journal of Medical Internet Research (JMIR)*, *4*(1), e10573, Accessed October 18, 2020.

Kattamis, C. A., Kyriazakou, M., & Chaidas, S. (1969). Favism. Clinical and biochemical data. *Journal of Medical Genetics*, *6*, 34–41.

KFMC (King Fahad Medical City). (2020). Poison control department. Available from https://www.kfmc.med.sa/EN/Patient/Poison-Control/Pages/default.aspx. Accessed December 5, 2020.

Khalaf. (2006, September 12). 700 people suffer from food poisoning. Blog. Available from https://ajloun.blogspot.com/2006/09/700-people-suffer-from-food-poisoning.html. Accessed December 8, 2020.

Khuri-Bulos, N. A., Khalaf, M. A., Shehabi, A., & Shami, K. (1994). Foodhandler-associated Salmonella outbreak in a university hospital despite routine surveillance cultures of kitchen employees. *Infection Control and Hospital Epidemiology*, *15*, 311–314.

Korzeniewski, K. (2009). Prevalence of infectious diseases in the population of United Nations soldiers in Lebanon. *International Journal of Health Science*, *2*(1), 147–153.

LaBudde, R. A. (1998, October 27). Food poisoning, biscuits – Egypt (Mansoura): RFI 981025175331 ProMED. Archive Number: 19981030.2114. Available from http://www.promedmail.org. Accessed September 4, 2020.

Lami, F. H., Radhi, F., Al Dahhan, S., Hashim, R. A., Mahmood, H., Araj, R., & Arbaji, A. (2019). Knowledge, attitude, and practices of food handlers on food safety and personal hygiene during Arbaeenia Mass Gathering, Baghdad, Iraq, 2014: Cross-sectional study. *JMIR Public Health and Surveillance.*, *5*(4), e10922. Available from https://doi.org/10.2196/10922, Published online 2019 Oct 9; PMCID: PMC6811768; Accessed October 18, 2020.

Mark and others. (2020). Mass food poisoning. Twofortyeightam. Available from https://248am.com/mark/news/mass-food-poisoning/. Accessed August 13, 2020.

Maslamani, Y. A., Al Mazroa, M. A., & Nooh, R. M. (2011). Foodborne disease outbreak among construction workers, Ha'il, Saudi Arabia, February 2011. *Saudi Epidemiology Bulletin*, *18* (2), 21–23. Available from C:/Users/todde/Downloads/Bulletin%20(V18)-2%202011.pdf. Accessed September 8, 2020.

Masriya, A. (2013, April 30). Egypt: Azhar's food poisoning cases rise to 161 – MOH. *AllAfrica*. Available from https://allafrica.com/stories/201305010321.html. Accessed September 4, 2020.

Masudi, F. (2014, November 11). Food poisoning cases could be higher than reported. *Gulf News*. Available from https://gulfnews.com/uae/health/food-poisoning-cases-could-be-higher-than-reported-1.1411035. Accessed August 24, 2020.

Memish, Z. A., Zumla, A., Alhakeem, R. F., Assiri, A., Turkestan, I. A., Al Harby, K. D., … Al-Tawfiq, J. A. (2014). Hajj: Infectious disease surveillance and control. *Lancet*, *383* (9934), 2073–2082. Available from https://doi.org/10.1016/S0140-6736(14)60381-0, June 14 Epub May 20, 2014. PMID: 24857703; PMCID: PMC7137990.

Mousavi, J., & Jafari, F. (2016). Prevalence of diseases in pilgrims referring to Iranian clinics in Iraq. *International Journal of Travel Medicine and Global Health*, *4*(1), 31–33. Available from https://doi.org/10.20286/ijtmgh-040131.

Myers, M. (2018, July 25). Army looking into food poisoning outbreak at Kuwait base. *Army Times*. Available from https://www.armytimes.com/news/your-army/2018/07/25/army-looking-into-food-poisoning-outbreak-at-kuwait-base/. Accessed August 13, 2020.

Nashef, N. A. (2018). Linking household food insecurity with food safety knowledge and practices of Syrian refugee mothers: Findings from a pilot study in the Bekaa Region, Lebanon.

Thesis 2018. American University of Beirut. Available from https://scholarworks.aub.edu.lb/bitstream/handle/10938/21382/st-6803.pdf?sequence = 1. Accessed August 23, 2020.

Park, N. Y., Ro, E. Y., Jo, H. J., Park, K. S., & Yoon, K. S. (2014). Effect of packaging and temperature on survival kinetics of Campylobacter jejuni on precooked chicken breast. *Journal of Food Science*, *34*(4), 371–379.

Rahimi, S. (2007, October 28). Scores hospitalised in food poisoning scare. *Arab Business*. Available from https://www.arabianbusiness.com/scores-hospitalised-in-food-poisoning-scare-53411.html. Accessed October 18, 2020.

Rejimon, K. (2015, August 31). 20 admitted to hospital in Oman for food poisoning, restaurant shut down. *Times of Oman*. Available from https://timesofoman.com/article/66695/Oman/20-admitted-to-hospital-in-Saham-for-food-poisoning-restaurant-shut-down. Accessed September 8, 2020.

Robesyn, E., Micalessi, M. I., Quoilin, S., Naranjo, M., & Thomas, I. (2011). Cluster of hepatitis A cases among travellers returning from Egypt, Belgium, September through November 2008. *Euro Surveillance: Bulletin Europeen sur les Maladies Transmissibles = European Communicable Disease Bulletin*, *14*(3), 19095. Available from https://doi.org/10.2807/ese.14.03.19095-en.

Saljila. (2011, October 6). 1,663 cases of food-borne diseases in Dubai. *Khaleej Times*. Available from https://www.khaleejtimes.com/lifestyle/health-fitness/1-663-cases-of-food-borne-diseases-in-dubai. Accessed August 24, 2020.

Sane, J., MacDonald, E., Vold, L., Gossner, C., & Severi, E.on behalf of the International Outbreak Investigation Team. (2015). Multistate foodborne hepatitis A outbreak among European tourists returning from Egypt – Need for reinforced vaccination recommendations, November 2012 to April 2013. *Euro Surveillance: Bulletin Europeen sur les Maladies Transmissibles = European Communicable Disease Bulletin*, *20*(4), 21018. Available from https://doi.org/10.2807/1560-7917.ES2015.20.4.21018.

Sangar, A. (2017, June 13). Over 820 Mosul IDPs suffering from food poisoning in Erbil. Kurdistan 24. Available from https://www.kurdistan24.net/en/news/c00ca1e3-6e09-4b3a-af4f-915e102f3b86. Accessed August 6, 2020.

Santacruz, S. (2015, May 14). Jail sentences and deportation for Qatar food poisoning. *Australian Food Safety News*. Available from https://www.foodsafety.com.au/news/jail-sentences-and-deportation-for-qatar-food-poisoning. Accessed September 13, 2020.

Sawalha, A. F. (2008). Poison Control and the Drug Information Center: The Palestinian experience. *Israel Medical Association Journal*, *10*(11), 757–760.

Schachtel, J. Report: 45 ISIS Fighters Killed by Poisoned Ramadan Meal (breitbart.com). July 8, 2015. https://www.breitbart.com/national-security/2015/07/08/report-45-isis-fighters-killed-by-poisoned-ramadan-meal/ Accessed August 12, 2021.

SFDA. (2020). The Saudi Food and Drug Authority. Available from https://www.sfda.gov.sa/en#nav-food. Accessed October 18, 2020.

Sreeraman, V. R. (2007, August 14). Jordan bans sandwiches over Salmonella outbreak. *Med India*. Available from https://www.medindia.net/news/jordan-bans-sandwiches-over-salmonella-outbreak-24964-1.htm. Accessed September 5, 2020.

Staff. (2019, September 26). Dubai closes restaurant after 15 affected by salmonella outbreak. *Gulf Business*. Available from https://gulfbusiness.com/dubai-closes-restaurant-15-affected-salmonella-outbreak/. Accessed August 24, 2020.

Taha, R. R., Alghalibi, S. M., & Saeed Saleh, M. G. (2013). Salmonella spp. in patients suffering from enteric fever and food poisoning in Thamar city, Yemen. *Eastern Mediterranean Health Journal*, *19*(1), 88–93.

Todd, E. C. D. (2017a). Foodborne disease in the Middle East. In A. Badran, S. Murad, E. Baydoun, & N. Daghir (Eds.), *Water, energy & food sustainability in the Middle East* (pp. 389–440). Cham, New York: Springer.

Todd, E. C. D. (2017b). Foodborne disease and food control in the Gulf states. *Food Control, 73* (Part B), 341–366.

UAE (United Arab Emirates). (2020). Food safety. Available from https://u.ae/en/information-and-services/health-and-fitness/food-safety-and-health-tips#: ~ :text = The%20law%20imposes%20strict%20penalties%20on%20those%20found,and%20a%20fine%20of%20up%20to%20AED%20500%2C000. Accessed September 11, 2020.

Vaidya, S. K., (2013, January 9). 300 oil company contractors suffer food poisoning in Oman. *Gulf News Oman.* Available from https://gulfnews.com/world/gulf/oman/300-oil-company-contractors-suffer-food-poisoning-in-oman-1.1129768. Accessed September 8, 2020.

Walker, L. (2014, December 1). Amid growing complaints, SCH launches food poisoning hotline in Qatar. *Doha News.* Available from https://www.dohanews.co/amid-growing-complaints-sch-launches-food-poisoning-hotline-qatar/. Accessed September 13, 2020.

Weill, F., Domman, D., Njamkepo, E., et al. (2019). Genomic insights into the 2016–2017 cholera epidemic in Yemen. *Nature, 565*, 230–233. Available from https://doi.org/10.1038/s41586-018-0818-3.

Whitehead, F. (2015, April 2). Water scarcity in Yemen: the country's forgotten conflict. *The Guardian.* Available from https://www.theguardian.com/global-development-professionals-network/2015/apr/02/water-scarcity-yemen-conflict. Accessed December 8, 2020.

WHO (World Health Organization). (2009). Interim planning considerations for mass gatherings in the context of pandemic (H1N1) 2009 influenza. Available from https://www.who.int/csr/resources/publications/swineflu/h1n1_mass_gatherings/en/. Accessed October 18, 2020.

WHO (World Health Organization). (2019). World directory of poisons centres. Available from https://www.who.int/gho/phe/chemical_safety/poisons_centres_text/en/#: ~ :text = World%20directory%20of%20poisons%20centres%20Situation%20as%20of,information%20centre%20started%20in%201949%20in%20the%20Netherlands. Accessed December 5, 2020.

Zmeter, C., Tabaja, H., Sharara, A. I., & Kanj, S. S. (2018). Non-O1, non-O139 Vibrio cholerae septicemia at a tertiary care center in Beirut, Lebanon; a case report and review. *Journal of Infection and Public Health, 11*(5), 601–604.

Chapter 3

Foodborne infections in the Middle East

Ihab Habib[1,2,3] and Mohamed Yousif Ibrahim Mohamed[1]
[1]Department of Veterinary Medicine, College of Agriculture and Veterinary Medicine, United Arab of Emirates University, Al Ain, United Arab Emirates, [2]Department of Environmental Health, High Institute of Public Health, Alexandria University, Alexandria, Egypt, [3]Centre for Biosecurity and One Health, School of Veterinary Medicine, Murdoch University, Perth, Australia

3.1 Foodborne infections—a global and regional challenge

Globally, foodborne pathogens continue to be a significant challenge to food safety and international trade. In Europe and many other countries, foodborne infection is a major public health concern (ECDC, 2017). According to the European Centre for Disease Prevention and Control (ECDC) and Zoonoses Reports of the European Food Safety Authority (EFSA), the incidence of human cases infected with *Campylobacter jejuni* surpassed salmonellosis in the last 10 years (ECDC, 2012, 2018). In the United States, *C. jejuni* has been reported as the most common pathogen causing foodborne illnesses, followed by *Listeria* and *Salmonella*. Also, in the United States, the Foodborne Diseases Active Surveillance Network (FoodNet) of the Centre for Disease Control and Prevention reported that the incidence of foodborne-attributed hospitalization caused by campylobacteriosis and salmonellosis was increasing over the years (Huang et al., 2017).

According to the WHO (2015), the Middle East and North Africa (MENA) region reported the third-highest estimated burden of foodborne disease per population and came just after the African and the South-East Asian regions. That study of the WHO also estimated that 70% of the MENA region's foodborne disease burden is caused by Escherichia *coli*, nontyphoidal *Salmonella* (NTS), *Campylobacter*, and *Norovirus* spp. (WHO, 2015), stressing the severe burden caused by pathogens involved in causing foodborne infections. In the Middle East, the true incidence of foodborne infections is difficult to determine since there are limited systematic surveillance efforts to detect sporadic cases, outbreaks, and to provide isolates that

Food Safety in the Middle East. DOI: https://doi.org/10.1016/B978-0-12-822417-5.00005-2

could be used for source attribution and risk assessment at national and regional levels. In addition to the lack of reliable data on the occurrences of pathogens and infections, the situation of antimicrobial resistance (AMR) in bacteria causing foodborne infections is not fully understood across the Middle East region, despite some reports indicating varying trends at the human–food interface (Harb, O'Dea, Abraham, & Habib, 2019; Moujaber et al., 2017; Rafei, Hawli, Osman, Dabboussi, & Hamze, 2020). In this review chapter, we collate updated knowledge on the epidemiology of four important pathogens commonly causing foodborne infections in humans in the Middle East, and these are NTS, *Campylobacter*, *Listeria monocytogenes*, and *Brucella*. We used PubMed, Science Direct, Scopus, Web of Science, and Google Scholar to collect the available research papers about foodborne infections in various food types throughout the Middle East. We also searched for resources like postgraduate thesis and reports that include details about foodborne pathogens in the Middle East.

This chapter aims at elucidating—(1) background knowledge, (2) recent updates on the prevalence of the four concerned pathogens (NTS, *Campylobacter*, *L. monocytogenes*, and *Brucella*) in the food chain in the Middle East and highlight available evidence on public health burden and the status of AMR among the concerned four pathogens. It is important to note that some other chapters within this book will cover complementary aspects to what we are exploring in this chapter, such as—aspects of foodborne outbreaks (Chapter 2: Overview on Food Safety in the Middle East) and foodborne intoxication and toxico-infection (Chapter 4: Foodborne Intoxications and Toxico-infections in the Middle East).

3.2 Nontyphoidal *Salmonella* in the food chain in the Middle East

NTS are Gram-negative, rod-shaped bacteria within the family *Enterobacteriaceae*. NTS are among the most common foodborne zoonotic pathogens affecting humans worldwide (Fernández, Guerra, & Rodicio, 2018; Kirk et al., 2015). These microbes are mostly transmitted to humans by ingesting contaminated food of animal origin, mainly beef meat, poultry meat, pork, milk, and eggs, and contacting with animals, including reptiles and turtles (ECDC, 2017; Sodagari et al., 2020). Nevertheless, other foods, including vegetables and fruits contaminated with animal feces, have also been involved in salmonellosis outbreaks in humans (Nguyen et al., 2021). The incubation period for NTS infection is between 6 and 72 hours, with median incubation periods of 3 days (Eikmeier, Medus, & Smith, 2018). NTS usually causes mild-to-moderate self-limiting gastroenteritis, characterized by abdominal, diarrhea, vomiting, cramps, fever, and nausea, and severe disease resulting in death does occur (Harb et al., 2019). With recurrent infection, the NTS can spread beyond the intestine, giving rise to focal or invasive infections, mainly in immunocompromised patients, the elderly, or children. Ciprofloxacin and extended-spectrum cephalosporins are the most frequently used antibiotics for treating invasive salmonellosis infections in humans, especially children and the elderly (Zhu et al., 2017). Over the past decades, the increase of multidrug-resistant (MDR) forms of Salmonella enterica in food-producing animals has been an emerging problem worldwide, likely due to the widespread use of common antimicrobials in poultry and animal husbandry for therapeutics, prophylaxis, and growth promotion (Sodagari et al., 2020).

Measuring the prevalence of NTS in food products is important to quantify the risk of foodborne *Salmonella* infections in humans in the Middle East. According to a recent meta-analysis study by Al-Rifai, Chaabna, Denagamage, and Alali (2019), the pooled prevalence of NTS in the human population in the MENA region was estimated at 6.6% [95% confidence interval (CI): 5.4%–7.9%]. In 2020 Rafei and colleagues conducted a systematic review and meta-analysis to summarize current data on national and regional specific NTS prevalence in foods in the MENA region. The pooled prevalence of NTS was 8.8% (95% CI: 7.0%–10.8%). The pooled prevalence of NTS in animal-sourced foods was 9.0% (95% CI: 6.8–11.4) based on studies from 13 countries. Furthermore, the pooled prevalence of NTS in fishery products and in plant-sourced foods (in six countries) was 22.9% (95% CI: 13.8%–33.4%) and 0.4% (95% CI: 0.0%–1.9%), respectively. Their study noted that *Salmonella typhimurium* (28.0%), *Salmonella enteritidis* (23.6%), and *Salmonella kentucky* (20.3%) were the most frequently reported serotypes in the tested food commodities in the MENA region. There is a scarcity of understanding of the magnitude of NTS in the food chain in the Arab countries. Additionally, not much work has been done at the molecular characterization level to address the source attribution of such an important pathogen in the food chain in the Middle East (Harb et al., 2018).

Table 3.1 summarizes the published research depicting NTS prevalence rates in foods in the Middle East in recent years. In Egypt, in the Kafr El-Sheikh governorate, a study reported NTS occurrence in 4% (2/50) of imported frozen beef liver (Kirrella, Deeb, & Abdallah, 2017). Another study in Egypt detected higher rates of *Salmonella* at 60% (37/62) and 64% (14/20) in chicken parts and skin, respectively, whereas none of the tested table eggs samples ($n = 60$) were positive for *Salmonella* (Abdel-Maksoud et al., 2015). In Iraq, Harb et al. (2018) reported the occurrence of *Salmonella* in 16% (16/100) of imported frozen chicken carcasses. The results summarized in Table 3.1 show a varying trend in the rates of *Salmonella* detection in the various Middle East, which might be attributed to the variability in the utilized laboratory methods, as well as variability in food sample types (animal-sourced vs plant-sourced) and their origin (local vs imported). Nonetheless, the collective descriptive results summarized in Table 3.1 affirm that NTS is present in food products consumed in the Middle East.

Given the abundant detection of NTS in various food commodities (Table 3.1), there is a need to strengthen national and regional surveillance efforts for AMR in NTS in our food chain (Pande, Gole, McWhorter, Abraham, & Chousalkar, 2015). In the primary production of animal-sourced

TABLE 3.1 The occurrence of nontyphoidal *Salmonella* (*NTS*) in foods in the Middle East.

Country	References	Tested food samples (no.)	% of NTS positive samples	Serotypes (%)
Egypt	Kirrella et al. (2017)	Frozen beef liver ($n = 50$)	4	—
	Moawad et al. (2017)	Fresh poultry ($n = 60$)	10	*Enteritidis* (13.3), *typhimurium* (60.0), *kentucky* (6.7).
		Frozen poultry ($n = 30$)	3.3	
		Fresh beef ($n = 60$)	11.7	
		Frozen beef ($n = 30$)	3.3	
	Abaza (2017)	Fresh vegetables and ready-to-eat salads ($n = 121$)	0	—
	Tarabees, Elsayed, Shawish, Basiouni, and Shehata (2017)	Raw chicken meat ($n = 100$)	5	*typhimurium* (60.0), *enteritidis* (40.0).
	Abdel-Aziz (2016)	Poultry products ($n = 75$)	6.6	*enteritidis* (40), *typhimurium* (40), *kentucky* (20)
	Amin and El Rahman (2015)	Fresh chicken meat ($n = 200$)	3.5	*enteritidis* (14.3), *typhimurium* (71.4), *kentucky* (14.3).
		Ready-to-eat chicken meat ($n = 100$)	0	
	Abdel-Maksoud et al. (2015)	Raw egg yolk ($n = 30$)	0	*enteritidis* (3.1), *typhimurium* (0), *kentucky* (41.5), other types (55.4)
		Egg shell ($n = 30$)	0	
		Mixed chicken meat samples ($n = 62$)	60	
		Chicken skin ($n = 22$)	64	

(*Continued*)

TABLE 3.1 (Continued)

Country	References	Tested food samples (no.)	% of NTS positive samples	Serotypes (%)
	Abd-Elghany, Sallam, Abd-Elkhalek, and Tamura (2015)	Chicken carcasses ($n=50$)	16	*enteritidis* (37.4), *typhimurium* (30.1), *kentucky* (10.8), *muenster* (8.4), *virchow* (4.8), *anatum* (4.8), *haifa* (1.2), other types (2.4)
	Ahmed and Shimamoto (2014)	Frozen beef ($n=160$)	0.5	*enteritidis* (32.1), *typhimurium* (41.5), *infantis* (20.8)
		Fresh beef ($n=80$)	1.9	
		Beef carcasses ($n=240$)	2.5	
		Chicken breast ($n=160$)	0.25	
		Chicken legs ($n=160$)	1.5	
		Raw milk (buffalo) ($n=240$)	1	
		Raw milk (cow) ($n=240$)	0.5	
		Cheese (Kareish) ($n=120$)	0.4	
		Cheese (Domiati) ($n=120$)	0.1	
		Yogurt ($n=80$)	0	
	Hassanein et al. (2011)	Frozen chicken breast fillets ($n=25$)	52	*enteritidis* (100)
		Frozen chicken legs ($n=25$)	36	*enteritidis* (100)
		Minced frozen meats ($n=25$)	20	*kentucky* (100)

(Continued)

TABLE 3.1 (Continued)

Country	References	Tested food samples (no.)	% of NTS positive samples	Serotypes (%)
Iraq	Harb et al. (2018)	Frozen chicken ($n = 100$)	16	*enteritidis* (12.5), *typhimurium* (50.0), *kentucky* (6.3), *newport* (6.3), *muenchen* (6.3), *hadar* (12.5).
	Mohammed (2018)	Uncooked hamburger ($n = 10$)	50	—
	Abid (2016)	Fresh sheep and beef meat ($n = 50$)	4.5	—
Jordan	Momani, Janakat, and Khatatbeh (2018)	Eggs ($n = 25$)	12	—
	Obaidat and Bani Salman (2017)	Fresh fish from Yemen ($n = 110$)	6.4	—
	Al-Groom (2017)	Presliced imported cheddar cheese ($n = 100$)	10	—
			0.08	
	Osaili et al. (2014)	Chicken shawarma ($n = 301$)	1	—
		Roasted chicken ($n = 157$)	0.6	
		Chicken burgers ($n = 20$)	0	
		Beef kubba ($n = 115$)	0.9	
	Nimri, AL-Dahab, and Batchoun (2014)	Chicken shawarma ($n = 80$)	13.8	*choleraesuis* (100)
		Beef shawarma ($n = 20$)	5	

(Continued)

TABLE 3.1 (Continued)

Country	References	Tested food samples (no.)	% of NTS positive samples	Serotypes (%)
	Omar et al. (2011)	Raw milk ($n = 20$) White soft cheeses Fresh ($n = 20$)	0 0	—
		Labaneh ($n = 20$)	0	
	Malkawi and Gharaibeh (2003)	Fresh and frozen beef, lamb, and poultry meat ($n = 300$)	31	—
Lebanon	Kassaify, Najjar, Toufeili, and Malek (2010)	*Qishta'a* (heat-coagulated milk) ($n = 31$)	42	—
Palestine	Khatib and Mitwalli (2009)	Raw milk, yogurt ($n = 155$)	0	—
		Pasteurized milk ($n = 235$)	0	
		Concentrated yogurt, salt ($n = 170$)	0	
		Cheese and cooked cheese ($n = 109$)	0	
Saudi Arabia	Elhadi (2014)	Fish from Thailand ($n = 98$)	44.9	—
		Fish from Vietnam ($n = 25$)	52	
		Fish from Bahrain ($n = 35$)	31.4	
		Fish from India ($n = 50$)	28	
		Fish from Myanmar ($n = 15$)	46.7	
	Iyer et al. (2013)	Frozen meat and fresh meat ($n = 60$)	25	—

(Continued)

TABLE 3.1 (Continued)

Country	References	Tested food samples (no.)	% of NTS positive samples	Serotypes (%)
	Khiyami, Noura, Busaeed, and Sher (2011)	West region ($n = 40$)	0	—
		East region ($n = 40$)	20	
		North region ($n = 40$)	0	
		South region ($n = 40$)	7.5	
		Center region ($n = 40$)	2.5	
	Hassan, Altalhi, Gherbawy, and El-Deeb (2011)	Fresh vegetables ($n = 68$)	0	—
	Al-Dughaym and Altabari (2010)	Chicken ($n = 100$)	1	*arizona* (100)
	Nasser (2008)	Coffee beans ($n = 31$)	0	—

foods, there has been an increase in the usage of the traditional first-line drugs sulfonamides, chloramphenicol, ampicillin, tetracycline, and streptomycin and that caused the emergence and development of resistant NTS due to selective pressure (Mohamed-Yousif et al., 2014). According to a study in Saudi Arabia by Badahdah and Aldagal (2018), among 150 strains of *S. enteritidis* that were isolated from local chickens, there was frequent resistance to streptomycin (55.8%), chloramphenicol (58.5%), neomycin (58.9%), and sulfamethoxazole (73.5%). In Egypt, according to Hassan, Salam, and Abdel-Latef (2016), 55% of *Salmonella* serotypes isolated from broilers showed resistance to nalidixic acid, and 89.3% were found resistant to tetracycline. Because AMR of NTS is associated with the increase in the costs of the healthcare system, morbidity, and mortality, determination of AMR profiles should be regarded as an important part of NTS surveillance in reference to food safety and public health laboratories in the Middle East.

Implementation of evidence-based food safety systems in the Middle East region will help better manage exposure to NTS—a step that will help lessen the public health burden of NTS infections in the region. NTS gastroenteritis's global burden is estimated to be around 94 million infections, with a death estimate of 155,000 and an average incidence rate of 1.14 episodes/100,000 inhabitants (WHO, 2018). This reflects the disease's enormous burden in both industrialized and developing countries (Kirk et al., 2015). For the WHO-defined East Mediterranean region, the median incidence rate of NTS is 1610 illnesses, with 0.6 deaths per 100,000 persons (Farag et al., 2016). The rate of salmonellosis incidence varies between countries across the Middle East and is influenced largely by the absence of systematic, harmonized national and regional surveillance and reporting systems. According to a recent systematic review and meta-analysis on the prevalence of enteric NTS in humans in the Arab countries, the highest pooled *Salmonella* prevalence measures were in Morocco (17.9%, 95% CI: 5.7%−34.8%, 1997−2012), Tunisia (10.2%, 95% CI: 4.3%−18.0%, 1988−2009), and Sudan (9.2%, 95% CI: 6.5%−12.2%, 2006−8), while the lowest were in Jordan (1.1%, 95% CI: 0.1%−3.0%, 1993−2010), Oman (1.2%, 95% CI: 1.2%−1.3%, 1998−2002), and Palestine (1.2%, 95% CI: 0.4%−2.1%, 1999−2011) (Rifai et al., 2019). Several published studies indicate that the most widely reported serovars associated with acute diarrheal disease across the Middle East are the *Salmonella* serovar *typhimurium* and *Salmonella* serovar *enteritidis* (Ramadan, Unni, Hablas, & Rizk, 1992; Ranjbar et al., 2011; Taha, Alghalibi, & Saleh, 2013). Similar to the Middle East pattern, *S. typhimurium*, followed by *S. enteritidis*, has also been reported as being the top-ranked serovar (involved in human diarrheal illnesses) across Africa, North America, and Oceania (Australia and New Zealand) (Hendriksen et al., 2011). On the other hand, *S. enteritidis* is more frequently reported than *S. typhimurium* in human clinical isolates in Asia, Latin America, and Europe (Galanis et al., 2006). The variation in NTS serovars' diversity among foods and humans is dynamic, and it is not surprising to capture variations between countries across the Middle East. Such variations could be explained by several factors impacting NTS levels in food, animals, and the environment, which play a major role in human exposure to infection. Among these factors are food-animal production practices, climate, the environmental spread of specific serotypes, and the extent of vaccination programs in food animals. The public health burden of NTS in the Middle East and several published research data in recent years (Table 3.1) stress the need to prioritize NTS in future preventative health plans in Arab countries.

3.3 *Campylobacter* sp. in the food chain in the Middle East

The WHO report on the global burden of foodborne diseases concluded that foodborne transmission is considered the most important route for

Campylobacter infection in the Middle East and globally (WHO, 2015). *Campylobacter* sp. are microaerophilic, Gram-negative bacteria, spirally curved, motile rods with polar flagella, and intestinal commensals of mammals and birds (Man et al., 2010; Pielsticker, Glünder, & Rautenschlein, 2012). They are slow-growing organisms that require selective media containing charcoal and various antibiotics, such as cephalothin, to suppress competing fecal microflora (Chon et al., 2012). They are microaerophilic bacteria that require oxygen for growth but at lower levels than regular atmospheric air, and, as such, *Campylobacter* species grow best at 5%–10% oxygen and 10% carbon dioxide (Kendall, Barrero-Tobon, Hendrixson, & Kelly, 2014; Lynch, Cagney, McDowell, & Duffy, 2010). *C. jejuni* and *Campylobacter coli* are thermotolerant (growing best at 42°C) (Chon et al., 2012), while other *Campylobacter* species (such as *Campylobacter fetus*) are not (Kienesberger et al., 2011). *C. jejuni* and *C. coli* are the key causes of human campylobacteriosis, a very widely recognized foodborne illness that can be transmitted to humans through the consumption of improperly cooked meat, especially chicken meat, contaminated milk and water, and contact with farm animals such as poultry and livestock (Hansson, Sandberg, Habib, Lowman, & Engvall, 2018). Human campylobacteriosis is characterized by watery or bloody diarrhea, abdominal pain, cramps, fever, malaise, and vomiting (Mohamed-Yousif et al., 2019). The incubation period is usually between 2 and 5 days but can range from 1 to 10 days (Awofisayo-Okuyelu et al., 2017). This illness is more dangerous in young children who are more prone to dehydration and loss of nutrients, such as sodium and protein, due to diarrheal illness (Gundogdu & Wren, 2020). Although antibiotics therapy is not generally indicated in most campylobacteriosis cases, treatment can decrease the duration and reduce the symptoms if initiated early in severe cases that warrant antimicrobial intervention (Hansson et al., 2018). Macrolides (specifical erythromycin) and fluoroquinolones (specifical ciprofloxacin) are considered the first and second choice of antimicrobials, respectively, for the management of severe human *Campylobacter* infections.

Recent studies showed that *Campylobacter* sp. is widely presented in several Middle East food products (Abushahba, Ahmed, Ibrahim, & Mosa, 2018; Ghaffoori, 2017; Yehia & Al-Dagal, 2014), as presented in Table 3.2. Much of the published research on *Campylobacter* in the Middle East is centered around poultry-sourced products (mainly chicken meat), followed by few studies in dairy products and other foods (Table 3.2). According to Ghaffoori (2017), in Iraq, the prevalence of *C. jejuni* in broiler chicken carcasses ($n = 20$) was as high as 60%. In Saudi Arabia, *Campylobacter* sp. was detected 5% (1/20) in retail unwashed eggshells that were sampled from retail at Al-Taif city (Bahobail, Hassan, & El-Deeb, 2012). In Egypt, *C. coli* was frequently isolated in 46.7% of chicken carcasses ($n = 30$) surveyed at Assiut city (Abdel-Aziz & Abd-Allah, 2017). Other studies in Egypt isolated *Campylobacter* sp. from raw milk (El-Sharoud, 2009; El-Zamkan &

TABLE 3.2 The occurrence of *Campylobacter* spp. in foods in the Middle East.

Country	References	Types of food samples (no.)	*Campylobacter* sp. %	*C. jejuni* %	*C. coli* %	Other species
Egypt	Abushahba et al. (2018)	Broiler ($n=101$)	16.8	—	4	—
		Slaughterhouses ($n=104$)	24	—	3.9	—
	Abdel-Aziz and Abd-Allah (2017)	Fresh chicken meat products ($n=30$)	53.3	46.7	46.7	—
		Frozen chicken meat products ($n=30$)	53.3	46.7	40	—
		Chicken burger ($n=15$)	0	0	0	—
		Chicken nuggets ($n=15$)	13.3	13.3	13.3	—
	El-Zamkan and Hameed (2016)	Raw milk ($n=50$)	22	20	20	2
		Kareish cheese ($n=50$)	34	14	14	20
		Yoghurt ($n=50$)	18	8	8	10
	El-Tawab et al. (2015)	Skin ($n=39$)	30.8	12.8	17.9	*C. lari* (17.9) *C. hyointestinalis* (0)
		Thigh meat ($n=39$)	38.5	17.9	20.5	*C. lari* (20.5), *C. hyointestinalis* (1)

(*Continued*)

TABLE 3.2 (Continued)

Country	References	Types of food samples (no.)	*Campylobacter* sp. %	*C. jejuni* %	*C. coli* %	Other species
		Breast meat ($n = 39$)	41	33.3	5.1	*C. lari* (5.1), *C. hyointestinalis* (2.7)
	El-Sharoud (2009)	Raw milk ($n = 50$)	—	4	—	—
		Laban Rayeb ($n = 25$)	—	0	—	—
		Stored Domiati cheese ($n = 39$)	—	0	—	—
		Fresh Domiati cheese ($n = 38$)	—	11	—	—
		Zabady ($n = 25$)	—	0	—	—
		Ras cheese ($n = 25$)	—	0	—	—
		Kariesh cheese ($n = 25$)	—	0	—	—
Iraq	Kanaan and Khashan (2018)	Retail frozen chicken meat ($n = 40$)	75	25	50	—
	Ghaffoori (2017)	Broiler chicken carcasses ($n = 20$)	—	60	—	—
	Motlak (2016)	Broiler carcasses ($n = 280$)	—	49.6	—	—

Jordan	Alaboudi, Malkawi, Osaili, Abu-Basha, and Guitian (2020)	Broiler chicken carcasses ($n = 177$)	31.6	17	—	—
	Neves et al. (2019)	Broiler chicken ($n = 50$)	—	30	—	—
		($n = 92$)				
	Osaili, Al-Nabulsi et al. (2012), Osaili, Alaboudi, and Al-Akhras (2012)	Live and dressed chicken ($n = 140$)	40	—	—	—
Qatar	Abu-Madi, Behnke, Sharma, Bearden, and Al-Banna (2016)	Chicken skin (400)	36.5	29.3	—	—
Saudi Arabia	Yehia and Al-Dagal (2014)	Chicken product ($n = 99$)	—	52.3		—
	Bahobail et al. (2012)	Unwashed egg shell ($n = 20$)	5	—	—	—

Hameed; 2016). Table 3.2 elaborates further on the recent studies on *Campylobacter* prevalence in various foods in the Middle East region. It is worth highlighting that there are very few studies on *Campylobacter* in the food chain in the Gulf Cooperation Council (GCC) countries. Such gap in research in the GCC countries should be considered urgently, as it is estimated that 2%–28% of diarrheal cases in the Arabian Gulf countries are attributed to infection caused by *Campylobacter* (Al-Freihi et al., 1993). Another critical gap is the gap in quantitative (counts/numbers) surveillance efforts for *Campylobacter* in the chicken meat supply across all Arab countries, despite the availability of several qualitative (presence/absence) surveillance data. The percentage of *Campylobacter*-contaminated poultry carcasses varies from country to country; it can be as low as 15%, as in Iceland, and as high as 90%, as in the United States (Hansson et al., 2018). Future research in the Middle East should conduct more quantitative surveillances as these form the base for developing quantitative risk assessment (QRA) and management plans for *Campylobacter* at national or regional levels. There are no QRA efforts that have been published in relation to *Campylobacter* in the chicken meat supply across the Middle East (Habib et al., 2020).

According to the WHO, AMR in *Campylobacter* has shown increasing resistance to erythromycin and fluoroquinolones in many parts of the World (WHO, 2013a). Such increase appears to be associated with the use of these antimicrobials in poultry and livestock production systems (Coker, Isokpehi, Thomas, Amisu, & Obi, 2002). In Egypt, the resistance of *C. jejuni* and *C. coli* to ampicillin, streptomycin, chloramphenicol, erythromycin, and tetracycline, isolated from foods of animals origin, especially poultry, showed to be more than 50% (in isolates characterized in several studies) (Hassanain, 2011; Street, 2015; Wasfy et al., 2000). According to a recent study in Iraq by Kanaan, Mohammed, and Ahmad (2020), the rates of resistance of *C. jejuni* and *C. coli* toward tetracycline and erythromycin was up to 90%, yet lower rates of resistance were recognized toward enrofloxacin and gentamicin, up to 30%. These results stress the need to investigate further the mechanism of AMR and the spread of resistance genes in *Campylobacter* sp. harboring food sources, notably chicken meat, in the Middle East. The World Health Organization (WHO) declared *Campylobacter* as one of the 12 bacteria that pose the greatest threat to human health because it is resistant to antibiotics. In the United Arab Emirates (UAE), Sonnevend et al. (2006) investigated the antibiotic sensitivity and the serotype and molecular type distribution of 41 *C. jejuni* strains isolated from diarrheal patients in a hospital of Al Ain (a major city in Abu Dhabi, UAE). While all strains were sensitive to erythromycin, 35 isolates (85.4%) exhibited resistance to ciprofloxacin (Sonnevend et al., 2006). These results point that the local incidence of fluoroquinolone resistance among *C. jejuni* was the highest reported worldwide. Infection with an antimicrobial-resistant *Campylobacter* strain may lead to a suboptimal antimicrobial treatment outcome or even treatment failure (Jumaa & Neringer, 2005).

Although campylobacteriosis is a well-recognized problem in the Middle East countries, there are limited surveillance programs for *Campylobacter* in the region. Nationally representative prevalence and quantitative data of *Campylobacter* per gram of chicken are not currently available across the Middle East, notably the Arabian Gulf countries. Such data are required to fill a gap in assessing the microbial safety of chicken meat and could be used as an input for further development of QRA of *Campylobacter* in the Middle East.

3.4 *Listeria* sp. and *Listeria monocytogenes* in the food chain in the Middle East

Foodborne infection caused by *L. monocytogenes* is a severe public health problem worldwide and in the Middle East. Contamination of fresh produce and food of animal origin with *L. monocytogenes* could occur at primary production or postprocessing stages (Bahobail et al., 2012). *L. monocytogenes* and *Listeria* spp. are a group of Gram-positive bacteria, nonsporulating rods that have no capsule, facultatively anaerobic, and are motile at 10°C–25°C (Moumita, Das, Patnaik, Balasubramanian, & Jayabalan, 2019; Pan, Zhang, Cheng, & Sun, 2020; Schlech & Acheson, 2000). *Listeria* can multiply at a broad range of temperature (0°C–45°C) and pH (pH 4.5–9), and in high salt concentrations (10% NaCl) (Magalhães et al., 2016; Redfern & Verran, 2017). *Listeria* consists of 17 species: *Listeria seeligeri, L. monocytogenes, Listeria aquatica, Listeria cornellensis, Listeria ivanovii, Listeria welshimeri, Listeria marthii, Listeria booriae, Listeria innocua, Listeria grayi, Listeria fleischmannii, Listeria newyorkensis, Listeria rocourtiae, Listeria weihenstephanensis, Listeria grandensis, Listeria floridensis*, and *Listeria riparia*. Only *L. monocytogenes* causes foodborne disease in humans, and *L. ivanovii* is only associated with animal infection. *Listeria* has been isolated from an assortment of food origins, including meat, seafood, dairy products, vegetables, water, plants, soil, and feces of asymptomatic human and animal carriers (Chen et al., 2019; Guévremont, Lamoureux, Génénreux, & Côté, 2017; Lasagabaster, Jiménez, Lehnherr, Miranda-Cadena, & Lehnherr, 2020; Maury et al., 2019). Globally, listeriosis (due mainly to *L. monocytogenes* strain) causes approximately 23,150 sicknesses per year and a fatality rate of 5463 deaths per year; Listeriosis could be severe among the elderly, pregnant women, and immunocompromised persons (Bahrami, Baboli, Schimmel, Jafari, & Williams, 2020; da Silva et al., 2020). Consumption of contaminated food products accounts for an estimated 99% of all human listeriosis cases (Miceli & Settanni, 2019). The listeriosis incubation period is between 3 and 70 days (Angelo, Jackson, Wong, Hoekstra, & Jackson, 2016). Clinical symptoms of listeriosis (from a few days up to about 3–4 weeks) manifest as septicemia, meningitis, meningoencephalitis, prenatal infection, abortion, and gastroenteritis (Inoue et al., 2017; Koopmans et al., 2018; Rezaei, Kazemi Pour, Vandyousefi, Rokhbakhsh Zamin, & Irajian, 2018; Turner et al., 2017). *L. monocytogenes* infections are accountable for the highest hospitalization rates among all foodborne pathogens and have also been linked to large outbreaks of human illness worldwide (King, Huh, Shenai, Brooks, & Brooks, 2018; Reda, Abdel-Moein, Hegazi, Mohamed, & Abdel-Razik, 2016).

L. monocytogenes has been isolated from food of animal origin and food of nonanimal origin in across the Middle East. Few studies have been conducted in the GCC. However, in Egypt, meat and meat products have been the focus of several studies on the detection of *L. monocytogenes* from food animals, slaughterhouses, supermarkets, and rural areas (Abdel-Malek, Ali, Moemen, Mohamed, & Elsayh, 2010; El-Naenaeey, Abdelwahab, Merwad, & Abdou, 2019; Ismaiel, Ali, & Enan, 2014) (Table 3.3). Yehia, Ibraheim, and Hassanein (2016) detected *L. monocytogenes* in raw beef, raw chicken, raw fish, and raw camel milk from the wholesale poultry market located in Riyadh city in Saudi Arabia, as detailed in Table 3.3. While there are several reports on *L. monocytogenes* in animal-sourced foods, fewer are published on *L. monocytogenes* in plant-sourced foods in the Middle East. Mohamed, Abdelmonem, and Amin (2018) reported the occurrence of MDR *L. monocytogenes* at 14.2% (47/331) in vegetables (okra, carrot, green beans, artichoke, Molokia, spinach, green peas, strawberry, grape leaves, broad bean, broccoli, grape, peach, salad, mixed vegetables, pomegranates, and cauliflowers) purchased from various local retail stands in Egyptian markets. Information on the serotypes and strains circulating in the Middle East and the GCC Arab region is widely lacking or limited.

Identification of possible pathways of *L. monocytogenes* and their AMR profile throughout the food chain, from farm-to-fork, will be of added value to the risk management of human illnesses in Arab countries (Osman, Kappell, Fox, Orabi, & Samir, 2020). In Jordon, Osaili, Alaboudi, and Nesiar (2011) detected AMR in *L. monocytogenes* isolates ($n = 51$) toward tetracycline and tilmicosin (9.8% each) in ready-to-eat chicken products. A recent study in Egypt by Aziz and Mohamed (2020) reported nine *L. monocytogenes* isolates from meat showing high resistance to penicillin, ampicillin, and tetracycline. The isolates in that study also showed resistance to erythromycin (66.6%), amoxicillin–clavulanic (55.5%), vancomycin (22.2%), and sulfamethoxazole/trimethoprim (11.1%). The high level of resistance to ampicillin is a real cause for concern considering that ampicillin is the drug of choice in empirical listeriosis therapy. Added to that, the occurrence of MDR *L. monocytogenes* isolates is an issue of public health concern that alarms the necessity for surveillance programs on antibiotic resistance evolution at the human–food interface. Food contamination by *L. monocytogenes* is not uncommon in the Middle East. Although considered

TABLE 3.3 The occurrence of *Listeria* spp. in foods in the Middle East.

Country	References	Types of food sample (no.)	*Listeria* spp. %	*L. monocytogenes* %	Other *Listeria* spp. %
Egypt	Dapgh et al. (2020)	Soft cheese ($n = 155$)	14.2	4.5	*L. innocua* (9.7).
	El-Naenaeey et al. (2019)	Milk of dairy cows ($n = 200$)	19	4	*L. ivanovii* (6), *L. innocua* (2), *L. grayi* (3), *L. welshimeri* (4)
	Mahmoud, Karmi, and Maky (2019)	Minced meat ($n = 20$)	50	15	*L. ivanovii* (10), *L. welshimeri* (5), *L. innocua* (20), *L. seeligeri* (0), *L. grayi* (0).
		Kofta ($n = 20$)	70	20	*L. ivanovii* (5), *L. welshimeri* (10), *L. innocua* (14), *L. seeligeri* (10), *L. grayi* (5).
		Sausage ($n = 20$)	35	10	*L. ivanovii* (10), *L. welshimeri* (5), *L. innocua* (10), *L. seeligeri* (0), *L. grayi* (0).
		Burger ($n = 20$)	60	15	*L. ivanovii* (15), *L. welshimeri* (10), *L. innocua* (10), *L. seeligeri* (5), *L. grayi* (5).
		Luncheon ($n = 20$)	40	10	*L. ivanovii* (10), *L. welshimeri* (10), *L. innocua* (5), *L. seeligeri* (5), *L. grayi* (0).
		Pastirma ($n = 20$)	25	5	*L. ivanovii* (10), *L. welshimeri* (0), *L. innocua* (5), *L. seeligeri* (5), *L. grayi* (0).
	Mohamed et al. (2018)	Vegetable ($n = 331$)	—	14.2	—

(Continued)

TABLE 3.3 (Continued)

Country	References	Types of food sample (no.)	*Listeria* spp. %	*L. monocytogenes* %	Other *Listeria* spp. %
	Tahoun et al. (2017)	Raw milk, milking equipment, and hand swabs ($n = 300$)		23	*L. innocua* (3.3)
	Mohamed et al. (2016)	Beef burgers ($n = 50$)	—	32%	—
		Minced meat ($n = 25$)	—	4%	—
		Luncheon ($n = 25$)	—	4%	—
	Meshref, Zeinhom, and Abdel-Atty (2015)	Raw milk ($n = 51$)	27.5	3.9	*L. ivanovii* (3.9), *L. innocua* (9.8), *L. seeligeri* (5.9), *L. grayi* (2), *L. welshimeri* (2).
		Kareish cheese ($n = 51$)	13.73	2	*L. ivanovii* (2), *L. innocua* (2), *L. seeligeri* (6.5), *L. grayi* (0), *L. welshimeri* (2).
		Burger ($n = 50$)	8	0	*L. ivanovii* (2), *L. innocua* (0), *L. seeligeri* (0), *L. grayi* (4). *L. welshimeri* (2).
		Butter ($n = 31$)	6.5	0	*L. ivanovii* (3.2), *L. innocua* (0), *L. seeligeri* (0), *L. grayi* (0), *L. welshimeri* (3.2).
	Ismaiel et al. (2014)	Frozen lean beef ($n = 30$)	13.3	3.3%	*L. ivanovii* (6.7), *L. grayi* (3.3), *L. innocua* (3.3), *L. seeligeri* (3.3), *L. welshimeri* (0).

		Raw milk ($n = 30$)	6.7	0	*L. ivanovii* (3.3), *L. grayi* (3.3), *L. innocua* (0), *L. seeligeri* (3.3), *L. welshimeri* (3.3).
	Abdel-Malek et al. (2010)	Minced frozen beef ($n = 25$)	32	4	*L. ivanovii* (0), *L. innocua* (28), *L. welshimeri* (0), *L. seeligeri* (0), *L. grayi* (0), *L. murrayi* (0).
		Luncheon ($n = 25$)	32	8	*L. ivanovii* (4), *L. innocua* (0), *L. welshimeri* (8), *L. seeligeri* (8), *L. grayi* (4), *L. murrayi* (0).
		Frozen chicken leg ($n = 25$)	52	0	*L. ivanovii* (12), *L. innocua* (8), *L. welshimeri* (8), *L. seeligeri* (0), *L. grayi* (16), *L. murrayi* (0).
		Frozen chicken fillet ($n = 25$)	56	8	*L. ivanovii* (12), *L. innocua* (12), *L. welshimeri* (12), *L. seeligeri* (0), *L. grayi* (8), *L. murrayi* (4).
Iraq	Al-Mashhadany (2019)	Red meat ($n = 375$)	—	13.9	—
	Al-Brefkani and Mammani (2019)	Frozen chicken ($n = 309$)	—	8.7	—
		Fresh red meat ($n = 167$)	—	6	—
	Al-Ali et al. (2018)	Gallbladder of sheep ($n = 150$)	—	4	—
		Gallbladder of cattle ($n = 150$)	—	1.3	—
	Ahmed, Tayeb, Ameen, Merza, and Sharif (2017)	Cheese ($n = 50$)	—	2	—
		Minced meat ($n = 50$)	—	14	—

(*Continued*)

TABLE 3.3 (Continued)

Country	References	Types of food sample (no.)	*Listeria* spp. %	*L. monocytogenes* %	Other *Listeria* spp. %
		Frozen chicken ($n=50$)	—	8	—
Jordan	Al-Nabulsi et al. (2015)	Raw and processed meat ($n=270$)	—	24.4	*L. ivanovii* (27), *L. grayi* (8.9), *L. seeligeri* (3.7), *L. welshimeri* (2.2), *L. innocua* (6.3)
	Osaili et al. (2014)	Ready-to-eat meat Products ($n=1028$)	—	2	—
	Osaili, Al-Nabulsi et al. (2012), Osaili, Alaboudi, and Al-Akhras (2012)	White cheese ($n=350$)	27.1	11.1	*L. grayi* (6.9%), *L. innocua* (2%), *L. ivanovii* (4%), *L. seeligeri* (2%), and *L. welshimeri* (0.3%)
	Osaili et al. (2011)	RTE chicken shawarma ($n=30$)	—	13.3	*L. ivanovii* (66.7), *L. grayi* (6.6), *L. seeligeri* (3.3), *L. welshimeri* (0).
		Fresh broiler chicken ($n=160$)		9.4	*L. ivanovii* (30), *L. grayi* (5), *L. seeligeri* (2.5), *L. welshimeri* (0.6).
		RTE chicken burger ($n=30$)	—	76.7	*L. ivanovii* (10), *L. grayi* (0), *L. seeligeri* (0), *L. welshimeri* (0).
		RTE chicken sausage ($n=30$)	—	30	*L. ivanovii* (6.7), *L. grayi* (0), *L. seeligeri* (0), *L. welshimeri* (3.3).
		Mortadella ($n=30$)		0	*L. ivanovii* (0), *L. grayi* (0), *L. seeligeri* (0), *L. welshimeri* (0).

	Awaisheh (2010)	RTE beef meat ($n = 120$)	—	19.2	*L. innocua* (24), *L. welshimeri* (14.2).
		Ready-to-eat poultry meat ($n = 120$)	—	15	*L. innocua* (23), *L. welshimeri* (15.8).
Saudi Arabia	Yehia et al. (2016)	Raw beef ($n = 10$)	50	0	*L. innocua* (10), *L. seeligeri* (10), *L. welshimeri* (20), *L. grayi* (10), *L. ivanovii* (0).
		Raw chicken ($n = 10$)	50	20%	*L. innocua* (10), *L. seeligeri* (10), *L. welshimeri* (0), *L. grayi* (0), *L. ivanovii* (10).
		Raw fish ($n = 10$)	30	0%	*L. innocua* (0), *L. seeligeri* (10), *L. welshimeri* (10), *L. grayi* (10), *L. ivanovii* (0).
		Raw camel milk ($n = 10$)	20	0%	*L. innocua* (0), *L. seeligeri* (0), *L. welshimeri* (0), *L. grayi* (10), *L. ivanovii* (0).
	Bahobail et al. (2012)	Unwashed egg shell ($n = 20$)	10	—	—
Syria	Al-Mariri, Younes, and Ramadan (2013)	Cow milk ($n = 345$)	70	6.7	*L. innocua* (3.2), *L. ivanovi* (2), *L. gravi* (0.9), *L. welshimeri* (1.4).
		Sheep milk ($n = 225$)	30	5.3	*L. innocua* (1.8), *L. ivanovi* (2.2), *L. gravi* (0.4), *L. welshimeri* (1.3).

a rare clinical pathogen, this microorganism has a very high mortality rate, particularly among infants, children, and the elderly. Outbreaks of sporadic listeriosis cases have serious public health and economic implications that need to be curtailed through effective food safety management systems.

Some studies have been conducted in the Middle East on *L. monocytogenes* at the human–food animal interface, notably in high-risk human groups. In Egypt, El-Gohary et al. (2018) detected *Listeria* spp. in 11.1% (1/9) of stool samples from cases of aborted women in the Dakahlia governorate. El-Naenaeey et al. (2019) also isolated *L. monocytogenes* from 4% (8/200) of stools from healthy pregnant Egyptian women. Their study detected *inl*A and *inl*B genes in all isolates, indicating the potential virulence of such isolates. There is a need for strengthening the surveillance systems of foodborne zoonoses in general, and for *L. monocytogenes* in particular, in the Middle East. National food safety agencies should urge risk-based microbiological standards and strike a balance between meeting realistic and achievable limits for the industry while ensuring adequate protection. Individual countries across the Middle East should also realize the importance of national surveillance and audit their existing food testing facilities to identify their limitations and improve their workflow to be up to far with international norms.

3.5 *Brucella* spp. in the food chain in the Middle East

Brucella spp. are elective intracellular coccobacillus that belongs to the α2-Proteobacteriacea family (Neta et al., 2010). The genus *Brucella* is categorized as a Gram-negative, intracellular, facultative bacterium, and nonmotile (Abedi et al., 2020; Moreno, Cloeckaert, & Moriyón, 2002). *Brucella abortus* and *Brucella melitensis* are considered the most important human brucellosis species and may also be frequently found in cattle, goats, and sheep, as also being favored hosts, respectively (Abedi et al., 2020). Furthermore, two *Brucella* species isolated from marine mammals, *Brucella pinnipedialis* and *Brucella ceti*, can also cause brucellosis in humans (Foster, Osterman, Godfroid, Jacques, & Cloeckaert, 2007). Notably, *Brucella canis*, *Brucella neotomae*, and *Brucella ovis* pathogens of dogs, desert rats, and sheep have a comparatively lower rate and are not associated with human brucellosis (Godfroid et al., 2005). According to the WHO, millions of people become sick annually because of food-sourced zoonosis, and brucellosis is among the most investigated zoonosis (WHO, 2013b). Human brucellosis is considered a life-threatening illness. Among the most critical zoonosis diseases caused by *Brucella* sp. is Mediterranean fever or Malta fever (Xavier, Paixao, den Hartigh, Tsolis, & Santos, 2010). The incubation period of brucellosis is usually 2–4 weeks up to several months, and the duration of the disease's symptoms ranged from 3 weeks to 2 months. The symptoms of Mediterranean fever in humans are fever, anorexia, malaise, headache, arthralgia, myalgia, and backache that may later cause chronic disease affecting different organs and tissues (Abedi et al., 2020; Hizel et al., 2007; Kato et al., 2007). The indirect or direct contact with infected animals and the consumption of contaminated milk or milk products could result in pathogen transmission to humans (Pereira et al., 2020). The disease in domestic animals most often occurs as a chronic infection that results in orchitis and epididymitis in males or placentitis and abortion in pregnant females (Ren, Hou, Zhao, Wang, & Peng, 2020). Furthermore, the disease's acute clinical signs in domestic animals may also decrease dairy products' production (Abedi et al., 2020). The thermal process of milk can reduce the population of this *Brucella* spp. However, accidental failures in the pasteurization process or postproduction contamination of products could provide suitable conditions for the organisms' growth (Moslemi et al., 2018). For instance, *B. melitensis* can grow in infected unpasteurized milk stored up to 5 and 9 days at 4°C and −20°C, respectively (Abedi et al., 2020).

Brucellosis is considered a public health and economic problem in the MENA, Mediterranean region, India, Southern and Central Asia, and Central and South America (Lai et al., 2017). The EFSA has reported that the annual occurrence rate of brucellosis in humans is 0.3 cases per million. In contrast, among numerous developed countries, the occurrence may reach more than 1000 cases per million (ECDC, 2014). In Arab countries, there is a variation between and within-country in the reporting of human brucellosis due to socioeconomic and demographic factors and the application of surveillance systems and animal-based control programs. A systematic review of human and animal brucellosis in the Middle East supported the widespread presence of *Brucella* in the region (Wernery, 2014). Fifteen countries had at least one occurrence of *B. melitensis*, and 9 reported *B. abortus*. Four studies gave reliable estimates of brucellosis in ruminants of 2%−10% in individual animals and up to 50% for flocks, while only one study, in Egypt, reported on human brucellosis with an estimated annual incidence of 64−70/100,000 persons between 2002 and 2003 (Musallam, Abo-Shehada, Hegazy, Holt, & Guitian, 2016).

In several countries across the Arab countries, the traditional customs such as the drinking of unpasteurized milk (particularly camel milk) and consuming dairy products made from unpasteurized milk, along with the popularity of pastoralism, contribute to the foodborne and occupational transmission of *Brucella* in humans (Bagheri Nejad, Krecek, Khalaf, Hailat, and Arenas-Gamboa, 2020). *Brucella* spp. have been detected in milk and milk products in various countries in the Middle East. In Iraq, drinking raw milk is concerned as a significant source for human infection with *Brucella* sp., as numerous studies have isolated the organism from the milk (Abbas & Aldeewan, 2009; Al-Sanjary, Mohammed, & Dahl, 2014; Turgay & Ahmed, 2016) and traditional cheese (Akbarmehr, 2011; Khalil & Fadihl, 2016; Talei, 2010) (Table 3.4). As indicated in Table 3.4, molecular techniques

TABLE 3.4 The occurrence of *Brucella* spp. in foods in the Middle East.

Country	References	Type of food sample (no.)	Isolation procedure	Species (%)
Egypt	Aman, Al-Hawary, Helmy, and El-Gushi (2020)	Raw milk ($n=200$)	RT-PCR	*Brucella* spp. (2.5)
	El-Diasty et al. (2016)	Raw cow and buffalo milk ($n=205$)	PCR	*B. abortus* (6.3)
	Wareth, Melzer, Elschner, Neubauer, and Roesler (2014)	Raw cow milk ($n=215$)	RT-PCR	*Brucella* spp. (17.7)
	Abdel-Razik et al. (2008)	Cattle milk ($n=32$)	PCR	*Brucella* spp. (18.8)
		Buffalo' milk ($n=30$)	PCR	*Brucella* spp. (13.3)
		Sheep' milk ($n=30$)	PCR	*Brucella* spp. (20)
	Samaha, Al-Rowaily, Khoudair, and Ashour (2009)	Cattle milk ($n=1966$)	Culture	*Brucella* spp. (5.4)
		Buffalo' milk ($n=1337$)	Culture	*Brucella* spp. (4.11)
		Sheep' milk ($n=813$)	Culture	*Brucella* spp. (5.4)
		Goat milk ($n=366$)	Culture	*Brucella* spp. (3.6)
	Hamdy and Amin (2002)	Cattle milk ($n=52$)	PCR	*Brucella* spp. (55.8)
		Sheep' milk ($n=21$)	PCR	*Brucella* spp. (47.6)
		Goat milk ($n=18$)	PCR	*Brucella* spp. (72.2)
		Camel milk ($n=12$)	PCR	*Brucella* spp. (8.3)

(*Continued*)

TABLE 3.4 (Continued)

Country	References	Type of food sample (no.)	Isolation procedure	Species (%)
Iraq	Khalil and Fadihl (2016)	Traditional cheese (Gibin Al-Arab) ($n=50$)	Culture	*B. melitensis* (8), *B. abortus* (4).
	Al-Sanjary et al. (2014)	Raw sheep milk ($n=50$)	PCR	*B. melitensis* (68)
	Akbarmehr (2011)	Traditional cheese ($n=1000$)	Culture and biochemical tests	*B. melitensis* (0.7), *B. abortus* (1.5)
	Talei (2010)	Traditional cheese ($n=100$)	Culture	*B. abortus* (8)
	Abbas and Aldeewan (2009)	Raw cow milk ($n=120$)	Culture	*B. abortus* (7.5), *B. melitensis* (2.5), *B. ovis* (0).
		Raw buffalo milk ($n=120$)	Culture	*B. abortus* (11.7), *B. melitensis* (4.6), *B. ovis* (0).
		Raw sheep milk ($n=180$)	Culture	*B. abortus* (5.6), *B. melitensis* (9.4), *B. ovis* (2.2)
Kuwait	El-Gohary, Mohamed, and Al-Sherida (2016)	Raw cow milk ($n=4671$)	Buffered Acidified Plate Antigen Test (BAPAT)	*Brucella* spp. (7.3)
Lebanon	Alwan (2005)	Milk products ($n=164$)	PCR	*B. abortus* (3.7)
Saudi Arabia	Khan et al. (2018)	Raw camel milk ($n=80$)	PCR	*B. melitensis* (22)
Syria	Al-Mariri (2015)	Raw cow milk ($n=2372$)	PCR	*Brucella* spp. (25)

have been widely deployed in several studies investigated *Brucella* sp. in dairy products across the Middle East. Several researchers could have preferred using molecular detection methods, given the critical biosafety requirements needed for handling *Brucella* culture, such as the need for a high level of biosafety (Level 3) that is not common in most food testing laboratories. Limited studies in the Middle East looked at the AMR of *Brucella* isolates in foods. In Lebanon, Alwan (2005) detected a high level of resistance of *B. abortus* isolates ($n = 8$) to streptomycin and ciprofloxacin in 66.7% each and gentamicin in 50% of the isolates recovered from Lebanese dairy products (Table 3.4). In Egypt, the detection of *Brucella* spp. was reported in raw milk from cows, buffalo, and sheep (Abdel-Razik, Ismail, Youssef, & Hashad, 2008) (Table 3.4). A recent study in Egypt by Khan et al. (2020) has also detected *Brucella* sp. from camels at 15.5% (59/381). In Saudi Arabia, Khalifa, Alshaikh, Aljumaah, Jarelnabi, and Hussein (2018) detected *Brucella* sp. in 16.7% (63/378) from camels. In some of the Arab countries camels serve as a vital source of milk and meat for local consumption. It is crucial to monitor milk and meat from camels for contamination with *Brucella* spp. It is also critical to screen for *Brucella* contamination in the animals' farm environment, milk handlers, and dairy workers.

It is important to note that in countries where food hygiene practices prevent foodborne brucellosis, the disease is mostly occupational (Mohammed, Shigidy, & Al juboori, 2013). Control of brucellosis in humans depends on the control of livestock brucellosis by combining vaccination campaigns and testing-and-slaughter approaches of infected animals and better farm biosecurity and hygiene (FAO, 2010). Given the vast number of small noncommercial farms and the enduring popularity among locals, especially in GCC countries, it is not clear how to implement a *Brucella* management strategy in livestock in that region. The popularity of small noncommercial livestock farms throughout the Arab countries is unique and will stifle any efforts of control that aim to eliminate *Brucella* infection from livestock in the region. To take a significant step forward toward mitigation of brucellosis burden in the region, the implementation of health education and public awareness campaigns supported by One Health approach is urgent and is hoped to lead to lasting change in current disease situations in Arab countries (Aligol, Nasirzadeh, Bakhtiari, & Eslami, 2014).

3.6 Conclusions

Foodborne infections caused by bacterial pathogens are a common cause of human illness, with a substantial burden resulting in economic loss and public health consequences. *Salmonella*, *Campylobacter*, *L. monocytogenes*, and *Brucella* have been frequently detected in various food types. The current evidence presented in this chapter points out that the detection of these bacterial pathogens is frequent in animal- and plant-origin foods. These bacteria may access the human food chain from primary production up to final products' final consumption. These bacterial pathogens are currently a significant concern for public health due to the emergence of MDR strains. Despite reports on the prevalence of foodborne bacteria in foods of animal origin, animals, and humans, the burden of these pathogens in foods of animal origin is still not well studied. The associated risk factors are not clearly identified, and the incidence of human infections from foodborne exposure is not well documented. The literature evidence presented in this chapter stresses that *Salmonella*, *Campylobacter*, *L. monocytogenes*, and *Brucella* continue to challenge food safety and public health in the Arab countries. Thus we recommend the following: (1) Coordinated surveillance and monitoring system for foodborne pathogens should be done to design an informed control and prevention strategies against these pathogens at national and regional levels across the Arab countries; (2) the epidemiological information regarding risk factors and incidence of human infections associated with foodborne infection should be established and well documented at the national level; (3) awareness of the public should be developed based on pieces of evidence stemmed from a scientific risk analysis of bacterial pathogens causing foodborne infection; (4) it is crucial to utilize the state-of-art molecular level characterization (e.g., whole-genome sequencing) to implement better prevention and control strategies across the Arab countries.

References

Abaza, A. (2017). Bacteriological assessment of some vegetables and ready-to-eat salads in Alexandria, Egypt. *Journal of Egyptian Public Health Association, 92*(3), 177–187.

Abbas, B., & Aldeewan, A. (2009). Occurrence and epidemiology of *Brucella* spp. in raw milk samples at Basrah province, Iraq. *Bulgarian Journal of Veterinary Medicine, 12*(2), 136–142.

Abdel-Aziz, N. M. (2016). Detection of *Salmonella* species in chicken carcasses using genus specific primer belong to invA gene in Sohag city, Egypt. *Veterinary World, 9*(10), 1125.

Abdel-Aziz, D., & Abd-Allah, S. (2017). Incidence of *Campylobacter* species in wholesale chicken carcasses and chicken meat products in Assiut city, Egypt. *International Food Research Journal, 24*(6), 2660–2665.

Abd-Elghany, S., Sallam, K., Abd-Elkhalek, A., & Tamura, T. (2015). Occurrence, genetic characterization and antimicrobial resistance of *Salmonella* isolated from chicken meat and giblets. *Epidemiology & Infection, 143*(5), 997–1003.

Abdel-Malek, A. M., Ali, S. F. H., Moemen, R. H., Mohamed, A., & Elsayh, K. I. (2010). Occurrence of *Listeria* species in meat, chicken products and human stools in Assiut city, Egypt with PCR use for rapid identification of *Listeria monocytogenes*. *Veterinary World, 3*(8), 353.

Abdel-Maksoud, M., Abdel-Khalek, R., El-Gendy, A., Gamal, R. F., Abdelhady, H. M., & House, B. L. (2015). Genetic characterisation of multidrug-resistant *Salmonella enterica* serotypes isolated from poultry in Cairo, Egypt. *African Journal of Laboratory Medicine, 4*(1), 1–7.

Abdel-Razik, K., Ismail, E., Youssef, H., & Hashad, M. (2008). Diagnosis of brucellosis in dairy animals using nested polymerase chain reaction. *International Journal of Dairy Science, 3*, 55–62.

Abedi, A.-S., Hashempour-Baltork, F., Alizadeh, A. M., Beikzadeh, S., Hosseini, H., Bashiry, M., & Sarlak, Z. (2020). The prevalence of Brucella spp. in dairy products in the Middle East region: A systematic review and meta-analysis. *Acta Tropica*, *202*, 105241.

Abid, A. J. (2016). Conventional and molecular approaches in bacterial contamination detection for meat samples. *International Journal of PharmTech Research*, *9*(3), 212–218.

Abu-Madi, M., Behnke, J. M., Sharma, A., Bearden, R., & Al-Banna, N. (2016). Prevalence of virulence/stress genes in *Campylobacter jejuni* from chicken meat sold in Qatari retail outlets. *PLoS One*, *11*(6), e0156938.

Abushahba, M. F., Ahmed, S. O., Ibrahim, A. A., & Mosa, H. A. (2018). Prevalence of zoonotic species of *Campylobacter* in broiler chicken and humans in Assiut governorate, Egypt. *Approaches in Poultry, Dairy & Veterinary Sciences*, *3*, 1–9.

Ahmed, M. A., & Shimamoto, T. (2014). Isolation and molecular characterization of *Salmonella enterica, Escherichia coli* O157: H7 and Shigella spp. from meat and dairy products in Egypt. *International Journal of Food Microbiology*, *168*, 57–62.

Ahmed, S., Tayeb, B., Ameen, A., Merza, S., & Sharif, Y. (2017). Isolation and molecular detection of *Listeria monocytogenes* in minced meat, frozen chicken and cheese in Duhok province, Kurdistan region of Iraq. *Journal of Food: Microbiology, Safety & Hygiene*, *2*(1), 118.

Akbarmehr, J. (2011). The prevalence of *Brucella abortus* and *Brucella melitensis* in local cheese produced in Sarab city, Iran and its public health implication. *African Journal of Microbiology Research*, *5*(12), 1500–1503.

Alaboudi, A. R., Malkawi, I. M., Osaili, T. M., Abu-Basha, E. A., & Guitian, J. (2020). Prevalence, antibiotic resistance and genotypes of *Campylobacter jejuni* and *Campylobacter coli* isolated from chickens in Irbid governorate, Jordan. *International Journal of Food Microbiology*, *327*, 108656.

Al-Ali, H. J., Abd Al-Rodhan, M., Al-Hilali, S. A., Al-Charrakh, A. H., Al-Mohana, A. M., & Hadi, Z. J. (2018). Molecular detection of serotype groups of *Listeria monocytogenes* isolated from gallbladder of cattle and sheep in Iraq. *Veterinary World*, *11*(4), 431.

Al-Brefkani, A. M. T., & Mammani, I. M. A. (2019). Characterisation of *Listeria monocytogenes* from food and human clinical samples at Duhok, Kurdistan Region of Iraq. *Journal of Pure and Applied Microbiology*, *13*(4), 2215–2226.

Al-Dughaym, A., & Altabari, G. (2010). Safety and quality of some chicken meat products in Al-Ahsa markets-Saudi Arabia. *Saudi Journal of Biological Sciences*, *17*(1), 37–42.

Al-Freihi, H., Twum-Danso, K., Sohaibani, M., Bella, H., El-Mouzan, M., & Sama, K. (1993). The microbiology of acute diarrhoeal disease in the eastern province of Saudi Arabia. *East African Medical Journal*, *70*(5), 267–269.

Al-Groom, R. (2017). Extant of microbial contamination of cheddar cheese from markets and restaurants in Amman-Jordan. *Journal of Pure and Applied Microbiology*, *11*(3), 1427–1433.

Aligol, M., Nasirzadeh, M., Bakhtiari, M. H., & Eslami, A. A. (2014). The effects of education on promoting knowledge, beliefs and preventive behaviors on brucellosis among women: Applying a health belief model. *Jundishapur Journal of Health Sciences*, *6*(2), 343–349.

Al-Mariri, A. (2015). Isolation of *Brucella melitensis* strains from Syrian bovine milk samples. *Bulgarian Journal of Veterinary Medicine*, *18*(1), 40–48.

Al-Mariri, A., Younes, A., & Ramadan, L. (2013). Prevalence of *Listeria* spp. in raw milk in Syria. *Bulgarian Journal of Veterinary Medicine*, *16*(2), 112–122.

Al-Mashhadany, D. A. (2019). Occurrence and antibiogram of *Listeria monocytogenes* isolates from retail meat shops at Erbil City, Kurdistan Region, Iraq. *Italian Journal of Food Safety*, *8*(4), 8451.

Al-Nabulsi, A. A., Osaili, T. M., Awad, A. A., Olaimat, A. N., Shaker, R. R., & Holley, R. A. (2015). Occurrence and antibiotic susceptibility of *Listeria monocytogenes* isolated from raw and processed meat products in Amman, Jordan. *CyTA – Journal of Food, 13*(3), 346–352.

Al-Rifai, H. R., Chaabna, K., Denagamage, T., & Al-Ali, W. Q. (2019). Prevalence of enteric non-typhoidal *Salmonella* in humans in the Middle East and North Africa: A systematic review and meta-analysis. *Zoonoses and Public Health, 66*(7), 701–728.

Al-Sanjary, R. A., Mohammed, H. A., & Dahl, M. O. (2014). Using polymerase chain reaction technique (PCR) for detection *Brucella melitensis* in aborted ewes' milk in Nineveh, Iraq. *Assiut Veterinary Medical Journal, 60*(140), 155–159.

Alwan, N. H. (2005). *Isolation, molecular characterization and antimicrobial resistance of Brucella and Listeria species in representative Lebanese foods*. Department of Biology, American University of Beirut.

Aman, I. M., Al-Hawary, I. I., Helmy, N. M., & El-Gushi, A. M. (2020). Detection of Brucella organisms from Egyptian raw milk using cultural and molecular techniques. *Kafrelsheikh Veterinary Medical Journal, 18*(2), 14–19. Available from https://doi.org/10.21608/kvmj.2020.39842.1007.

Amin, H. S., & El Rahman, A. E.-R. A. A. (2015). Molecular characterization of *Salmonella enterica* isolated from chicken meat and its products by multiplex PCR. *Alexandria Journal for Veterinary Sciences, 46*(1), 155–160.

Angelo, K. M., Jackson, K. A., Wong, K. K., Hoekstra, R. M., & Jackson, B. R. (2016). Assessment of the incubation period for invasive listeriosis. *Clinical Infectious Diseases, 63*(11), 1487–1489.

Awaisheh, S. (2010). Incidence and contamination level of *Listeria monocytogenes* and other *Listeria* spp. in ready-to-eat meat products in Jordan. *Journal of Food Protection, 73*(3), 535–540.

Awofisayo-Okuyelu, A., Hall, I., Adak, G., Hawker, J., Abbott, S., & McCarthy, N. (2017). A systematic review and meta-analysis on the incubation period of campylobacteriosis. *Epidemiology & Infection, 145*(11), 2241–2253.

Aziz, S., & Mohamed, M. (2020). Prevalence, virulence genes, and antimicrobial resistance profile of *Listeria monocytogenes* isolated from retail poultry shops in Beni-Suef city, Egypt. *Journal of advanced veterinary and animal research*, 7(4), 710–717. Available from https://doi.org/10.5455/javar.2020.g472

Badahdah, S. A., & Aldagal, M. M. (2018). Antibiotic resistance in *Salmonella* spp. isolated from local chickens in Saudi Arabia. *International Journal of Food Science and Nutrition Engineering, 8*(5), 127–130. Available from https://doi.org/10.5923/j.food.20180805.03.

Bagheri Nejad, R., Krecek, R. C., Khalaf, O. H., Hailat, N., & Arenas-Gamboa, A. M. (2020). Brucellosis in the Middle East: Current situation and a pathway forward. *PLoS Neglected Tropical Diseases, 14*(5), e0008071.

Bahobail, A. A. S., Hassan, S. A., & El-Deeb, B. A. (2012). Microbial quality and content aflatoxins of commercially available eggs in Taif, Saudi Arabia. *African Journal of Microbiology Research, 6*(13), 3337–3342.

Bahrami, A., Baboli, Z. M., Schimmel, K., Jafari, S. M., & Williams, L. (2020). Efficiency of novel processing technologies for the control of *Listeria monocytogenes* in food products. *Trends in Food Science & Technology, 96*, 61–78.

Chen, M., Cheng, J., Zhang, J., Chen, Y., Zeng, H., Xue, L., & Wu, H. (2019). Isolation, potential virulence, and population diversity of *Listeria monocytogenes* from meat and meat products in China. *Frontiers in Microbiology, 10*, 946.

Chon, J.-W., Hyeon, J.-Y., Lim, J.-H., Kim, J.-H., Song, K.-Y., & Seo, K.-H. (2012). Improvement of modified charcoal-cefoperazone-deoxycholate agar by supplementation with a high concentration of polymyxin B for the detection of *Campylobacter jejuni* and *C. coli* in chicken carcass rinse. *Applied and Environmental Microbiology*, *78*(5), 1624–1626.

Coker, A. O., Isokpehi, R. D., Thomas, B. N., Amisu, K. O., & Obi, C. L. (2002). Human campylobacteriosis in developing countries1. *Emerging Infectious Diseases*, *8*(3), 237.

Dapgh, A. N., ELGedawy, A., Abouelhag, H. A., Mansour, A. S., Gaber, E., & Farahat, E. (2020). Advanced identification and characterization of *Listeria* species in Egyptian local soft cheese. *South Asian Journal of Research in Microbiology*, *8*(2), 11–18.

da Silva, D. A., Vallim, D., Rosas, C., de Mello, V., Brandão, M., & de Filippis, I. (2020). Genetic diversity of *Listeria monocytogenes* serotype 1/2a strains collected in Brazil by multi-virulence-locus sequence typing. *Letters in Applied Microbiology*. Available from https://doi.org/10.1111/lam.13413.

ECDC. (2012). The European Union summary report on antimicrobial resistance in zoonotic and indicator bacteria from humans, animals and food in 2010. *EFSA Journal*, *10*, 1–233.

ECDC. (2014). The European Union summary report on trends and sources of zoonoses, zoonotic agents and food-borne outbreaks in 2012. *EFSA Journal*, *12*(2), 3547.

ECDC. (2017). The European Union summary report on trends and sources of zoonoses, zoonotic agents and food-borne outbreaks in 2016. *EFSA Journal*, *15*(12), e05077.

ECDC. (2018). The European Union summary report on trends and sources of zoonoses, zoonotic agents and food-borne outbreaks in 2017. *EFSA Journal*, *16*(12), e05500.

Eikmeier, D., Medus, C., & Smith, K. (2018). Incubation period for outbreak-associated, non-typhoidal salmonellosis cases, Minnesota, 2000–2015. *Epidemiology & Infection*, *146*(4), 423–429.

El-Diasty, M. M., Ahmed, H. A., Sayour, A. E., El Hofy, F. I., Tahoun, A. B., & Shafik, S. M. (2016). Seroprevalence of *Brucella* spp. in cattle, molecular characterization in milk, and the analysis of associated risk factors with seroprevalence in humans, Egypt. *Vector-Borne and Zoonotic Diseases*, *16*(12), 758–764.

El-Gohary, A., Mohamed, A., & Al-Sherida, Y. (2016). Seroprevalence of brucellosis and typing of *Brucella melitensis* biovar 2 in lactating cows in Kuwait. *Journal of Advanced Veterinary and Animal Research*, *3*(3), 229–235.

El-Gohary A. H., Mohamed A. A., Ramadan H. H., & Abuhatab E. A. (2018). Zoonotic and Molecular Aspects of Listeria Species Isolated From Some Farm Animals at Dakahlia Province in Egypt. *AJVS*, 58(1), 208–214.

Elhadi, N. (2014). Prevalence and antimicrobial resistance of *Salmonella* spp. in raw retail frozen imported freshwater fish to Eastern Province of Saudi Arabia. *Asian Pacific Journal of Tropical Biomedicine*, *4*(3), 234–238.

El-Naenaeey, E.-S., Abdelwahab, A., Merwad, A., & Abdou, H. (2019). Prevalence of *Listeria* species in dairy cows and pregnant women with reference to virulotyping of *Listeria monocytogenes* in Egypt. *Zagazig Veterinary Journal*, *47*(3), 248–258.

El-Sharoud, W. M. (2009). Prevalence and survival of *Campylobacter* in Egyptian dairy products. *Food Research International*, *42*(5–6), 622–626.

El-Tawab, A., Ashraf, A., El Hofy, F. I., Ammar, A. M., Ahmed, H. A., & Hefny, A. A. (2015). Bacteriological and molecular identification of *Campylobacter* species in chickens and humans, at Zagazig city, Egypt. *Benha Veterinary Medical Journal*, *28*(1), 17–26.

El-Zamkan, M. A., & Hameed, K. G. A. (2016). Prevalence of *Campylobacter jejuni* and *Campylobacter coli* in raw milk and some dairy products. *Veterinary World*, *9*(10), 1147.

FAO. (2010). *Brucella melitensis in Eurasia and the Middle East*. FAO.

Farag, E., Garcell, H. G., Ganesan, N., Ahmed, S. N. N., Al-Hajri, M., Al Thani, S. M. H. J., & Al-Romaihi, H. E. (2016). A retrospective epidemiological study on the incidence of salmonellosis in the State of Qatar during 2004–2012. *Qatar Medical Journal*, *2016*(1), 3.

Fernández, J., Guerra, B., & Rodicio, M. R. (2018). Resistance to carbapenems in non-typhoidal *Salmonella enterica* serovars from humans, animals and food. *Veterinary Sciences*, *5*(2), 40.

Foster, G., Osterman, B. S., Godfroid, J., Jacques, I., & Cloeckaert, A. (2007). *Brucella ceti* sp. nov. and *Brucella pinnipedialis* sp. nov. for *Brucella* strains with cetaceans and seals as their preferred hosts. *International Journal of Systematic and Evolutionary Microbiology*, *57*(11), 2688–2693.

Galanis, E., Wong, D. M. L. F., Patrick, M. E., Binsztein, N., Cieslik, A., Chalermchaikit, T., & Wegener, H. C. (2006). Web-based surveillance and global Salmonella distribution, 2000–2002. *Emerging Infectious Diseases*, *12*(3), 381.

Ghaffoori, M. H. (2017). Prevalence of *Campylobacter jejuni* in chicken meat marketed in Baghdad province. *International Journal of Advanced Research in Biological Sciences*, *4*(6), 1–11.

Godfroid, J., Cloeckaert, A., Liautard, J.-P., Kohler, S., Fretin, D., Walravens, K., & Letesson, J.-J. (2005). From the discovery of the Malta fever's agent to the discovery of a marine mammal reservoir, brucellosis has continuously been a re-emerging zoonosis. *Veterinary Research*, *36*(3), 313–326.

Guévremont, E., Lamoureux, L., Généreux, M., & Côté, C. (2017). Irrigation water sources and time intervals as variables on the presence of *Campylobacter* spp. and *Listeria monocytogenes* on romaine lettuce grown in muck soil. *Journal of Food Protection*, *80*(7), 1182–1187.

Gundogdu, O., & Wren, B. W. (2020). Microbe profile: *Campylobacter jejuni*–survival instincts. *Microbiology (Reading, England)*, *166*(3), 230–232.

Habib, I., Harb, A., Hansson, I., Vågsholm, I., Osama, W., Adnan, S., & Boqvist, S. (2020). Challenges and opportunities towards the development of risk assessment at the consumer phase in developing countries—The case of *Campylobacter* cross-contamination during handling of raw chicken in two middle eastern countries. *Pathogens*, *9*(1), 62.

Hamdy, E. R. M., & Amin, A. (2002). Detection of *Brucella* species in the milk of infected cattle, sheep, goats and camels by PCR. *The Veterinary Journal*, *163*(3), 299–305.

Hansson, I., Sandberg, M., Habib, I., Lowman, R., & Engvall, E. O. (2018). Knowledge gaps in control of *Campylobacter* for prevention of campylobacteriosis. *Transboundary and Emerging Diseases*, *65*, 30–48.

Harb, A., Habib, I., Mezal, E. H., Kareem, H. S., Laird, T., O'Dea, M., & Abraham, S. (2018). Occurrence, antimicrobial resistance and whole-genome sequencing analysis of *Salmonella* isolates from chicken carcasses imported into Iraq from four different countries. *International Journal of Food Microbiology*, *284*, 84–90.

Harb, A., O'Dea, M., Abraham, S., & Habib, I. (2019). Childhood diarrhoea in the eastern Mediterranean region with special emphasis on non-typhoidal Salmonella at the human–food interface. *Pathogens*, *8*(2), 60.

Hassan, A. R. H. A., Salam, H. S., & Abdel-Latef, G. K. (2016). Serological identification and antimicrobial resistance of *Salmonella* isolates from broiler carcasses and human stools in Beni-Suef, Egypt. *Beni-Suef University Journal of Basic and Applied Sciences*, *5*(2), 202–207.

Hassan, A. S., Altalhi, A. D., Gherbawy, Y. A., & El-Deeb, B. A. (2011). Bacterial load of fresh vegetables and their resistance to the currently used antibiotics in Saudi Arabia. *Foodborne Pathogens and Disease*, *8*(9), 1011–1018.

Hassanain, N. A. (2011). Antimicrobial resistant *Campylobacter jejuni* isolated from humans and animals in Egypt. *Global Veterinaria*, *6*(2), 195–200.

Hassanein, R., Ali, S. F. H., El-Malek, A., Mohamed, A., Mohamed, M. A., & Elsayh, K. I. (2011). Detection and identification of *Salmonella* species in minced beef and chicken meats by using multiplex PCR in Assiut city. *Veterinary World*, *4*(1), 112–146.

Hendriksen, R. S., Vieira, A. R., Karlsmose, S., Lo Fo Wong, D. M., Jensen, A. B., Wegener, H. C., & Aarestrup, F. M. (2011). Global monitoring of *Salmonella* serovar distribution from the World Health Organization global foodborne infections network country data bank: Results of quality assured laboratories from 2001 to 2007. *Foodborne Pathogens and Disease*, *8*(8), 887–900.

Hizel, K., Guzel, O., Dizbay, M., Karakus, R., Senol, E., Arman, D., & Ulutan, F. (2007). Age and duration of disease as factors affecting clinical findings and sacroiliitis in brucellosis. *Infection*, *35*(6), 434–437.

Huang, L., Xu, Y.-B., Xu, J.-X., Ling, J.-Y., Chen, J.-L., Zhou, J.-L., & Du, Q.-P. (2017). Antibiotic resistance genes (ARGs) in duck and fish production ponds with integrated or non-integrated mode. *Chemosphere*, *168*, 1107–1114.

Inoue, T., Itani, T., Inomata, N., Hara, K., Takimoto, I., Iseki, S., & Shimada, Y. (2017). *Listeria monocytogenes* septicemia and meningitis caused by *Listeria enteritis* complicating ulcerative colitis. *Internal Medicine*, *56*(19), 2655–2659.

Ismaiel, A. A.-R., Ali, A. E.-S., & Enan, G. (2014). Incidence of *Listeria* in Egyptian meat and dairy samples. *Food Science and Biotechnology*, *23*(1), 179–185.

Iyer, A., Kumosani, T., Yaghmoor, S., Barbour, E., Azhar, E., & Harakeh, S. (2013). *Escherichia coli* and *Salmonella* spp. in meat in Jeddah, Saudi Arabia. *Journal of Infection in Developing Countries*, *7*(11), 812–818.

Jumaa, P., & Neringer, R. (2005). A survey of antimicrobial resistance in a tertiary referral hospital in the United Arab Emirates. *Journal of Chemotherapy*, *17*(4), 376–379.

Kanaan, G., Mohammed, M. H., & Ahmad, F. (2020). Antimicrobial resistance of *Campylobacter jejuni* from poultry meat in local markets of Iraq. *Plant Archives*, *20*(1), 410–415.

Kanaan, M., & Khashan, H. T. (2018). Prevalence of multidrug resistant thermotolerant species of *Campylobacter* in retail frozen chicken meat in Baghdad province. *Current Research in Microbiology and Biotechnology*, *6*(1), 1431–1440.

Kassaify, Z., Najjar, M., Toufeili, I., & Malek, A. (2010). Microbiological and chemical profile of Lebanese qishta [heat-coagulated milk]. *EMHJ-Eastern Mediterranean Health Journal*, *16*(9), 926–931.

Kato, Y., Masuda, G., Itoda, I., Imamura, A., Ajisawa, A., & Negishi, M. (2007). Brucellosis in a returned traveler and his wife: probable person-to-person transmission of *Brucella melitensis*. *Journal of Travel Medicine*, *14*(5), 343–345.

Kendall, J. J., Barrero-Tobon, A. M., Hendrixson, D. R., & Kelly, D. J. (2014). Hemerythrins in the microaerophilic bacterium *Campylobacter jejuni* help protect key iron–sulphur cluster enzymes from oxidative damage. *Environmental Microbiology*, *16*(4), 1105–1121.

Khalifa, A. L. I., Alshaikh, M., Aljumaah, R., Jarelnabi, A., & Hussein, M. F. (2018). Serological prevalence of abortifacient agents in female Mijaheem camels (*Camelus dromedarius*) in Saudi Arabia. *Journal of Animal Research*, *8*(3), 335–343.

Khalil, I. I., & Fadihl, S. J. (2016). Investigation of *Brucella* spp. from locally produced cheeses in Baquba city, Iraq. *Diyala Journal for Pure Science*, *12*(4-part 1), 83–90.

Khan, T. S., Ahmad, J., Wahab, R., Hirad, A. H., Musarrat, J., & Bahkali, A. H. (2018). An improved method of DNA preparation for PCR-based detection of *Brucella* in raw camel milk samples from Riyadh region and its comparison with immunological methods. *Journal of Food Safety*, *38*(1), e12381.

Khan, U. A., Sayour, A. E., Melzer, F., El-Soally, S. A. G. E., Elschner, M. C., & Roesler, U. (2020). Seroprevalence and molecular identification of *Brucella* spp. in camels in Egypt. *Microorganisms*, *8*(7), 1035.

Khatib, Al. I. A., & Mitwalli, Al. S. M. (2009). Microbiological quality and sample collection policy for dairy products in Ramallah and Al-Bireh district, Palestine. *EMHJ-Eastern Mediterranean Health Journal*, *15*(3), 709–716.

Khiyami, M., Noura, A.-F., Busaeed, B., & Sher, H. (2011). Food borne pathogen contamination in minimally processed vegetable salads in Riyadh, Saudi Arabia. *Journal of Medicinal Plants Research*, *5*(3), 444–451.

Kienesberger, S., Trummler, C. S., Fauster, A., Lang, S., Sprenger, H., Gorkiewicz, G., & Zechner, E. L. (2011). Interbacterial macromolecular transfer by the *Campylobacter fetus* subsp. Venerealis type IV secretion system. *Journal of Bacteriology*, *193*(3), 744–758.

King, M. T., Huh, I., Shenai, A., Brooks, T. M., & Brooks, C. L. (2018). Structural basis of VHH-mediated neutralization of the food-borne pathogen *Listeria monocytogenes*. *Journal of Biological Chemistry*, *293*(35), 13626–13635.

Kirk, M. D., Pires, S. M., Black, R. E., Caipo, M., Crump, J. A., Devleesschauwer, B., & Hald, T. (2015). World Health Organization estimates of the global and regional disease burden of 22 foodborne bacterial, protozoal, and viral diseases, 2010: A data synthesis. *PLoS Medicine*, *12*(12), e1001921.

Kirrella, G. A., Deeb, A. M., & Abdallah, R. M. I. (2017). Safety of frozen liver for human consumption. *Journal of Food and Drug Analysis*, *25*(3), 520–524.

Koopmans, M. M., Engelen-Lee, J., Brouwer, M. C., Jaspers, V., Man, W. K., Seron, M. V., & van de Beek, D. (2018). Characterization of a *Listeria monocytogenes* meningitis mouse model. *Journal of Neuroinflammation*, *15*(1), 1–11.

Lai, S., Zhou, H., Xiong, W., Gilbert, M., Huang, Z., Yu, J., & Li, Y. (2017). Changing epidemiology of human brucellosis, China, 1955–2014. *Emerging Infectious Diseases*, *23*(2), 184.

Lasagabaster, A., Jiménez, E., Lehnherr, T., Miranda-Cadena, K., & Lehnherr, H. (2020). Bacteriophage biocontrol to fight *Listeria* outbreaks in seafood. *Food and Chemical Toxicology*, *145*, 111682.

Lynch, O. A., Cagney, C., McDowell, D. A., & Duffy, G. (2010). A method for the growth and recovery of 17 species of *Campylobacter* and its subsequent application to inoculated beef. *Journal of Microbiological Methods*, *83*(1), 1–7.

Magalhães, R., Ferreira, V., Brandão, T. R., Palencia, R. C., Almeida, G., & Teixeira, P. (2016). Persistent and non-persistent strains of *Listeria monocytogenes*: A focus on growth kinetics under different temperature, salt, and pH conditions and their sensitivity to sanitizers. *Food Microbiology*, *57*, 103–108.

Mahmoud, H., Karmi, M., & Maky, M. (2019). Occurrence and characterization of *Listeria* species isolated from processed meat in Qena, Egypt. *Zagazig Veterinary Journal*, *47*(3), 267–276.

Malkawi, H. I., & Gharaibeh, R. (2003). Multiplex PCR for the direct detection of *Salmonella enterica* from chicken, lamb and beef food products. *Journal of Basic Microbiology: An International Journal on Biochemistry, Physiology, Genetics, Morphology, and Ecology of Microorganisms*, *43*(4), 328–336.

Man, S. M., Kaakoush, N. O., Leach, S. T., Nahidi, L., Lu, H. K., Norman, J., & Mitchell, H. M. (2010). Host attachment, invasion, and stimulation of proinflammatory cytokines by

Campylobacter concisus and other non-*Campylobacter jejuni Campylobacter* species. *Journal of Infectious Diseases*, *202*(12), 1855–1865.

Maury, M. M., Bracq-Dieye, H., Huang, L., Vales, G., Lavina, M., Thouvenot, P., & Lecuit, M. (2019). Hypervirulent *Listeria monocytogenes* clones' adaption to mammalian gut accounts for their association with dairy products. *Nature Communications*, *10*(1), 1–13.

Meshref, A., Zeinhom, M., & Abdel-Atty, N. S. (2015). Occurrence and distribution of *Listeria* species in some Egyptian foods. *Alexandria Journal for Veterinary Sciences*, *46*(1), 42–47.

Miceli, A., & Settanni, L. (2019). Influence of agronomic practices and pre-harvest conditions on the attachment and development of *Listeria monocytogenes* in vegetables. *Annals of Microbiology*, *69*(3), 185–199.

Moawad, A. A., Hotzel, H., Awad, O., Tomaso, H., Neubauer, H., Hafez, H. M., & El-Adawy, H. (2017). Occurrence of *Salmonella enterica* and *Escherichia coli* in raw chicken and beef meat in northern Egypt and dissemination of their antibiotic resistance markers. *Gut Pathogens*, *9*(1), 57.

Mohamed, I. R., Abdelmonem, M. A., & Amin, H. M. (2018). Virulence and antimicrobial susceptibility profile of *Listeria monocytogenes* isolated from frozen vegetables available in the Egyptian market. *African Journal of Microbiology Research*, *12*(9), 218–224.

Mohamed, Y., Reda, W. W., Abdel-Moein, K., Abd El-Razik, K. A., Barakat, A. M., & Hegazi, A. G. (2016). Prevalence and phylogenetic characterization of *Listeria monocytogenes* isolated from processed meat marketed in Egypt. *Journal of Genetic Engineering and Biotechnology*, *14*(1), 119–123.

Mohamed-Yousif, I. M., Abdul-Aziz, S., Jalila, A., Khairani-Bejo, S., Puan, C. L., Bitrus, A. A., ... Awad, E. A. (2014). *Occurrence of Campylobacter in wild bird, and chickens and ducks in selected Malaysian farms*. Universiti Putra Malaysia.

Mohamed-Yousif, I. M., Jalila, A., Abdul-Aziz, S., Zakaria, Z., Rashid Khan, A., & Awad, E. A. (2019). Occurrence of antibiotic resistant *C. jejuni* and *E. coli* in wild birds, chickens, environment and humans from Orang Asli Villages in Sungai Siput, Perak, Malaysia. *American Journal of Animal and Veterinary Sciences*, *14*(3), 158–169. Available from https://doi.org/10.3844/ajavsp.2019.158.169.

Mohammed, A. M., Shigidy, M. T., & Al juboori, A. Y. (2013). Sero-prevalence and epidemiology of brucellosis in camels, sheep and goats in Abu Dhabi Emirate. *International Journal of Animal and Veterinary Advances*, *5*(2), 82–86.

Mohammed, S. J. (2018). Quality and quantity microbial assessment of the mobile restaurants (caravans) in Baghdad. *Journal of Pharmaceutical Sciences and Research*, *10*(9), 2354–2355.

Momani, A. 1 W., Janakat, S., & Khatatbeh, M. (2018). Bacterial contamination of table eggs sold in Jordanian markets. *Pakistan Journal of Nutrition*, *17*(1), 15–20.

Moreno, E., Cloeckaert, A., & Moriyón, I. (2002). *Brucella* evolution and taxonomy. *Veterinary Microbiology*, *90*(1–4), 209–227.

Moslemi, E., Soltandalal, M. M., Beheshtizadeh, M. R., Taghavi, A., Kheiri Manjili, H., Mahmoudi Lamouki, R., & Izadi, A. (2018). Detection of *Brucella* spp. in dairy products by real-time PCR. *Archives of Clinical Infectious Diseases*, *13*(1), e12673.

Motlak, A. (2016). *Campylobacter jejuni* carriage of broiler carcasses at slaughter-house as "an important parameter of food hygiene". *Kufa Journal for Veterinary Medical Sciences*, *7*(2), 48–55.

Moujaber, E., Grace., Osman, M., Rafei, R., Dabboussi, F., & Hamze, M. (2017). Molecular mechanisms and epidemiology of resistance in *Streptococcus pneumoniae* in the Middle East region. *Journal of Medical Microbiology*, *66*(7), 847–858.

Moumita, S., Das, B., Patnaik, A., Balasubramanian, P., & Jayabalan, R. (2019). *Genomics and proteomics features of* Listeria monocytogenes food molecular microbiology (pp. 124–139). CRC Press.

Musallam, I., Abo-Shehada, M., Hegazy, Y., Holt, H., & Guitian, F. (2016). Systematic review of brucellosis in the Middle East: Disease frequency in ruminants and humans and risk factors for human infection. *Epidemiology & Infection, 144*(4), 671–685.

Nasser, L. A. (2008). Mycoflora, mycotoxins, bacteriological analysis and molecular assay of some bacterial species from coffee beans in Saudi Arabia. *Bulletin of Pharmaceutical Sciences. Assiut, 31*(2), 345–373.

Neta, A. V. C., Mol, J. P., Xavier, M. N., Paixão, T. A., Lage, A. P., & Santos, R. L. (2010). Pathogenesis of bovine brucellosis. *The Veterinary Journal, 184*(2), 146–155.

Neves, M., Malkawi, I., Walker, M., Alaboudi, A., Abu-Basha, E., Blake, D., & Crotta, M. (2019). The transmission dynamics of *Campylobacter jejuni* among broilers in semi-commercial farms in Jordan. *Epidemiology & Infection, 147*, e134.

Nguyen, T. K., Bui, H. T., Truong, T. A., Lam, D. N., Ikeuchi, S., Ly, L. K. T., & Hayashidani, H. (2021). Retail fresh vegetables as a potential source of *Salmonella* infection in the Mekong Delta, Vietnam. *International Journal of Food Microbiology, 341*, 109049.

Nimri, L., AL-Dahab, F. A., & Batchoun, R. (2014). Foodborne bacterial pathogens recovered from contaminated shawarma meat in northern Jordan. *Journal of Infection in Developing Countries, 8*(11), 1407–1414.

Obaidat, M. M., & Bani Salman, A. E. (2017). Antimicrobial resistance percentages of *Salmonella* and *Shigella* in seafood imported to Jordan: Higher percentages and more diverse profiles in *Shigella*. *Journal of Food Protection, 80*(3), 414–419.

Omar, S. S., Dababneh, B. F., Qatatsheh, A., Abu-Romman, S., Hawari, A. D., & Aladaileh, S. (2011). The incidence of *Listeria* species and other indicator bacteria in some traditional foods sold in Karak city, Jordan. *Journal of Food, Agriculture and Environment, 9*(2), 79–81.

Osaili, T. M., Alaboudi, A. R., & Al-Akhras, R. R. (2012). Prevalence and antimicrobial susceptibility of *Campylobacter* spp. in live and dressed chicken in Jordan. *Foodborne Pathogens and Disease, 9*(1), 54–58.

Osaili, T. M., Alaboudi, A. R., & Nesiar, E. A. (2011). Prevalence of *Listeria* spp. and antibiotic susceptibility of *Listeria monocytogenes* isolated from raw chicken and ready-to-eat chicken products in Jordan. *Food Control, 22*(3–4), 586–590.

Osaili, T. M., Al-Nabulsi, A. A., Shaker, R. R., Jaradat, Z. W., Taha, M., Al-Kherasha, M., & Holley, R. (2014). Prevalence of *Salmonella* serovars, *Listeria monocytogenes*, and *Escherichia coli* O157: H7 in Mediterranean ready-to-eat meat products in Jordan. *Journal of Food Protection, 77*(1), 106–111.

Osaili, T. M., Al-Nabulsi, A. A., Taha, M. H., Al-Holy, M. A., Alaboudi, A. R., Al-Rousan, W. M., & Shaker, R. R. (2012). Occurrence and antimicrobial susceptibility of *Listeria monocytogenes* isolated from brined white cheese in Jordan. *Journal of Food Science, 77*(9), M528–M532.

Osman, K. M., Kappell, A. D., Fox, E. M., Orabi, A., & Samir, A. (2020). Prevalence, pathogenicity, virulence, antibiotic resistance, and phylogenetic analysis of biofilm-producing *Listeria monocytogenes* isolated from different ecological niches in Egypt: Food, humans, animals, and environment. *Pathogens, 9*(1), 5.

Pan, Y., Zhang, Y., Cheng, J.-H., & Sun, D.-W. (2020). Inactivation of *Listeria monocytogenes* at various growth temperatures by ultrasound pretreatment and cold plasma. *LWT, 118*, 108635.

Pande, V. V., Gole, V. C., McWhorter, A. R., Abraham, S., & Chousalkar, K. K. (2015). Antimicrobial resistance of non-typhoidal *Salmonella* isolates from egg layer flocks and egg shells. *International Journal of Food Microbiology*, *203*, 23–26.

Pereira, C. R., Cotrim de Almeida, J. V. F., Cardoso de Oliveira, I. R., Faria de Oliveira, L., Pereira, L. J., Zangerônimo, M. G., & Dorneles, E. M. S. (2020). Occupational exposure to Brucella spp.: A systematic review and meta-analysis. *PLoS Neglected Tropical Diseases*, *14*(5), e0008164.

Pielsticker, C., Glünder, G., & Rautenschlein, S. (2012). Colonization properties of *Campylobacter jejuni* in chickens. *European Journal of Microbiology and Immunology*, *2* (1), 61–65.

Rafei, R., Hawli, M., Osman, M., Dabboussi, F., & Hamze, M. (2020). Distribution of emm types and macrolide resistance determinants among group A streptococci in the Middle East and North Africa. *Journal of Global Anticmicrobial Resistance*, *22*, 334–348.

Ramadan, F., Unni, A., Hablas, R., & Rizk, M. (1992). *Salmonella*-induced enteritis. Clinical, serotypes and treatment. *The Journal of the Egyptian Public Health Association*, *67*(3–4), 357–367.

Ranjbar, R., Giammanco, G. M., Farshad, S., Owlia, P., Aleo, A., & Mammina, C. (2011). Serotypes, antibiotic resistance, and class 1 integrons in *Salmonella* isolates from pediatric cases of enteritis in Tehran, Iran. *Foodborne Pathogens and Disease*, *8*(4), 547–553.

Reda, W. W., Abdel-Moein, K., Hegazi, A., Mohamed, Y., & Abdel-Razik, K. (2016). *Listeria monocytogenes*: An emerging food-borne pathogen and its public health implications. *Journal of Infection in Developing Countries*, *10*(02), 149–154.

Redfern, J., & Verran, J. (2017). Effect of humidity and temperature on the survival of *Listeria monocytogenes* on surfaces. *Letters in Applied Microbiology*, *64*(4), 276–282.

Ren, J., Hou, H., Zhao, W., Wang, J., & Peng, Q. (2020). Administration of exogenous progesterone protects against *Brucella abortus* infection-induced inflammation in pregnant mice. *The Journal of Infectious Diseases*. Available from https://doi.org/10.1093/infdis/jiaa722.

Rezaei, M., Kazemi Pour, N., Vandyousefi, J., Rokhbakhsh Zamin, F., & Irajian, G. (2018). Distribution and characterization of dominant serovars of *Listeria monocytogenes* strains isolated from spontaneous human abortion in Tehran. *International Journal of Medical Laboratory*, *5*(4), 294–302.

Samaha, H., Al-Rowaily, M., Khoudair, R. M., & Ashour, H. M. (2009). Multicenter study of brucellosis in Egypt. *Emerging Infectious Diseases*, *14*(12), 1916–1968. Available from https://doi.org/10.3201/eid1412.071452.

Schlech, W. F., III, & Acheson, D. (2000). Foodborne listeriosis. *Clinical Infectious Diseases*, *31*(3), 770–775.

Sodagari, H. R., Habib, I., Shahabi, M. P., Dybing, N. A., Wang, P., & Bruce, M. (2020). A review of the public health challenges of *Salmonella* and turtles. *Veterinary Sciences*, *7*(2), 56.

Sonnevend, A., Rotimi, V. O., Kolodziejek, J., Usmani, A., Nowotny, N., & Pál, T. (2006). High level of ciprofloxacin resistance and its molecular background among *Campylobacter jejuni* strains isolated in the United Arab Emirates. *Journal of Medical Microbiology*, *55*(11), 1533–1538.

Street, D. (2015). Prevalence of virulence genes and antimicrobial resistance patterns of *Campylobacter* species isolated from chicken in Egypt. *Asian Journal of Poultry Science*, *9* (4), 250–261.

Taha, R., Alghalibi, S., & Saleh, M. (2013). *Salmonella* spp. in patients suffering from enteric fever and food poisoning in Thamar city, Yemen. *EMHJ-Eastern Mediterranean Health Journal*, *19*(1), 88–93.

Tahoun, A. B., Abou Elez, R. M., Abdelfatah, E. N., Elsohaby, I., El-Gedawy, A. A., & Elmoslemany, A. M. (2017). *Listeria monocytogenes* in raw milk, milking equipment and dairy workers: Molecular characterization and antimicrobial resistance patterns. *Journal of Global Antimicrobial Resistance, 10*, 264–270.

Talei, B. A. A. A. B. (2010). Isolation, identification and biotyping of *Brucella* spp. from milk product at Basrah province. *Basrah Journal of Veterinary Research, 9*(1), 152–162.

Tarabees, R., Elsayed, M. S., Shawish, R., Basiouni, S., & Shehata, A. A. (2017). Isolation and characterization of *Salmonella enteritidis* and *Salmonella typhimurium* from chicken meat in Egypt. *Journal of Infection in Developing Countries, 11*(04), 314–319.

Turgay, O., & Ahmed, C. (2016). The prevalence of brucellosis in goat and sheep milk samples in Duhok district. *The Indian Veterinary Journal, 14*, 3–14.

Turner, L. H., Kinder, J. M., Wilburn, A., D'Mello, R. J., Braunlin, M. R., Jiang, T. T., & Way, S. S. (2017). Preconceptual Zika virus asymptomatic infection protects against secondary prenatal infection. *PLoS Pathogens, 13*(11), e1006684.

Wareth, G., Melzer, F., Elschner, M. C., Neubauer, H., & Roesler, U. (2014). Detection of Brucella melitensis in bovine milk and milk products from apparently healthy animals in Egypt by real-time PCR. *Journal of Infection in Developing Countries, 8*(10), 1339–1343.

Wasfy, M. O., Oyofo, B. A., David, J. C., Ismail, T. F., El-Gendy, A. M., Mohran, Z. S., & Peruski, L. F., Jr (2000). Isolation and antibiotic susceptibility of *Salmonella, Shigella*, and *Campylobacter* from acute enteric infections in Egypt. *Journal of Health, Population, and Nutrition, 18*(1), 33–38.

Wernery, U. (2014). Zoonoses in the Arabian Peninsula. *Saudi Medical Journal, 35*(12), 1455.

WHO. (2013a). *Global tuberculosis report 2013*. World Health Organization.

WHO. (2013b). Integrated disease surveillance and response. In *AFENET pre-conference workshop, Addis Ababa-Ethiopia*. Available from https://www.msh.org/resources/integrated-disease-surveillance-and-response-afenet-2013-workshop-report

WHO. (2015). *WHO estimates of the global burden of foodborne diseases: Foodborne disease burden epidemiology reference group 2007–2015*. World Health Organization.

WHO. (2018). *Salmonella* (non-typhoidal). Available from https://www.who.int/en/news-room/fact-sheets/detail/salmonella-(non-typhoidal) Accessed January 5, 2021.

Xavier, M. N., Paixao, T. A., den Hartigh, A. B., Tsolis, R. M., & Santos, R. L. (2010). Pathogenesis of Brucella spp. *The Open Veterinary Science Journal, 4*(1), 109–118.

Yehia, H. M., & Al-Dagal, M. M. (2014). Prevalence of *Campylobacter jejuni* in chicken produced by major poultry companies in Saudi Arabia. *International Journal of Food Contamination, 1*(1), 2.

Yehia, H. M., Ibraheim, S. M., & Hassanein, W. A. (2016). Prevalence of *Listeria* species in some foods and their rapid identification. *Tropical Journal of Pharmaceutical Research, 15* (5), 1047–1052.

Zhu, Y., Lai, H., Zou, L., Yin, S., Wang, C., Han, X., & Zhou, K. (2017). Antimicrobial resistance and resistance genes in *Salmonella* strains isolated from broiler chickens along the slaughtering process in China. *International Journal of Food Microbiology, 259*, 43–51.

Chapter 4

Foodborne intoxications and toxicoinfections in the Middle East

Wageh Sobhy Darwish[1], Waleed Rizk El-Ghareeb[2], Abdullah F. Alsayeqh[3] and Alaa Eldin M.A. Morshdy[1]
[1]Food Control Department, Faculty of Veterinary Medicine, Zagazig University, Zagazig, Egypt, [2]Department of Public Health, College of Veterinary Medicine, King Faisal University, Al-Ahsa, Saudi Arabia, [3]Veterinary Medicine, College of Agriculture and Veterinary Medicine, Qassim University, Buraidah, Saudi Arabia

4.1 Staphylococcal foodborne intoxication

Staphylococcal food poisoning (SFP) is one of the most common foodborne diseases and results from the ingestion of staphylococcal enterotoxins (SEs) preformed in food by enterotoxigenic strains of *Staphylococcus* spp., particularly *S. aureus* (Hennekinne, De Buyser, & Dragacci, 2012).

4.1.1 General characteristics

Staphylococci are widespread microorganisms, they occur in a wide variety of mammals and birds, as well as on most surfaces. *S. aureus* is a commensal and opportunistic pathogen, and humans are considered the main source associated with SFP (Le Loir, Baron, & Gautier, 2003). *S. aureus* are Gram-positive cocci, non-motile, non-capsular, non-sporulating microbe. Cell division occurs in more than one level, so that cells form irregular clumps resembling bunches of grapes (Staphyo in Greek = grape). *S. aureus* are facultative anaerobes, but grow rapidly under aerobic conditions. They are coagulase, thermonuclease, and haemolysin positive, grow at low a_w and high NaCl content of about 15%. *S. aureus* species are present in the nose, throat, hair and skin of healthy individuals. They are abundant in cuts, browses and abscesses. In addition, they can be transmitted via clothes, utensils and equipment (Scott & Bloomfield, 1990). Waste water, sewage, soil and dust are among the possible sources for the transmission of the

Food Safety in the Middle East. DOI: https://doi.org/10.1016/B978-0-12-822417-5.00001-5

bacterium or its related toxins (Darwish et al., 2018). *S. aureus* can survive in the presence of high concentrations of salt and sugar, and grows best multiplying rapidly between 7°C and 48.5°C with an optimum temperature of 30°C–37°C (Chaibenjawong & Foster, 2011). Some strains of *Staphylococcus* (coagulase and thermostable nuclease positive *S. aureus*) are capable of producing highly heat stable toxin. Normal cooking temperatures will not destroy the toxin produced by this bacterium. *S. aureus* produces seven different protein exotoxins designated as A, B, C1, C2, C3, D and E. Several foodstuffs, including: Milk and dairy products, meat and meat products, poultry and egg, potato, tuna and chicken salad, cream and food with mayonnaise, macaroni and bakery products have been implicated in *S. aureus* food poisoning (Al-Nabulsi et al., 2020; Darwish et al., 2018) (Fig. 4.1).

4.1.2 Pathogenicity and symptoms

The mechanisms of the intoxication by SEs are not clearly known. However, it is assumed that SEs directly affect intestinal epithelium and vagus nerve and that lead to stimulation of the emetic center (Kadariya, Smith, & Thapaliya, 2014). The incubation period of *S. aureus* foodborne intoxication is 2–4 h with a range 30 min to 8 h. The symptoms appear rapidly, in many

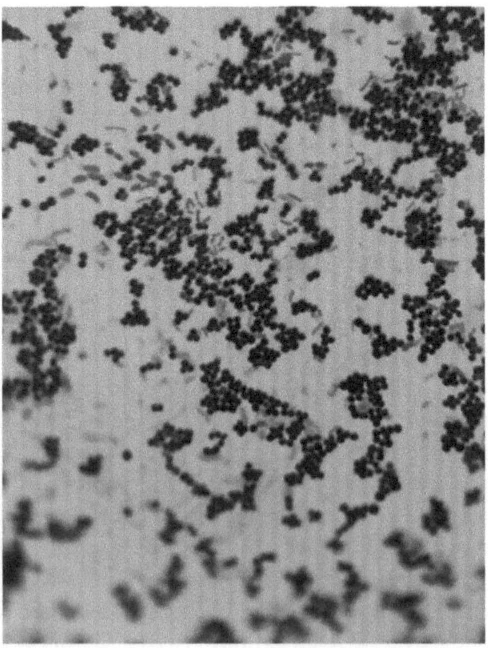

FIGURE 4.1 *Staphylococcus aureus.*

cases they are acute and that depends on susceptibility of the individual to the staphylococcus toxins, the amount of the contaminated food eaten, amount of toxin in food and the general health (immune system) condition of the patient. The most frequent symptoms are nausea, vomiting, abdominal cramps and prostration, weakness and chills. In severe cases headache, muscle cramping, and transient changes in pulse and blood pressure. However, complete recovery may take 2 days or longer in severe cases (Le Loir et al., 2003). Enterotoxins of *S. aureus* are the most probable causes of communal food poisoning, as a toxic dose of less than 1.0 μg in contaminated food, is sufficient to produce symptoms of staphylococcal intoxication. This toxin level is reached when *S. aureus* populations exceed 100,000 CFU/g (Hennekinne et al., 2012). The complications of the disease are very rare and death due to *S. aureus* is seldom, although such cases have occurred among the elderly, infants and severely debilitated persons.

4.2 Prevalence of *S. aureus* and its enterotoxins in the food in the Middle East

The sources and occurrence of *S. aureus*, and Staphylococcus enterotoxins (SEs) in the Middle-Eastern countries are summarized in Table 4.1.

4.2.1 Egypt

Several studies were conducted in Egypt to screen the incidence of *Staphylococcal* spp. in different food matrices retailed in Egypt. Zeinhom, Abdel-Latef, and Jordan (2015) reported that 12% of milk, 12% cheese, and 17% of hand swab samples from milk and cheese handlers in Beni-Suef province were positive for coagulase positive *S. aureus*. Out of the identified isolates 25%, 33%, and 31%, respectively, contained the genes for *Staphylococcus* enterotoxin type B (SEB). Al-Ashmawy, Sallam, Abd-Elghany, Elhadidy, and Tamura (2016) investigated the prevalence of methicillin-resistant *Staphylococcus aureus* (MRSA) and their toxin-producing genes in dairy products sold in Mansoura city. MRSA was detected in 75%, 65%, 40%, 50%, and 35% in raw milk, Damietta cheese, Kareish cheese, ice cream, and yogurt samples, respectively. Interestingly, genes encoding α-hemolysin and SE types A, B, and C (SEA, SEB, and SEC) were detected in all isolates. Production of SE was dependent on the initial *S. aureus* counts and the optimal temperatures for SEA production ranged between 36°C and 48°C (Sabike, Fujikawa, Sakha, & Edris, 2014). Furthermore, Shawish and Al-Humam (2016) studied the prevalence rates of *S. aureus* in retailed meat products in Egypt. The results revealed that the presence rates of *S. aureus* in minced meat, beef burger, beef sausage, beef kofta, and beef luncheon were 38%, 22%, 30%, 32%, and 12%, respectively. Similarly, the rate (%) of the enterotoxigenic *S. aureus* present in the

TABLE 4.1 Prevalence of *S. aureus* and its toxins in the foods in the Middle East.

Country	Food matrix or samples' source	Staph. or toxin type	References
Egypt	Milk, cheese, milk and cheese handlers' hand swabs	SEB	Zeinhom et al. (2015)
	Raw milk, Damietta cheese, Kareish cheese, ice cream, and yogurt	MRSA, SEA, SEB, and SEC	Al-Ashmawy et al. (2016)
	Chicken meat products, food handlers	SEA, SED	El Bayomi et al. (2016)
	Minced meat, beef burger, beef sausage, beef kofta, and beef luncheon	SEs	Shawish and Al-Humam (2016)
	Chicken giblets, washing waste water	MRSA, SEA, SEB, SEC, SED	Darwish et al. (2018)
	Fish	SEA, SEB, SED	Hussein et al. (2019)
	Meat products	MRSA	Morshdy et al. (2019)
	Chicken livers	MRSA, SEB	Abolghait et al. (2020)
Kuwait	Restaurant works	SEA, SEB, SEC, SED	Al-Bustan et al. (1996)
	Restaurant works	SEA, SEB, SEC	Udo et al. (1999)
Saudi Arabia	Meat, egg, milk, and dairy products	*S. aureus*	Haque et al. (1987)
	Food poisoning patients	*S. aureus*	Kurdi et al. (1998)
	Camel milk	SEs	Yehia et al. (2019)
	Camel meat	MRSA	El-Ghareeb et al. (2019)
Jordan	Shawarma meat	*S. aureus*	Nimri et al. (2014)
	Imported fish	SEA, SHE, SEI	Obaidat et al. (2015)

(Continued)

TABLE 4.1 (Continued)

Country	Food matrix or samples' source	Staph. or toxin type	References
	Bulk milk	MRSA	Obaidat et al. (2018)
Lebanon	workers in a pastry factory	*S. aureus*	Hamzé et al. (2008)
	Kishk, shanklish, and baladi cheese	*S. aureus*	Zouhairi et al. (2012)
	Food handlers	MRSA	Osman et al. (2019)
	Fish	*S. aureus*	Jisr et al. (2020)
	Red meat, poultry, and dairies	*S. aureus*	Kharroubi et al. (2020)
Occupied Palestinian Territory	Cooked and raw foods	*S. aureus*	Al-Khatib et al. (2004)
	Dairy products	*S. aureus*	Al-Khatib and Al-Mitwalli (2009)
Iraq	Lamb carcasses and refrigerated ground lamb	*S. aureus*	Ali et al. (1982)
	Milk samples	SEC, SED	Abbar et al. (1986)

MRSA, Methicillin-resistant *Staphylococcus aureus*; *SE*, staphylococcal enterotoxin; *SEA*, *Staphylococcus* enterotoxin type A; *SEB*, *Staphylococcus* enterotoxin type B; *SEC*, *Staphylococcus* enterotoxin type C; *SED*, *Staphylococcus* enterotoxin type D.

examined minced meat, beef burger, beef sausage, beef kofta, and beef luncheon was 16%, 8%, 8%, 6%, and 2%, respectively. Besides, Morshdy, Darwish, Salah El-Dien, and Khalifa (2019) isolated multidrug-resistant *S. aureus* from retailed meat products in Zagazig city, Sharkia Governorate.

Fish might serve as potential reservoirs for enterotoxigenic *S. aureus*. Hussein et al. (2019) reported that the prevalence rates of *S. aureus* enterotoxin genes in fish ranged from 4% to 36% and *S. aureus* count ranged from 2 to 4 $\log_{10}$ CFU/g. The enterotoxins SED, SEA, and SEB genes in *S. aureus* isolates were detected with 40%, 26.6%, and 20%, respectively. Chicken meat products may also present other potential sources of enterotoxigenic *S.*

aureus. For instances, El Bayomi et al. (2016) recorded that 37.5% of chicken product samples were positive for *S. aureus*, whereas hand swabs taken from meat handlers revealed that 18 (60%) were positive. Additionally, 10.4% were positive for each of the SEA and SED genes. Moreover, Darwish et al. (2018) demonstrated that chicken giblets are potential sources for the transmission of MRSA and the heat-resistant SEs to people. SEA had the highest frequency among SEs in MRSA isolates. In addition, Abolghait, Fathi, Youssef, and Algammal (2020) isolated MRSA strains from broiler chicken livers. The isolates initiated SEB production in experimentally contaminated chicken livers within 24 h of storage at temperatures over 8°C. SEB was maximally produced at 24°C with MRSA counts of $7.3 \times 103 \pm 1.2 \times 10^3$ CFU/g sample homogenate.

4.2.2 Kuwait

Limited studies were conducted on the prevalence of *S. aureus* and their toxins in foods in Kuwait. Al-Bustan, Udo, and Chugh (1996) screened the nasal carriage of *S. aureus* among 500 restaurant workers in Kuwait city. About 27% of them carried *S. aureus* and 86.6% of the *S. aureus* produced SEs. Twenty-eight percent produced SEA, 28.5% produced SEB, 16.4% produced SEC, and 3.5% produced SED. Furthermore, the same group of researchers isolated Coagulase negative *S. aureus* from the restaurant workers in Kuwait city, and SEA, SEB, and /or SEC were produced by 6% of the isolates (Udo, Al-Bustan, Jacob, & Chugh, 1999).

4.2.3 Saudi Arabia

In Saudi Arabia, Haque et al. (1987) reported that *S. aureus* was implicated in 59.6% of the food poisoning cases among children admitted to children hospital in Riyadh City (capital of Saudi Arabia). The major food items consumed by children were meat, egg, milk, and dairy products. Kurdi, Kamball, Muhammad, and al-Zahrani (1998) reported that *S. aureus* was also responsible for 41% of food poisoning cases reported to the Ministry of Health, Riyadh, KSA, during the period 1990–1992. Hassan, Altalhi, Gherbawy, and El-Deeb (2011) isolated *S. aureus* from raw vegetables distributed in Saudi markets at 11.8%. Limited studies were conducted in Saudi Arabia to investigate the prevalence, the risk factors, and genetic distribution of MRSA isolated from healthy and clinical human and animal cases. Yehia, Ismail, Hassan, Al-Masoud, and Al-Dagal (2019) reported abnormal heat resistant and enterotoxin-producing strain of *S. aureus* isolated from camel milk sold in Riyadh City. Furthermore, El-Ghareeb, Almathen, Fayez, and Alsultan (2019) recovered 20 *S. aureus*-positive isolates out of 187 camel meat samples (10.7% prevalence). Three were resistant to methicillin (1.6% prevalence), 35% of *S. aureus* isolates were resistant to β-lactam antibiotic. MRSA isolates were resistant to all antimicrobials tested, and 15% of the tested *S. aureus* strains were methicillin resistant. Besides, Yehia, Al-Masoud, Alarjani, and Alamri (2020) reported that pasteurized camel milk samples collected from retail markets in Saudi Arabia were contaminated with *S. aureus* at 10%; of these 20% were showed methicillin heat resistance.

4.2.4 Jordan

Al-Natour, Alaboudi, Al-Hatamelh, and Osaili (2012) observed that enterotoxigenic *S. aureus* can grow on the egg shell in feces, and *E. coli* O157:H7 facilitates the penetration of *S. aureus* into table eggs. *S. aureus* was also isolated at 8% from shawarma meat sandwiches served to public in Northern Jordan (Nimri, Abu Al-Dahab, & Batchoun, 2014). Furthermore, Obaidat, Salman, and Lafi (2015) isolated enterotoxigenic strains of *S. aureus* from imported fresh fish samples collected in Jordan. Most isolates carried SEA, SEG, and SEI genes. Besides, Obaidat, Bani Salman, and Roess (2018) determined the prevalence of MRSA in the bulk milk tanks collected from cattle, sheep, and goat dairy farms in Jordan. MRSA was detected in 31.8% of cattle, 29.8% of sheep, and 11.5% of goat dairy farms. Al-Nabulsi et al. (2020) studied the factors affecting the viability of *S. aureus* and enterotoxin production in white-brined cheese in Jordan. They isolated enterotoxin producing *S. aureus* from unsalted Ultra heat-treated (UHT) milk; while salt prevented the enterotoxin production. They also concluded that the use of starter cultures, salt at 15%, and low storage temperature at 10°C reduced the growth of *S. aureus*, and salt may have prevented enterotoxin production in white-brined cheese.

4.2.5 Lebanon

Hamzé, Naja, and Mallat (2008) found that 39% of the workers in a pastry factory in North Lebanon had nasal carriage of *S. aureus* in a study conducted in 2004. Furthermore, Osman et al. (2019) found a high prevalence (23.8%) of the nasal carriage of the MRSA among the food handlers in Tripoli (Northern Lebanon province). Zouhairi et al. (2012) isolated multidrug resistant *S. aureus* from three Lebanese dairy-based food products that are sometimes consumed raw, namely, "Kishk," "Shanklish," and "Baladi" (artisanal types) cheeses. Jisr et al. (2020) mentioned that *S. aureus* counts (1.75–1.87 $\log_{10}$ cfu/g) in the edible tissues of commonly consumed fish collected from the marine area of Tripoli were within the recommended threshold values ($>2 \log_{10}$ cfu/g). Furthermore, Kharroubi, Nasser, El-Harakeh, Sulaiman, and Kassem (2020) in a recent study reported that *S. aureus* was the causative agent for 12.8% of foods (rejected as being found unsafe) in Lebanon including: Red meat, poultry, and dairies.

4.2.6 Palestine

Al-Khatib et al. (2004) reported that 93.6% of cooked and raw foods collected from restaurants and sweet shops in the Ramallah and al-Bireh district within the Palestinian and international standards of *S. aureus*. Furthermore, Al-Khatib and Al-Mitwalli (2009) revealed that 1% of dairy products in Ramallah and Al-Bireh district, Palestine, was unacceptable because of contamination with *S. aureus*.

4.2.7 Iraq

Ali, Hoshyare, and Al-Delaimy (1982) revealed that *S. aureus* counts on the surfaces of the lamb carcasses and in the refrigerated ground lamb collected from various retail shops in Baghdad (capital of Iraq) ranged between 10^3 and 10^4 CFU/cm^2 or g. Besides, Abbar, Mohammed, and Arslain (1986) reported that five *S. aureus* strains that were isolated from milk samples in Iraq, produced SEC, and two strains produced SED genes.

4.2.8 Control measures of prevention of *S. aureus*

The effective means for the prevention and control of *S. aureus* in milk is pasteurization (71°C/15 s) before its cold storage at 4°C, as thermal treatment is very important process that will eliminate staphylococci bacteria, before toxin production. Proper sanitation of the food environments and proper personal hygiene of food handlers particularly hand washing before working with food or after touching any part of the body (nose, hair, mouth, skin, etc.) are effective means to minimize the risk of food poisoning by SEs. Food handlers with skin or respiratory diseases should be avoided from handling foods. Proper selection of raw material and ingredients is also effective means of decreasing the risk of *S. aureus*. Using chemical preservatives such as citric acid 0.4%–0.8% in a combination with proper refrigeration can inhibit the growth of *S. aureus* (Osaili et al., 2015). The use of starter culture in the cheese preparation, salt (15%), or preservation at low temperature (<10°C) will reduce the growth of *S. aureus* and prevent enterotoxin production (Al-Nabulsi et al., 2020). The application of Hazard Analysis Critical Control Point (HACCP) and good manufacturing practices (GMP) practices during food processing is highly encouraged.

4.3 Botulism

4.3.1 General characteristics

It is the disease caused by the ingestion of foods containing a potent neuroparalytic exotoxin produced by certain strains of *C. botulinum*. This disease was first reported in 1820 in Germany after hundreds of human cases suffered poisoning due to sausage consumption. The word botulinum is named after the Latin word for sausage, *botulus* (El-Bahnasawy, Aly, Abdel-Fattah, & Morsy, 2014). *C. botulinum* species are Gram-positive anaerobic spore-forming rod-shaped bacteria. There are seven serologically identified toxin-producing types of *C. botulinum*, namely A, B, C, D, E, F, and G. These types are species specific. For instance, types A, B, E, F, and G are responsible for the human botulism. However, types C and D cause the disease in the animals and birds. *C. botulinum* types A and B are indigenous to soils and manure as reported in several studies worldwide (Rasetti-Escargueil, Lemichez, & Popoff, 2019). *C. botulinum* type E is more confined to marine water environment and known as an aquatic organism as reported in studies from Japan, Finland, Russia, and the United States. Type F spores were isolated from a home-made liver paste, venison jerky in California, and from salmon caught in a Colombian river. Type G strain was isolated mainly from soil samples in Argentina. This type is not highly incriminated in food-poisoning as this type produces less neurotoxin than other types (Hielm, Bjorkroth, & Hyytia, 1998; Huss, 1980; Saito, 1990).

C. botulinum is divided into two categories proteolytic and nonproteolytic types. In general, the growth of both types requires amino acids, vitamins, and minerals. The organism can grow over a wide range of temperatures ranging between 10°C and 50°C for the proteolytic type, and between 3.3°C and 45°C for the nonproteolytic type (Jay, 2000). Proteolytic strains are much heat resistant than nonproteolytic types, with type A the most resistant followed by types F and B, respectively (Baker & Genigeorgis, 1990). The $D_{82.2°C}$ of 0.51 min was reported in crab meat for the vegetative cells (Jay, 2000). In another study, heating to an internal temperature of 80°C for 30 min would destroy the toxin if present (Imai, Oshita, & Hashimoto, 1990). Toxins of *C. botulinum* are heat-labile and can be destroyed by heating at 80°C for 10 min, or boiling for a few minutes. Radiation affects well the endospores of different strains of *C. botulinum* with D values of 1.1–2.5 kGy (Lambert, Smith, & Dodds, 1991). It is suggested that growth and toxin production of *C. botulinum* is favored in foods such as tomato juice of pH 4.8. However, in food matrices including whole shrimp and tomato paste acidified with acetic and citric acids (pH 4.2 and 4.6, respectively), either no growth, or no production of toxins were observed for *C. botulinum* E incubated in shrimp and tomato paste at 26°C for 6 weeks. Both proteolytic and nonproteolytic types showed similarity in their pH requirements (Dodds, 1994). Water activity (a_w) drastically affects the growth and toxin production of *C. botulinum*. Types A and B can grow well at a water activity (a_w) value of 0.94. It was previously reported that 10% salt and 50% glucose inhibit *C. botulinum* toxin production in smoked fish (Sperber, 1983). *C. botulinum* growth and toxin production are favored in the absence of other pathogens and that is easily achieved by heat treatment of foods. While the growth of *C. botulinum* is antagonized in the presence of other microorganisms such as lactic acid bacteria. In addition, the growth of *C. botulinum* A was inhibited in the presence of other bacteria such as *C. perfringens*, and *B. cereus* (Jay, 2000).

4.3.2 Pathogenicity and symptoms

C. botulinum forms neurotoxin within the organism and released upon autolysis. Botulinal toxins are the most toxic substances known. The human lethal dose is about 1 ng/kg body weight. Type A is more toxic than other types. Symptoms of botulism are produced orally or parenterally. The toxins are not completely activated by the gastric enzymes and acid, and might be protected by the other nontoxic substances attached. The toxin is then released into the blood stream, and it passes into the peripheral nervous system (Jay, 2000). The induction of the toxin activities first requires attachment to the ganglioside receptors, then blocks the release of acetyl and choline from the cholinergic nerve endings (Wieckowski, Kokai-Kun, & McClane, 1998).

Botulism occurs in humans due to the ingestion of already performed exotoxins in the food. Absorption of the toxin from the oral mucosa posttasting of foods was also recorded. All ages are susceptible to the disease. Development of symptoms after the ingestion of the spores is unknown in the adults. However, it was reported in infants less than 1 year old (Cagan, Peker, Dogan, & Caksen, 2010). The incubation period for the development of botulism symptoms ranged between 12 and 72 h, postingestion of contaminated foods. This syndrome is characterized by the lack of fever. The symptoms include nausea, constipation, dizziness, fatigue, dried mouth and throat, double vision, paralysis, respiratory failure, and death. The duration of the disease is 1–10 days depending on the dose of the toxin, immunity status, and age. The mortality rate of botulism is considered high (30%–65%). Death usually results from respiratory paralysis causing asphyxia or from secondary bronchopneumonia. Botulinal toxins cause paralysis by blocking the motor nerve terminals at the myoneuronal junction (Jackson, Mahon, Copeland, & Fagan, 2015). Early diagnosis and interference with the specific antisera favor the prognosis. The most important implicated foods are nonacid vegetables such as beans, spinach, asparagus, and corn. Fish, seafood, smoked fish, and verities of meat as ham, sausage, chicken, liver paste, dairies, milk powder are also involved. Botulism comes mainly from the consumption of either home-prepared or home-canned foods that lack hygienic preparation and did not receive enough heat treatment (Scalfaro, Auricchio, De Medici, & Anniballi, 2019). Therefore it is highly recommended to expose any suspected food to boiling temperature for several minutes ($>$10 min), which should be enough to destroy the botulinal toxins.

4.4 Incidence of botulism in the Middle East

In general, there are considerably few reports that have investigated the occurrence of botulism and the characteristics of the pathogen species in the Middle-Eastern countries. Here we would like to demonstrate and discuss the available literature about botulism and *C. botulinum* in these countries as shown in Table 4.2.

TABLE 4.2 Prevalence of botulinal toxins in food matrices in the Middle East.

Country	Food matrix	Organism or toxin type	References
Egypt	Un-eviscerated salted fish (faseikh)	E	Weber et al. (1993)
	Honey, fish products, meat products	*C. botulinum*	Ahmed et al. (2011)
Arabian Gulf countries	Commercially prepared honey	Infant botulism	van der Vorst et al. (2006)

4.4.1 Egypt

The first documented outbreak on *C. botulinum* in Cairo, Egypt, was recorded in 1991, and it was reported to the Ministry of Health in Egypt. In that outbreak, 91 patients were reported to have the symptoms of botulism with 18 (20%) of the patients died. The affected persons had a history of consumption of uneviscerated salted fish (faseikh), a common and popular salted fish in Egypt; this fish product was purchased from the same shop. Isolation of *C. botulinum* E and the type E botulinal toxin from the salted fish samples was confirmed (Weber et al., 1993). Furthermore, Ahmed, Badary, Mohamed, and Elkhawaga (2011) isolated *C. botulinum* at 26% in honey, 19% in fish products, and 21% in meat products were collected from Assiut city, Egypt.

4.4.2 Arabian Gulf countries

Few reports are available about the incidence of botulism in the Arabian Gulf area. For instance, van der Vorst, Jamal, Rotimi, and Moosa (2006) reported the first case of infant botulism (toxicoinfection) in Arabian Gulf states due to the consumption of contaminated commercially prepared honey. The 6-week-old infant had generalized weakness with acute flaccid paralysis and a history of honey consumption. Electromyogram examination revealed a decreased amplitude of compound muscle action potential in all motor nerves.

4.4.3 Control measures of *C. botulinum*

In order to prevent the contamination of canned food products with *C. botulinum*, efficient hygienic precautions should be followed during all steps of processing starting with the handling of the raw materials. Application of the GMP and HACCP principles are highly recommended in the food processing plants and these include the following: (1) Thorough thermal treatment of the canned food; (2) avoid any canned food with an apparent damage or bulged with air; (3) proper refrigeration of foods within 2 h after cooking; (4) boiling of home-processed foods before consumption; (5) proper selection of raw material and ingredients; and (6) sanitation of the food environments.

Continuous monitoring programs and surveillance systems to prompt the notification of the disease-suspected cases to the public health authorities is mandatory in order to prepare the ideal response. Educational and training courses are highly required to increase the awareness of the operators and the population for the disease management (Lami et al., 2019; Osaili et al., 2013).

4.5 *C. perfringens* toxicoinfection

4.5.1 General characteristics

C. perfringens is an anaerobic, Gram-positive, and nonmotile rod-shaped spore-forming organism. The colonies of *C. perfringens* appear as large, regular, round, and shiny colonies on agar plates. Moreover, the colonies of *C. perfringens* form a double zone of hemolysis on blood agar plates. *C. perfringens* is a ubiquitous organism that can grow at a variety of environments such as soil, intestinal tracts of humans and animals, vegetables, and other food matrices (Heredia & Labbé 2001). *C. perfringens* grows between 15°C and 50°C; the optimum temperature for the growth of *C. perfringens* ranges between 37°C and 45°C. *C. perfringens* can tolerate temperatures as low as 6°C (Brynestad & Granum, 2002). Spores of *C. perfringens* can germinate well at 10°C–54°C, or with slow cooling and reheating of contaminated foods (McClane, 2007). The bacterium can tolerate low oxygen up to a redox potential of +200 mV (Juneja, Marmer, & Miller, 1994). *C. perfringens* optimum pH is 6.0–7.0 and can tolerate pH in the range of 5.1–9.7 and a minimum water activity of 0.93 (Li & McClane, 2006).

4.5.2 Pathogenesis and symptoms

There are five types of *C. perfringens* (A, B, C, D, and E) based on the production of four major toxins (alpha, beta, epsilon, and iota toxins) and hydrolytic enzymes, including amylases, collagenase, DNAse, hemolysins, hyaluronidase, and lecithinase (Brynestad & Granum, 2002). A small percentage (1%–5%) of all *C. perfringens* isolates, mostly of type A, possesses an intestinally active enterotoxin (CPE) that is responsible for the characteristic gastrointestinal symptoms of *C. perfringens* type A illness (McClane, 2005). *C. perfringens* type C causes a rare but severe necrotic enteritis (Bates & Bodnaruk, 2003). The pathogenicity of *C. perfringens* type A illness involves the release of CPE into the small intestine, which is followed by a series of events involving: Binding with protein receptor, forming a protein complex that facilitates the insertion of CPE into the intestinal membrane and followed by a several biochemical and conformational changes will alter the permeability of the brush border membranes in the epithelial cells of the small intestine (García & Heredia, 2011; McClane, 1996). The required dose of the organism for toxin production in the small intestine is 10^6/g of food. The incubation period after the ingestion of the contaminated foods varies between 6 and 24 h. The disease symptoms involve watery diarrhea with severe abdominal pain, which disappears within 24 h or less; the vomiting and nausea are rare. The diarrhea flushes the toxin and the sporulating cells outside the body and subsequently lessens the disease. The fatality rate is relatively low at 0.05% (McClane, 2007). In very rare cases, intoxication occurs with preformed toxins in the food, resulting in earlier onset of the symptoms (Bates & Bodnaruk, 2003; McClane, 2007).

4.6 Prevalence of *C. perfringens* and its toxins in foods in the Middle East

There are to date only a limited number of studies that focused on the prevalence and characterization of *C. perfringens* in foods of the Middle East (Table 4.3).

TABLE 4.3 Prevalence of *C. perfringens* in food matrices in the Middle East.

Country	Food matrix	Organism or toxin type	References
Egypt	Dairy products	*C. perfringens*	El-Bassiony (1980)
	fish	*C. perfringens* A, C, E	Sabry et al. (2016)
	Chicken meat	*C. perfringens*	Hamad et al. (2020)
	Chicken carcasses	*C. perfringens* A	Gharieb et al. (2020)
Saudi Arabia	Shawarma	*C. perfringens*	Ayaz et al. (1986)
	Dessert, eggs, rice, and dairy products	*C. perfringens*	Haque et al. (1987)

4.6.1 Egypt

C. perfringens was detected in dairy products sold in markets of Assiut city (Egypt) as early as 1980 (El-Bassiony, 1980). Results revealed that the counts of *C. perfringens* were 76.4/mL, 170/g, 140/g, 42.9/g, 590/g, 2.9/g, 172.9/g, and 109/mL in the examined raw milk, hard and processed Damietta and Kareish (local) cheeses, yogurt, butter, and ice cream samples, respectively. However, El-Dengawy and Nassar (2001) could not isolate *C. perfringens* from the wild quail carcasses. It was also thought that local fish could be considered as a reservoir of *C. perfringens*, as this was isolated from fresh fish collected from aquaculture estuaries at 54.5% and from markets at 71%, respectively (Sabry, Abd El-Moein, Hamza, & Abdel Kader, 2016). Moreover, these authors identified *C. perfringens* A, which is positive former of the enterotoxin (CPE), and also *C. perfringens* types C and E from fresh fish. Besides, Hamad, Abdelmotilib, Darwish, and Zeitoun (2020) isolated *C. perfringens* at 30% from chicken meat collected from Alexandria retail markets and shops, with counts reached 3.71 ± 0.25 Log_{10} CFU/g. Similarly, toxin-producing *C. perfringens* A was isolated from chicken carcasses in Zagazig city (Gharieb et al., 2020).

4.6.2 Saudi Arabia

In Saudi Arabia, *C. perfringens* was isolated from shawarma (a popular ready-to-eat meat product available in the Middle East) collected from various fast-food restaurants in Riyadh city. The counts of *C. perfringens* ranged between < 10 and 10^6 CFU/g (Ayaz et al., 1986). Furthermore, Haque et al. (1987) reported that *C. perfringens* was implicated in 7.83% of the food-poisoning cases among children in Riyadh. The most common food items consumed by children were dessert, eggs, rice, and dairy products.

The lack of *C. perfringens* in foods of the Middle East may not necessarily be due to its nonexistence in the local foods, as also laboratory-based data are rather limited or not well documented in published journals. The anaerobic bacterium is also one of the water quality parameter criterions, and data are also lacking in the area, in general, therefore further studies are needed to monitor its potential presence in foods of the Middle East.

4.6.3 Control measures of *C. perfringens*

Adoption of strict hygienic measures, confirming personal hygiene during preparation, processing, and storage of the food, and avoiding cross-contamination with soil, intestinal tract contents, or excreta are considered among the recommended measures to avoid or halt food contamination with *C. perfringens*. Foods should be rapidly and properly cooled. Chemical preservatives such as organic acid salts as sodium citrate (0.5%–4.0%, Sabah, Juneja, & Fung, 2004), 1% sodium lactate, 1% sodium citrate, and 1% sodium acetate (Juneja & Thippareddi, 2004) decrease the risk of *C. perfringens* in foods. Using spices and essential oils such as thymol, carvacrol, cinnamaldehyde, and oregano is also an effective strategy to control the growth and germination of *C. perfringens* (Juneja, Thippareddi, & Friedman, 2006). The addition of the generally regarded as safe food additives such as mono sodium glutamates, sodium benzoate, and potassium sorbate to the food may alter the cold tolerance of *C. perfringens* (García & Heredia, 2011; Limón, Solis, García, & Heredia, 2007). Furthermore, Hamad et al. (2020) suggested the use of the probiotics strain *Lactobacillus rhamnosus* EMCC 1105 to inhibit the growth of *C. perfringens* in poultry meat. The use of different means of physical and chemical preservation of the food will be of help to introduce different stressors that halt *C. perfringens* growth in foods. The application of the principles of HACCP and GMP practices during the manufacture and processing of food is highly recommended. Furthermore, the adoption of efficient food safety training programs and training courses among food handlers will improve the food safety and microbiological qualities of food (Lami et al., 2019; Osaili et al., 2013). Besides, the enforcement of the management practices and food handler commitment will positively affect the food safety performance in the food manufacturing and processing facilities (Taha, Wilkins, Juusola, & Osaili, 2020).

4.7 *B. cereus* intoxication and toxicoinfection

4.7.1 General characteristics

B. cereus is a rod-shaped aerobic, spore-forming, and Gram-positive bacterium. *B. cereus* forms one endospore per cell. *B. cereus* has the ability to grow at extreme environmental conditions, as the spores are resistant to heat, cold, radiation, and disinfectants (Turnbull, 1996). *B. cereus* is usually isolated from the soil, plants, raw, and processed meat and meat products (Carlin et al., 2010; Ceuppens, Boon, & Uyttendaele, 2013). *B. cereus* spores can germinate and multiply in low acid humidity foods at a wide range of temperatures (4°C–55°C). However, the emetic *B. cereus* strains are unable to produce their toxin in the absence of oxygen or below 10°C (EFSA, 2005). *B. cereus* causes two food poisoning syndromes, namely, emetic and diarrheal syndromes (Stenfors Arnesen, Fagerlund, & Granum, 2008).

4.7.2 Pathogenesis and symptoms

Food poisoning with *B. cereus* occurs after the ingestion of foods contaminated with *B. cereus* (diarrheal type) or their toxins produced in the food (emetic type) if it is kept within the temperature danger zone (10°C–60°C) for several hours allowing *B. cereus* reaching $>10^6$ cells/g. Foods such as cooked meat, processed meat products, vegetables, rice and starchy food, and dairy products are encountered in *B. cereus* foodborne-related illness. The emetic form of *B. cereus* is characterized by a rapid onset as it occurs within 1–5 h postingestion of contaminated foods. Acute attack of nausea and vomiting are the main symptoms with the absence of diarrhea. Due to its rapid onset, and the similarity of the symptoms with *S. aureus* intoxications, emetic *B. cereus* intoxication is presumably underreported. *B. cereus* intoxication occurs due to the ingestion of the preformed heat-stable emetic enterotoxin (cereulide) (EFSA, 2005). The emetic syndrome is usually mild and rarely becomes fatal (Mahler et al., 1997). The emetic form is considered as a type of foodborne intoxication. The second form of *B. cereus*-related illnesses is a slow-onset diarrheal form, which is mainly characterized by severe diarrhea and manifested via the release of a heat-labile diarrheal enterotoxin. The major symptoms after an incubation period of 4–16 h, include watery, nonbloody diarrhea and abdominal pain. The symptoms last for 12–24 h. The diarrheal form is developed through the production of a number of enterotoxins in the intestinal tract (EFSA, 2005). These enterotoxins include hemolysin BL (HBL), non-hemolytic enterotoxin (NHE), and two forms of cytotoxin K (cytK) (cytK-1 and cytK-2) (Moravek et al., 2006). In this form, the number of the bacterium or spore is important and regarded as a type of foodborne illness.

4.8 Prevalence of *B. cereus* and its toxins in foods in the Middle East

There are scanty number of reports concerning the prevalence and characterization of *B. cereus* in the different food matrices in the Middle East (Table 4.4).

4.8.1 Egypt

In Egypt, several studies were conducted to investigate the prevalence of *B. cereus* and to detect the toxin-coding genes among the identified isolates. For instance, Shawish and Tarabees (2017) isolated *B. cereus* from minced meat, burger, sausage, kofta, and luncheon collected from Menofia and Cairo governorates at 22.5%, 30%, 25%, 37.5%, and 15%, respectively. Using PCR, HBL was detected in 18 out of 20 isolates (90%) while cytK enterotoxin-encoding genes detected in all isolates (100%) were have cytK. Besides, El-Aziz, Tartor, El-Aziz Gharib, and Ammar (2018) isolated *B. cereus* at 21.3% from raw meat and meat products with an average count of 6.7 ± 0.75 CFU/g. Furthermore, Osman et al. (2018) recovered 124 *Bacillus* isolates, 27 belonged to *B. cereus* out of 255 poultry and meat samples; the isolation of *B. cereus* was positively associated with the detection of the enterotoxin-coding genes. In addition, Sadek, Abdel-Rahman, Azab, Darwesh, and Hassan (2018) isolated *B. cereus* from 21.2% of milk-based

TABLE 4.4 **Prevalence of *B. cereus* and its related toxins in food matrices in the Middle East.**

Country	Food matrix	Organism or toxin type	References
Egypt	Minced meat, burger, sausage, kofta, and luncheon	*B. cereus, cytK,* HBL	Shawish and Tarabees (2017)
	Raw meat and meat products	*B. cereus*	El-Aziz et al. (2018)
	Poultry and meat	*B. cereus*	Osman et al. (2019)
	Wheat, rice, honey, milk-based fruits, vegetables	*B. cereus, cytK,* HBLA, NHEC	Sadek et al. (2018)
	Cheese	*B. cereus*	Al-Gamal et al. (2019)
	Milk powder and Ras-cheese	*B. cereus, cytK*	Abdeen et al. (2020)
Saudi Arabia	Tehineh	*B. cereus*	Ayaz et al. (1986)
	Rice, meat, and dairy products	*B. cereus*	Haque et al. (1987)
	Cooked rice	*B. cereus*	Al-Joudi (2007)
Jordan	Different food samples	*B. cereus, cytK,* HBLA, HBLC, HBLD, NHEA, NHEB, NHEC	Batchoun et al. (2011)
Oman	Food handlers	*B. cereus*	Al-Abri et al. (2011)

HBL, Hemolysin BL; *HBLA*, hemolysin BLA; *HBLC*, hemolysin BLC; *HBLD*, hemolysin BLD; *NHEA*, nonhemolytic enterotoxin A; *NHEB*, nonhemolytic enterotoxin B; *NHEC*, nonhemolytic enterotoxin C.

fruit, vegetables (15.7%), honey (17.2%), rice (14.1%), and wheat (12%). Among 45 isolates, 43 isolated harbored cytK toxin–coding gene; NHE type C (NHEC) was detected in 32 isolates; and HBL type A (HBLA) was detected in just five isolates. Al-Gamal et al. (2019) isolated *B. cereus* from retailed cheese in Egyptian markets at 3.3%. Similarly *B. cereus* was also recovered from milk powder and Ras-cheese retailed in Egypt at 6.9% and 8.5%, respectively. Furthermore, cytK-coding gene was detected in the positive milk powder and Ras-cheese samples at 55.5% and 83.3%, respectively (Abdeen, Hussien, Hadad, & Mousa, 2020).

4.8.2 Jordan

A limited number of studies focused on the prevalence of *B. cereus* in Jordan. Batchoun, Al-Sha'er, and Khabour (2011) collected 202 food samples from local markets and restaurants in Jordan, and investigated the prevalence rate of *B. cereus* in such samples. They recovered *B. cereus* from 23.3% (47) of the food samples. They further detected HBLA (40.4%), HBLC (36.5%), and HBLD (75%). The NHE types A, B, and C were detected at 61.5%, 92.3%, and 92.3% of the identified *B. cereus* isolates, respectively, while, cytK gene was detected in 53.8% of the isolates.

4.8.3 Saudi Arabia

In Saudi Arabia, Ayaz, Sawaya, and Al-Sogair (1986) screened the microbiological status of tehineh, a product obtained by the milling of dehulled and roasted white sesame seeds, manufactured in Saudi Arabia. *B. cereus* count in tehineh, ranged between <10 and 400 CFU/g. Furthermore, Haque et al. (1987) reported that *B. cereus* was implicated in 13.0% of the food poisoning cases among children in Riyadh. The most common food items consumed by children were cooked rice (a potential *B. cereus* toxin producer, especially if stored within the danger temperature zone and over a long time period or if in cases left over rice is not sufficiently being thermally heated) meat, and dairy products. It must be stated that, especially in Saudi Arabia or in neighboring countries, rice dishes (all forms) are one of the stable foods served in meals, accompanying almost all of the local dishes (e.g., "Kabsah") that are widely consumed in these areas.

In addition, Al-Joudi (2007) investigated an outbreak of foodborne diarrheal illness among soldiers in Mina area during Hajj. He suggested that the cause of this diarrheal illness is the consumption of cooked rice contaminated with *B. cereus* and/or *C. perfringens*.

4.8.4 Oman

In Oman, Al-Abri et al. (2011) investigated a report of foodborne gastroenteritis among 58 patients and their attendants in a referral hospital in Oman. They isolated a toxin-producing *B. cereus* strain from the feces of 3/12 (25%) patients and 19/25 (76%) of food handlers, and 35/61 (57%) of food samples from the hospital's kitchen. They highlighted the need for training of the food handlers and the rigorous enforcement of food hygiene and safety regulations.

4.8.5 Control measures of *B. cereus*

The major control measures to avoid the occurrence of *B. cereus* or its toxins in the various foods and/or food products are basically to control their storage temperature. It must be taken into consideration that the area of the Middle East, mostly the Gulf regions, supports a dry climate with high temperatures throughout the season, especially during the summer season (July-August); therefore it is absolutely necessary to maintain low-temperature storage, apply efficient hygienic measures, and implement sufficient control during handling of both raw or processed foods and food products during preparation and subsequent storage. Cooked foods should be consumed as soon as possible, and if it is necessary to be preserved, these should be stored below 4°C, or kept hot over 65°C. The number of *B. cereus* should be kept at the minimum, and preferably to be kept below 10^5/g during the entire chain of production. Efficient heat treatment for all food matrices and during the canning process of canned foods is critically important to ensure a complete destruction of the spores of *B. cereus*. Efficient sanitation and disinfection of all tools, utensils, and equipments during all the chain of production and processing of foods are necessary to minimize the numbers of *B. cereus* spores. Rapid cooling of foods is used to control the germination and growth of *B. cereus* spores. Targeting low pH, below 4.6, and the reduction of the water activity ($a_w > 0.92$) would inhibit *B. cereus*. Adoption of the HACCP and GMP principles during the production of food products would help to ensure safety of the final products. In addition, *B. cereus* surveillance and monitoring programs should be regularly conducted.

4.9 *E. coli* O157:H7 toxicoinfection

4.9.1 General characteristics

E. coli is a Gram's negative, facultative anaerobic, rod-shaped bacteria, which was initially discovered in 1884 by Theodor Escherich, a German–Austrian pediatrician. *E. coli* was officially recognized in 1958. *E. coli* is a diverse species that has many types and strains. Most of the *E. coli* strains are normal inhabitants of the intestinal tracts of the humans and animals and nonpathogenic. *E. coli* species are classified into groups and serotypes based on their cell wall antigenic structure either O (somatic) or H (flagellar) types. The O and H antigens are given numbers reflecting their serotypes. There are hundreds of *E. coli* serotypes; *E. coli* O157:H7 is the most prominent serotype with public health significance (Ray, 2004).

Generally, *E. coli* causes food poisoning when the food is contaminated with the fecal matter of the animals, birds, and humans, and the major illness is diarrhea. The diarrheagenic *E. coli* is classified into six pathogroups namely, enteropathogenic *E. coli*, enterotoxigenic *E. coli*, enterohemorrhagic *E. coli* or called shiga toxin–producing *E. coli* (STEC), also named verotoxigenic *E. coli*, enteroinvasive *E. coli*, enteroaggregative *E. coli*, and diffusely aggregative *E. coli*. Of these, STEC is the most well-known causative agent of diarrhea. *E. coli* O157:H7 is one major species of STEC that caused bloody diarrhea and hemolytic uremic syndrome (HUS) worldwide (Darwish, Saad Eldin, & Eldesoky, 2015). *E. coli* O157:H7 does not ferment sorbitol or have glucuronidase activity (Sallam, Mohammed, Ahdy, & Tamura, 2013). It grows well at 30°C–42°C, poorly grows at 44°C–45°C, and below 10°C. The bacteria can be destroyed at 64.3°C for 9.6 s and can resist pH of 4.5. Recently, Osaili et al. (2020) examined the behavior of *E. coli* O157:H7 in ground lean camel meat and their thermal inactivation. They recorded average D-values ranging between 1.8 and 0.067 min at 57.5°C–65°C. The *z*-values of *E. coli* O157:H7 strains were 4.6°C and 5.0°C.

4.9.2 Pathogenicity and symptoms

As mentioned earlier, *E. coli* O157:H7 belongs to the pathogroups of STEC because of its ability to produce shiga toxins (*stx*) through the transfer of the shiga toxin–coding genes by the means of *stx* phage. *E. coli* O157:H7 can produce two types of *stx*, namely *stx1*, and *stx2*. *E. coli* O157:H7 strains that produce *stx2* were mainly associated with very severe HUS hospitalized cases and might contain many variants such as *stx2a*, *stx2c*, and *stx2d*. The infective dose of *E. coli* O157:H7 is low, as around 100 bacterial cells can be enough to initiate the disease. Once the disease is initiated with the colonization of the bacterial cells into the intestinal wall via adherence to the intestinal epithelial cells and production of the toxins, they act either locally on the colon or absorbed into the blood stream causing destruction of the small blood vessels in the intestine, kidney, and brain. *E. coli* O157:H7 causes HUS, which involves kidney failure and 5%–6% fatality, hemorrhagic colitis, and thrombotic thrombocytopenic purpura. The symptoms appear after 3–9 days of incubation period and last for 4 days. The symptoms involve abdominal cramps, vomiting, watery or bloody diarrhea, with or without fever. The bloody diarrhea is present in about 35% of the cases due to the ulceration or the damage of the lining layer of the large intestine. Kidney failure might occur and it is a fatal outcome, particularly among children. Thrombotic thrombocytopenic purpura occurs because of the formation of a blood clot in the brain tissue, with symptoms such as seizures, coma, and death may follow. The associated foods with *E. coli* O157:H7 includes improperly cooked ground beef, lamb, meat products as sausage and burgers, poultry, and fish. Dairy products such as unpasteurized milk, butter, cheese are also involved. Green leafy vegetables such as lettuce, and spinach and unpasteurized fruit juices such as apple, and contaminated water are among the implicated food sources in *E. coli* O157:H7 food-poisoning outbreaks (Ray, 2004).

4.10 Prevalence of *E. coli* O157:H7 and its related shiga toxins in the food in the Middle East

A summary for the occurrence of *E. coli* O157:H7 in different food matrices in the Middle East is displayed in Table 4.5.

4.10.1 Egypt

Several surveillance studies were conducted in Egypt to screen the prevalence of *E. coli O157:H7* and stx in the Egyptian foodstuffs. For instance, Abdul-Raouf, Ammar, and Beuchat (1996) recovered *E. coli* O157:H7 at 6% of beef samples, 4% of chicken samples, 4% of lamb samples, and 6% of milk samples obtained from slaughterhouses, supermarkets, and farmer's homes in Egypt. Elhadidy and Mohammed (2013) examined 64 Kareish and 60 Damietta cheese samples from Egypt for the presence of STEC. They could isolate 14 *E. coli* strains that were positive for the presence of the *stx2* gene, either single or in association with the *stx1*. *E. coli* O157 was recovered from retailed beef products (ground beef, beef burger, and fresh beef) collected from Mansoura city, Egypt, at 13.8% (12 out of 87 examined samples). Of these, 26.7% were identified as nonsorbitol-fermenting *E. coli* O157:H7. Using PCR, *stx1* gene was detected in 46.7%; while, *stx2* gene was detected in 86.7% of the identified *E. coli* O157 strains (Sallam et al., 2013). In addition, Ahmed and Shimamoto (2014) examined bacteriologically 1600 meat and dairy product samples collected from street vendors, butchers, retail markets, and slaughterhouses in Egypt. They identified *E. coli* O157:H7 in 29 dairy product samples (3.6%) and in 25 meat product samples (3.1%). All *E. coli* O157:H7 isolates were positive for *stx1* and/or *stx2* virulence genes. Leafy greens sold at the retail markets of Alexandria city were found to be contaminated with *E. coli* O157 at 16.7% for the organic samples, and 71.4% for the conventional samples. Only 2 out of 28 strains were classified as *E. coli* O157:H7. Multiplex PCR confirmed the ability of 21.4% (6/28) of the *E. coli* O157 strains to produce *stx* (Khalil, Gomaa, & Khalil, 2015). Besides, Elafify et al. (2020) recovered 36 STEC isolates from 125 milk and dairy product samples from Mansoura city. Three isolates were identified as *E. coli* O157:H7 and 33 isolates belonged to different serotypes. Molecular characterization revealed that all isolates harbored *stx1* and/or *stx2* genes. In addition, 31 out of 36 (86.11%) isolates showed multidrug-resistant profiling. In addition, Hamed et al. (2017) collected 260 meat and dairy product samples from Giza, and 50 stool samples from diarrheal children at Embaba fever hospital. They recovered only two STEC-producing *E. coli* O157, one from minced meat and the other from one stool sample. Hassanien and Shaker (2020) found that 11.3% and 14.7% of milk products and stool samples collected from retail markets and diarrheal patients in Sohag city were positive for *E. coli* O157:H7. The isolates showed high antimicrobial resistance to ampicillin, gentamycin, and tetracycline.

TABLE 4.5 Prevalence of *E. coli* O157:H7 and Shiga toxins in food and other sample sources in the Middle East.

Country	Food matrix or sample source	Staph. or toxin type	References
Egypt	Beef, chicken, lamb, and milk	*E. coli* O157:H7	Abdul-Raouf et al. (1996)
	Cheese	*E. coli* O157:H7, *stx1*, *stx2*	Elhadidy & Mohammed (2013)
	Beef and beef products	*E. coli* O157:H7, *stx1*, *stx2*	Sallam et al. (2013)
	Beef and milk products	*E. coli* O157:H7, *stx1*, *stx2*	Ahmed and Shimamoto (2014)
	Leafy green produce	*E. coli* O157:H7, *stx*	Khalil et al. (2015)
	Milk and dairy products	*E. coli* O157:H7, *stx1*, *stx2*	Elafify et al. (2020)
	Milk, dairy products, and stool samples	*E. coli* O157:H7	Hamed et al. (2017)
	Milk products and stool samples	*E. coli* O157:H7	Hassanien and Shaker (2020)
Saudi Arabia	Meat and milk samples	*E. coli* O157:H7	Al-Zogibi et al. (2015)
	Meat and meat products	*E. coli* O157:H7, *stx*	Hessain et al. (2015)
	Beef meat samples	*E. coli* O157:H7, *stx2*, *eaeA*	Hemeg (2018)
Jordan	Beef cattle	*E. coli* O157:H7, *stx1*, *stx2*, *eaeA*, *hlyA*	Osaili et al. (2013)
	Shawarma	*E. coli* O157:H7	Nimri et al. (2014)
	Bulk tank milk, rectoanal swabs from cattle	*E. coli* O157:H7	Obaidat and Stringer (2019)
	Imported beef cattle	*E. coli* O157:H7	Obaidat (2020)
Lebanon	Shawarma and Lahm-bi-Ajeen (meat pies)	*E. coli*, *stx1*	Harakeh et al. (2005)

(*Continued*)

TABLE 4.5 (Continued)

Country	Food matrix or sample source	Staph. or toxin type	References
	Dairy products	*E. coli* O157:H7	Saleh et al. (2009)
Iraq	Stool samples from children	*E. coli* O157:H7	Shebib et al. (2003)

4.10.2 Saudi Arabia

Few reports investigated the prevalence of *E. coli* O157:H7 and *stx* in foodstuffs in Saudi Arabia. Al-Zogibi, Mohamed, Hessain, El-Jakee, and Kabli (2015) collected 540 milk samples from 5 dairy farms and 150 raw meat samples from different abattoirs in Riyadh. Their obtained results revealed that *E. coli* O157:H7 were detected at 4.81% and 4% from the examined milk and meat samples. Similarly, the overall isolation rate of *E. coli* O157:H7 was 2.97% from the retailed meat and meat products in the local markets of Riyadh city. *E. coli* O157:H7 was isolated from raw beef, chicken, and mutton at 2%, 2.5%, and 2.5%, respectively. The isolation rates in the meat products were ground beef (5%), beef burgers (10%), beef sausage (0%), ground chicken (5%), and chicken burgers 0.0%, respectively. Using multiplex PCR, *stx*-coding genes were detected in 27.3% and 45.5% of the identified *E. coli* O157:H7 isolates from meat and meat products, respectively (Hessain et al., 2015). Furthermore, Hemeg (2018) recovered five strains of *E. coli* O157:H7 from the examined beef meat samples. Using multiplex PCR, *stx2* and the intimin (*eaeA*) genes were detected in all recovered *E. coli* O157: H7 strains.

4.10.3 Jordan

In Jordan, Osaili et al. (2013) identified 50 *E. coli* O157:H7 isolates from beef cattle slaughtered at Amman abattoir. The virulence factors *eaeA* and hemolysin (*hlyA*) were detected in 22% of the isolates. The identified *E. coli* O157:H7 isolates harbored *stx1*, *stx*2, and both of *stx1* and *stx2*, at 60%, 12%, and 22%, respectively. Furthermore, Nimri et al. (2014) isolated *E. coli* at 28.3%, with six isolates of serotype O157:H7 from contaminated shawarma in Northern Jordan. Obaidat and Stringer (2019) confirmed the isolation of *E. coli* O157:H7 from bulk tank milk at 3.3%, and from rectoanal mucosal swabs at 2.3%. Samples were collected from 61 dairy cattle farms. Multidrug resistance (resistance to three or more classes of antimicrobials) was exhibited at 91.7% of the identified *E. coli* O157:H7. Furthermore, Obaidat (2020) reported that the prevalence rate of *E. coli* O157:H7 was 1.7% in the imported beef cattle at Jordan's major abattoir. Besides, 94.1% of the identified *E. coli* O157:H7 showed multidrug resistance profile.

4.10.4 Lebanon

In Lebanon, Harakeh et al. (2005) reported that 55% of shawarma and Lahm-bi-Ajeen (meat pies) collected as meat-based fast food were contaminated with *E. coli*. The coding gene for *stx1* was detected in 9 out of 12 *E. coli* isolates at PCR examination. Furthermore, Saleh et al. (2009) isolated two strains of *E. coli* O157:H7 from popular Lebanese dairy products (Kishk and baladi) at 2.7% for each product, which had been collected in the Beqaa Valley, in northeastern Lebanon. The two isolates showed drug resistance profiling.

4.10.5 Iraq

Shebib, Abdul Ghani, and Mahdi (2003) isolated *E. coli* O157:H7 from children with bloody diarrhea at 11.5%. Stool samples were collected from 200 children with different ages from two hospitals in Baghdad city, Iraq. All *E. coli* O157:H7 isolates were resistant to erythromycin, polymixin B, and vancomycin.

4.10.6 Control measures of *E. coli* O157:H7

Adoption of proper sanitation measures, efficient cooking, and heat treatment of meat and dairy products are among the recommended preventive and control measures of the occurrence of *E. coli* O157:H7 in food. Rapid and efficient freezing and storage of meat, meat products, fish, and poultry are also highly recommended. In addition, confirming personal hygiene during preparation, processing, and storage of the food, avoiding fecal-oral transmission, and preventing the cross-contamination with hides, soil, intestinal tract contents, or animal excreta are considered among the recommended measures to avoid or control food contamination with *E. coli* O157:H7 (Bosilevac et al., 2015). Application of the principles of HACCP and GMP practices during the manufacture and processing of food is also highly recommended. Furthermore, in the food industry, regular training programs, and courses among food handlers are of value to improve the food safety and microbiological qualities of food (Lami et al., 2019; Osaili et al., 2013).

References

Abbar, F. M., Mohammed, M. T., & Arslain, S. H. (1986). Selected biological properties of enterotoxigenic staphylococci isolated from milk. *Journal of Food Protection*, *49*(11), 871–873. Available from https://doi.org/10.4315/0362-028X-49.11.871.

Abdeen, E. E., Hussien, H., Hadad, G. A. E., & Mousa, W. S. (2020). Prevalence of virulence determinants among *Bacillus cereus* isolated from milk products with potential public health concern. *Pakistan Journal of Biological Sciences*, *23*(3), 206–212. Available from https://doi.org/10.3923/pjbs.2020.206.212.

Abdul-Raouf, U. M., Ammar, M. S., & Beuchat, L. R. (1996). Isolation of *Escherichia coli* O157:H7 from some Egyptian foods. *International Journal of Food Microbiology*, *29*(2–3), 423–426. Available from https://doi.org/10.1016/0168-1605(95)00076-3.

Abolghait, S. K., Fathi, A. G., Youssef, F. M., & Algammal, A. M. (2020). Methicillin-resistant Staphylococcus aureus (MRSA) isolated from chicken meat and giblets often produces staphylococcal enterotoxin B (SEB) in non-refrigerated raw chicken livers. *International Journal of Food Microbiology*, *328*, 108669. Available from https://doi.org/10.1016/j.ijfoodmicro.2020.108669.

Ahmed, A. M., & Shimamoto, T. (2014). Isolation and molecular characterization of *Salmonella enterica*, *Escherichia coli O157:H7* and Shigella spp. from meat and dairy products in Egypt. *International Journal of Food Microbiology*, *168–169*, 57–62. Available from https://doi.org/10.1016/j.ijfoodmicro.2013.10.014.

Ahmed, S. H., Badary, M. S., Mohamed, W. A., & Elkhawaga, A. A. (2011). Multiplex PCR for detection and genotyping of C. botulinum types A, B, E and F neurotoxin genes in some Egyptian food products. *Journal of American Science*, *7*(10), 176–190.

Al-Abri, S. S., Al-Jardani, A. K., Al-Hosni, M. S., Kurup, P. J., Al-Busaidi, S., & Beeching, N. J. (2011). A hospital acquired outbreak of Bacillus cereus gastroenteritis, Oman. *Journal of Infection and Public Health*, *4*(4), 180–186. Available from https://doi.org/10.1016/j.jiph.2011.05.003.

Al-Ashmawy, M. A., Sallam, K. I., Abd-Elghany, S. M., Elhadidy, M., & Tamura, T. (2016). Prevalence, molecular characterization, and antimicrobial susceptibility of methicillin-resistant *Staphylococcus aureus* isolated from milk and dairy products. *Foodborne Pathogens and Disease*, *13*(3), 156–162. Available from https://doi.org/10.1089/fpd.2015.2038.

Al-Bustan, M. A., Udo, E. E., & Chugh, T. D. (1996). Nasal carriage of enterotoxin-producing Staphylococcus aureus among restaurant workers in Kuwait City. *Epidemiology and Infection*, *116*(3), 319–322. Available from https://doi.org/10.1017/s0950268800052638.

Al-Gamal, M. S., Ibrahim, G. A., Sharaf, O. M., Radwan, A. A., Dabiza, N. M., Youssef, A. M., & El-Ssayad, M. F. (2019). The protective potential of selected lactic acid bacteria against the most common contaminants in various types of cheese in Egypt. *Heliyon*, *5*(3), e01362. Available from https://doi.org/10.1016/j.heliyon.2019.e01362.

Ali, S. H., Hoshyare, D. F., & Al-Delaimy, K. S. (1982). Microbial counts on surfaces of lamb carcasses and shelf-life of refrigerated ground lamb. *Journal of Food Protection*, *45*(11), 1013–1015. Available from https://doi.org/10.4315/0362-028X-45.11.1013.

Al-Joudi, A. S. (2007). An outbreak of foodborne diarrheal illness among soldiers in mina during hajj: The role of consumer food handling behaviors. *Journal of Family & Community Medicine*, *14*(1), 29–33.

Al-Khatib, I., Giacaman, R., Husseini, A., Ramlawi, A., Atiyya, I., & Salem, I. (2004). Microbiological quality of food samples from restaurants and sweet shops in developing countries: A case study from the occupied Palestinian territory. *International Journal of Environmental Health Research*, *14*(6), 443–452. Available from https://doi.org/10.1080/09603120400012835.

Al-Khatib, I. A., & Al-Mitwalli, S. M. (2009). Microbiological quality and sample collection policy for dairy products in Ramallah and Al-Bireh district, Palestine. *Eastern Mediterranean Health Journal, 15*(3), 709–716.

Al-Nabulsi, A. A., Osaili, T. M., AbuNaser, R. A., Olaimat, A. N., Ayyash, M., Al-Holy, M. A., . . . Holley, R. A. (2020). Factors affecting the viability of Staphylococcus aureus and production of enterotoxin during processing and storage of white-brined cheese. *Journal of Dairy Science, 103*(8), 6869–6881. Available from https://doi.org/10.3168/jds.2020-18158.

Al-Natour, M. Q., Alaboudi, A. R., Al-Hatamelh, N. A., & Osaili, T. M. (2012). *Escherichia coli O157:H7* facilitates the penetration of *Staphylococcus aureus* into table eggs. *Journal of Food Science, 77*(1), M29–M34. Available from https://doi.org/10.1111/j.1750-3841.2011.02483.x.

Al-Zogibi, O. G., Mohamed, M. I., Hessain, A. M., El-Jakee, J. K., & Kabli, S. A. (2015). Molecular and serotyping characterization of shiga toxogenic *Escherichia coli* associated with food collected from Saudi Arabia. *Saudi Journal of Biological Sciences, 22*(4), 438–442. Available from https://doi.org/10.1016/j.sjbs.2015.02.019.

Ayaz, M., Sawaya, W. N., & Al-Sogair, A. (1986). Microbiological quality of Tehineh manufactured in Saudi Arabia. *Journal of Food Protection, 49*(7), 504–506. Available from https://doi.org/10.4315/0362-028X-49.7.504.

Baker, D. A., & Genigeorgis, C. (1990). Predicting the safe storage of fresh fish under modified atmospheres with respect to Clostridium botulinum toxigenesis by modeling length of the lag phase of growth. *Journal of Food Protectection, 53*, 131–140.

Batchoun, R., Al-Sha'er, A. I., & Khabour, O. F. (2011). Molecular characterization of Bacillus cereus toxigenic strains isolated from different food matrices in Jordan. *Foodborne Pathogens and Disease, 8*(11), 1153–1158. Available from https://doi.org/10.1089/fpd.2011.0853.

Bates, J. R., & Bodnaruk, P. W. (2003). Clostridium perfringens. In A. D. Hocking (Ed.), *Foodborne microorganisms of public health significance* (6th ed., pp. 505–542). Waterloo: Australian Institute of Food Science and Technology Inc., Food Microbiology Group.

Bosilevac, J. M., Gassem, M. A., Al Sheddy, I. A., Almaiman, S. A., Al-Mohizea, I. S., Alowaimer, A., & Koohmaraie, M. (2015). Prevalence of *Escherichia coli O157:H7* and Salmonella in camels, cattle, goats, and sheep harvested for meat in Riyadh. *Journal of Food Protection, 78*(1), 89–96. Available from https://doi.org/10.4315/0362-028X.JFP-14-176.

Brynestad, S., & Granum, P. E. (2002). *Clostridium perfringens* foodborne infections. *International Journal of Food Microbiology, 74*, 195–202. Available from https://doi.org/10.1016/S0168-1605(01)00680-8.

Cagan, E., Peker, E., Dogan, M., & Caksen, H. (2010). Infant botulism. *The Eurasian Journal of Medicine, 42*(2), 92–94. Available from https://doi.org/10.5152/eajm.2010.25.

Carlin, F., Brillard, J., Broussole, V., Clavel, T., Duport, C., Jobin, M., . . . Nguyen-The, C. (2010). Adaptation of *Bacillus cereus*, a ubiquitous worldwide-distributed foodborne pathogen, to a changing environment. *Food Research International, 43*(7), 1885–1894.

Ceuppens, S., Boon, N., & Uyttendaele, M. (2013). Diversity of *Bacillus cereus* group strains is reflected in their broad range of pathogenicity and diverse ecological lifestyles. *FEMS Microbiology Ecology, 84*(3), 433–450.

Chaibenjawong, P., & Foster, S. J. (2011). Desiccation tolerance in Staphylococcus aureus. *Archives of Microbiology, 193*(2), 125–135. Available from https://doi.org/10.1007/s00203-010-0653-x.

Darwish, W. S., Atia, A. S., Reda, L. M., Elhelaly, A. E., Thompson, L. A., & Saad Eldin, W. F. (2018). Chicken giblets and wastewater samples as possible sources of methicillin-resistant Staphylococcus aureus: Prevalence, enterotoxin production, and antibiotic susceptibility. *Journal of Food Safety*, *38*(10), e12478. Available from https://doi.org/10.1111/jfs.12478.

Darwish, W. S., Saad Eldin, W. F., & Eldesoky, K. I. (2015). Prevalence, molecular characterization and antibiotic susceptibility of *Escherichia coli* isolated from duck meat and giblets. *Journal of Food Safety*, *35*, 410–415.

Dodds, K. L. (1994). Clostridium botulinum. In Y. H. Hui, J. R. Gorham, K. D. Murrell, et al. (Eds.), *Foodborne disease handbook* (1, pp. 97–131). New York: Marcel Dekker.

Elafify, M., Khalifa, H. O., Al-Ashmawy, M., Elsherbini, M., El Latif, A. A., Okanda, T., ... Abdelkhalek, A. (2020). Prevalence and antimicrobial resistance of Shiga toxin-producing *Escherichia coli* in milk and dairy products in Egypt. *Journal of Environmental Science and Health. Part. B, Pesticides, Food Contaminants, and Agricultural Wastes*, *55*(3), 265–272. Available from https://doi.org/10.1080/03601234.2019.1686312.

El-Aziz, N. K. A., Tartor, Y. H., El-Aziz Gharib, A. A., & Ammar, A. M. (2018). Propidium monoazide quantitative real-time polymerase chain reaction for enumeration of some viable but nonculturable foodborne bacteria in meat and meat products. *Foodborne Pathogens and Disease*, *15*(4), 226–234. Available from https://doi.org/10.1089/fpd.2017.2356.

El-Bahnasawy, M. M., Aly, N. Z., Abdel-Fattah, M. A., & Morsy, T. A. (2014). Botulism as a food poisoning: What is it? *Journal of the Egyptian Society of Parasitology*, *44*(1), 211–220. Available from https://doi.org/10.12816/0006461.

El-Bassiony, T. A. (1980). Occurrence of Clostridium perfringens in milk and dairy products. *Journal of Food Protection*, *43*(7), 536–537. Available from https://doi.org/10.4315/0362-028X-43.7.536.

El Bayomi, R. M., Ahmed, H. A., Awadallah, M. A., Mohsen, R. A., Abd El-Ghafar, A. E., & Abdelrahman, M. A. (2016). Occurrence, virulence factors, antimicrobial resistance, and genotyping of Staphylococcus aureus strains isolated from chicken products and humans. *Vector Borne and Zoonotic Diseases (Larchmont, N.Y.)*, *16*(3), 157–164. Available from https://doi.org/10.1089/vbz.2015.1891.

El-Dengawy, R. A., & Nassar, A. M. (2001). Investigation on the nutritive value and microbiological quality of wild quail carcasses. *Die Nahrung*, *45*(1), 50–54. Available from https://doi.org/10.1002/1521-3803(20010101)45:1 < 50::AID-FOOD50 > 3.0.CO;2-J.

El-Ghareeb, W. R., Almathen, F. S., Fayez, M. M., & Alsultan, R. A. (2019). Methicillin resistant *staphylococcus aureus* (MRSA) in camel meat: prevalence and antibiotic susceptibility. *Slovenian Veterinary Research*, *56*(Suppl. 22), 249–256. Available from https://doi.org/10.26873/SVR-764-2019.

Elhadidy, M., & Mohammed, M. A. (2013). Shiga toxin-producing *Escherichia coli* from raw milk cheese in Egypt: prevalence, molecular characterization and survival to stress conditions. *Letters in Applied Microbiology*, *56*(2), 120–127. Available from https://doi.org/10.1111/lam.12023.

European Food Safety Authority (EFSA). (2005). Opinion of the scientific panel on biological hazards on *Bacillus cereus* and other *Bacillus* spp in foodstuffs. *The EFSA Journal*, *175*, 1–48. Available from https://kopernio.com/viewer?doi = 10.2903%2Fj.efsa.2005.175&token = WzMxMzk2MTgsIjEwLjI5MDMvai5lZnNhLjIwMDUuMTc1Il0.
n9wkKv_zLQnwRiLNTD9JjHAQHnk.

García, S., & Heredia, N. (2011). *Clostridium perfringens*: A dynamic foodborne pathogen. *Food Bioprocess Technology*, *4*, 624–630. Available from https://doi.org/10.1007/s11947-009-0182-2.

Gharieb, R., Saad, M., Abdallah, K., Khedr, M., Farag, E., & Abd El-Fattah, A. (2020). Insights on toxin genotyping, virulence, antibiogram profiling, biofilm formation and efficacy of disinfectants on biofilms of *Clostridium perfringens* isolated from poultry, animals and humans. *Journal of Applied Microbiology*, *130*(3), 819–831. Available from https://doi.org/10.1111/jam.14838.

Hamad, G. M., Abdelmotilib, N. M., Darwish, A. M. G., & Zeitoun, A. M. (2020). Commercial probiotic cell-free supernatants for inhibition of *Clostridium perfringens* poultry meat infection in Egypt. *Anaerobe*, *62*, 102181. Available from https://doi.org/10.1016/j.anaerobe.2020.102181.

Hamed, O. M., Sabry, M. A., Hassanain, N. A., Hamza, E., Hegazi, A. G., & Salman, M. B. (2017). Occurrence of virulent and antibiotic-resistant Shiga toxin-producing *Escherichia coli* in some food products and human stool in Egypt. *Veterinary World*, *10*(10), 1233–1240. Available from https://doi.org/10.14202/vetworld.2017.1233-1240.

Hamzé, M., Naja, M., & Mallat, H. (2008). Analyses biologiques réalisées chez des travailleurs dans le secteur alimentaire au nord du Liban [Biological analysis of workers in the food sector in north Lebanon]. *Eastern Mediterranean Health Journal = La Revue de Sante de la Mediterranee Orientale = al-Majallah al-sihhiyah li-sharq al-mutawassit*, *14*(6), 1425–1434.

Haque, K. N., Ayaz, M., Al-Omair, A., Aunullah, A., Al-Swailam, M., & Bahakim, H. (1987). Food poisoning among children in Riyadh, Saudi Arabia. *Annals of Saudi Medicine*, *7*(1), 23–27.

Harakeh, S., Yassine, H., Gharios, M., Barbour, E., Hajjar, S., El-Fadel, M., ... Tannous, R. (2005). Isolation, molecular characterization and antimicrobial resistance patterns of Salmonella and *Escherichia coli* isolates from meat-based fast food in Lebanon. *The Science of the Total Environment*, *341*(1–3), 33–44. Available from https://doi.org/10.1016/j.scitotenv.2004.09.025.

Hassan, S. A., Altalhi, A. D., Gherbawy, Y. A., & El-Deeb, B. A. (2011). Bacterial load of fresh vegetables and their resistance to the currently used antibiotics in Saudi Arabia. *Foodborne Pathogens and Disease*, *8*(9), 1011–1018. Available from https://doi.org/10.1089/fpd.2010.0805.

Hassanien, A. A., & Shaker, E. M. (2020). Investigation of the effect of chitosan and silver nanoparticles on the antibiotic resistance of *Escherichia coli O157:H7* isolated from some milk products and diarrheal patients in Sohag city, Egypt. *Veterinary World*, *13*(8), 1647–1653. Available from https://doi.org/10.14202/vetworld.2020.1647-1653.

Hemeg, H. A. (2018). Molecular characterization of antibiotic resistant *Escherichia coli* isolates recovered from food samples and outpatient clinics, KSA. *Saudi Journal of Biological Sciences*, *25*(5), 928–931. Available from https://doi.org/10.1016/j.sjbs.2018.01.016.

Hennekinne, J. A., De Buyser, M. L., & Dragacci, S. (2012). *Staphylococcus aureus* and its food poisoning toxins: Characterization and outbreak investigation. *FEMS Microbiology Reviews*, *36*(4), 815–836. Available from https://doi.org/10.1111/j.1574-6976.2011.00311.x.

Heredia, N. L., & Labbé, R. G. (2001). Clostridium perfringens. In J. S. García-Alvarado, & R. G. Labbé (Eds.), *Guide to foodborne pathogens* (pp. 133–142). New York: John Wiley & Sons.

Hessain, A. M., Al-Arfaj, A. A., Zakri, A. M., El-Jakee, J. K., Al-Zogibi, O. G., Hemeg, H. A., & Ibrahim, I. M. (2015). Molecular characterization of *Escherichia coli O157:H7* recovered from meat and meat products relevant to human health in Riyadh, Saudi Arabia. *Saudi Journal of Biological Sciences*, *22*(6), 725–729. Available from https://doi.org/10.1016/j.sjbs.2015.06.009.

Hielm, S., Bjorkroth, J., & Hyytia, E. (1998). Prevalence of Clostridium botulinum in Finnish trout farms: Pulsed-field gel electrophoresis typing reveals extensive genetic diversity among type E isolates. *Applied and Environmental Microbiology*, *64*, 4161–4167.

Huss, H. H. (1980). Distribution of Clostridium botulinum. *Applied and Environmental Microbiology*, *39*, 764–769.

Hussein, M. A., Merwad, A. M. A., Elabbasy, M. T., Suelam, I. I. A., Abdelwahab, A. M., & Taha, M. A. (2019). Prevalence of enterotoxigenic *Staphylococcus aureus* and Shiga toxin producing *Escherichia coli* in fish in Egypt: Quality parameters and public health hazard. *Vector Borne and Zoonotic Diseases (Larchmont, N.Y.)*, *19*(4), 255–264. Available from https://doi.org/10.1089/vbz.2018.2346.

Imai, H., Oshita, K., & Hashimoto, H. (1990). Factors inhibiting the growth and toxin formation of *Clostridium botulinum* types A and B in "tsuyu" (Japanese noodle soup). *Journal of Food Protection*, *53*, 1025–1032.

Jackson, K. A., Mahon, B. E., Copeland, J., & Fagan, R. P. (2015). Botulism mortality in the USA, 1975–2009. *Botulinum Journal.*, *3*(1), 6–17. Available from https://doi.org/10.1504/TBJ.2015.078132.

Jay, J. M. (2000). *Modern food microbiology* (6th ed.). Gaithersburg, MD: Aspen Publishers, INC..

Jisr, N., Younes, G., El Omari, K., Hamze, M., Sukhn, C., & El-Dakdouki, M. H. (2020). Levels of heavy metals, total petroleum hydrocarbons, and microbial load in commercially valuable fish from the marine area of Tripoli, Lebanon. *Environmental Monitoring and Assessment*, *192*(11), 705. Available from https://doi.org/10.1007/s10661-020-08672-w.

Juneja, V., Marmer, B. S., & Miller, A. J. (1994). Growth and sporulation of *Clostridium perfringens* in aerobic and vacuum packaged cooked beef. *Journal of Food Protection*, *57*, 393–398.

Juneja, V. K., & Thippareddi, H. (2004). Control of *Clostridium perfringens* in a model roast beef by salts of organic acids during chilling. *Journal of Food Safety*, *93*, 155–163.

Juneja, V. K., Thippareddi, H., & Friedman, M. (2006). Control of Clostridium perfringens in cooked ground beef by carvacrol, cinnamaldehyde, thymol, or oregano oil during chilling. *Journal of Food Protection*, *69*, 1546–1555.

Kadariya, J., Smith, T. C., & Thapaliya, D. (2014). *Staphylococcus aureus* and staphylococcal food-borne disease: An ongoing challenge in public health. *Biomed Research International*, *2014*, 827965. Available from https://doi.org/10.1155/2014/827965.

Khalil, R. K., Gomaa, M. A., & Khalil, M. I. (2015). Detection of shiga-toxin producing *E. coli* (STEC) in leafy greens sold at local retail markets in Alexandria, Egypt. *International Journal of Food Microbiology*, *197*, 58–64. Available from https://doi.org/10.1016/j.ijfoodmicro.2014.12.019.

Kharroubi, S., Nasser, N. A., El-Harakeh, M. D., Sulaiman, A. A., & Kassem, I. I. (2020). First nation-wide analysis of food safety and acceptability data in Lebanon. *Foods*, *9*(11), 1717. Available from https://doi.org/10.3390/foods9111717.

Kurdi, T. S., Kamball, A. M., Muhammad, M. H. A., & al-Zahrani, M. A. (1998). Manuals for worker for food poisoning accidents. *Riyadh (KSA): Ministry of Health*, 1–27.

Lambert, A. D., Smith, J. P., & Dodds, K. L. (1991). Combined effect of modified atmosphere packaging and low-dose irradiation on toxin production by Clostridium botulinum in fresh pork. *Journal of Food Protection*, *54*, 94–101.

Lami, F., Radhi, F., Al Dahhan, S., Hashim, R. A., Mahmood, H., Araj, R., & Arbaji, A. (2019). Knowledge, attitude, and practices of food handlers on food safety and personal hygiene during arbaeenia mass gathering, Baghdad, Iraq, 2014: Cross-sectional study. *JMIR Public Health and Surveillance*, *i*(4), e10922. Available from https://doi.org/10.2196/10922.

Le Loir, Y., Baron, F., & Gautier, M. (2003). *Staphylococcus aureus* and food poisoning. *Genetics and Molecular Research: GMR*, *2*(1), 63–76.

Li, J., & McClane, B. A. (2006). Comparative effects of osmostic, sodium nitrite-induced and pH-induced stress on growth and survival of *Clostridium perfringens* Type A isolates carrying chromosomal or plasmid-borne enterotoxin genes. *Applied Environmental Microbiology*, *72*, 7620–7625.

Limón, J., Solis, L., García, S., & Heredia, N. (2007). Influence of GRAS substances on the acquisition of cold tolerance in C. perfringens. In *Proceedings of the annual conference of the vereinigung fur allgemeine mikrobiologie (VAAN)*, April 1–4, 2007, Osnarbruck, Germany.

Mahler, H., Pasi, A., Kramer, J. M., Schulte, P., Scoging, A. C., Bar, W., & Krahenbuhl, S. (1997). Fulminant liver failure in association with the emetic toxin of *Bacillus cereus*. *New England Journal of Medicine*, *336*, 1142–1148.

McClane, B. A. (1996). An overview of *Clostridium perfringens* enterotoxin. *Toxicon*, *34*, 1335–1343. Available from https://doi.org/10.1016/S0041-0101(96)00101-8.

McClane, B. A. (2005). Clostridial enterotoxins. In P. Durre (Ed.), *Handbook on Clostridia* (pp. 385–406). Boca Raton, FL: Taylor and Francis.

McClane, B. A. (2007). Clostridium perfringens. In M. Doyle, & L. Beuchat (Eds.), *Food microbiology, fundamentals and frontiers* (3rd ed., pp. 423–445). Washington, DC: American Society for Microbiology.

Moravek, M., Dietrich, R., Buerk, C., Broussolle, V., Guinebretiere, M. H., Granum, P. E., … Martlbauer, E. (2006). Determination of the toxic potential of *Bacillus cereus* isolates by quantitative enterotoxin analyses. *FEMS Microbiology Letters*, *257*(2), 293–298.

Morshdy, A. E. M. A., Darwish, W. S., Salah El-Dien, W. M., & Khalifa, S. M. (2019). Prevalence of multidrug-resistant *Staphylococcus aureus* and *Salmonella enteritidis* in meat products retailed in Zagazig City, Egypt. *Slovenian Veterinary Research*, *55*, 295–301.

Nimri, L., Abu Al-Dahab, F., & Batchoun, R. (2014). Foodborne bacterial pathogens recovered from contaminated shawarma meat in northern Jordan. *The Journal of Infection in Developing Countries*, *8*(11), 1407–1414. Available from https://doi.org/10.3855/jidc.4368.

Obaidat, M. M. (2020). Prevalence and antimicrobial resistance of Listeria monocytogenes, Salmonella enterica and *Escherichia coli* O157:H7 in imported beef cattle in Jordan. *Comparative immunology, microbiology and infectious diseases*, *70*, 101447. Available from https://doi.org/10.1016/j.cimid.2020.101447.

Obaidat, M. M., Bani Salman, A. E., & Roess, A. A. (2018). High prevalence and antimicrobial resistance of mecA Staphylococcus aureus in dairy cattle, sheep, and goat bulk tank milk in Jordan. *Tropical Animal Health and Production*, *50*(2), 405–412. Available from https://doi.org/10.1007/s11250-017-1449-7.

Obaidat, M. M., Salman, A. E., & Lafi, S. Q. (2015). Prevalence of Staphylococcus aureus in imported fish and correlations between antibiotic resistance and enterotoxigenicity. *Journal of Food Protection*, *78*(11), 1999–2005. Available from https://doi.org/10.4315/0362-028X.JFP-15-104.

Obaidat, M. M., & Stringer, A. P. (2019). Prevalence, molecular characterization, and antimicrobial resistance profiles of Listeria monocytogenes, Salmonella enterica, and *Escherichia coli* O157:H7 on dairy cattle farms in Jordan. *Journal of Dairy Science*, *102*(10), 8710–8720. Available from https://doi.org/10.3168/jds.2019-16461.

Osaili, T. M., Abu Jamous, D. O., Obeidat, B. A., Bawadi, H. A., Tayyem, R. F., & Subih, H. S. (2013). Food safety knowledge among food workers in restaurants in Jordan. *Food Control*, *31*(1), 145–150. Available from https://doi.org/10.1016/j.foodcont.2012.09.037.

Osaili, T. M., Alaboudi, A. R., & Rahahlah, M. (2013). Prevalence and antimicrobial susceptibility of *Escherichia coli* O157:H7 on beef cattle slaughtered in Amman abattoir. *Meat Science*, *93*(3), 463–468. Available from https://doi.org/10.1016/j.meatsci.2012.11.023.

Osaili, T. M., Al-Nabulsi, A. A., Dhanasekaran, D. K., Hasan, F., Rao, S., Fatima, H., ... Obaid, R. S. (2020). Growth behaviour and thermal inactivation of *E. coli O157:H7* and *Salmonella spp.* in ground lean camel meat. *International Journal of Food Microbiology*, *316*, 108423. Available from https://doi.org/10.1016/j.ijfoodmicro.2019.108423.

Osaili, T. M., Al-Nabulsi, A. A., Jaradat, Z., Shaker, R. R., Alomari, D. Z., Al-Dabbas, M. M., ... Holley, R. A. (2015). Survival and growth of Salmonella typhimurium, *Escherichia coli* O157:H7 and Staphylococcus aureus in eggplant dip during storage. *International Journal of Food Microbiology*, *198*, 37–42. Available from https://doi.org/10.1016/j.ijfoodmicro.2014.12.025.

Osman, M., Kamal-Dine, K., El Omari, K., Rafei, R., Dabboussi, F., & Hamze, M. (2019). Prevalence of Staphylococcus aureus methicillin-sensitive and methicillin-resistant nasal carriage in food handlers in Lebanon: A potential source of transmission of virulent strains in the community. *Access Microbiology*, *1*(6), e000043. Available from https://doi.org/10.1099/acmi.0.000043.

Rasetti-Escargueil, C., Lemichez, E., & Popoff, M. R. (2019). Public health risk associated with botulism as foodborne zoonoses. *Toxins (Basel)*, *12*(1), 17. Available from https://doi.org/10.3390/toxins12010017.

Ray, B. (2004). *Fundamental food microbiology* (3rd ed.), pp. 401–403). Washington, DC: CRC Press.

Sabah, J. R., Juneja, V. K., & Fung, D. Y. (2004). Effect of spices and organic acids on the growth of *Clostridium perfringens* during cooling of cooked ground beef. *Journal of Food Protection*, *67*, 1840–1847.

Sabike, I. I., Fujikawa, H., Sakha, M. Z., & Edris, A. M. (2014). Production of Staphylococcus aureus enterotoxin A in raw milk at high temperatures. *Journal of Food Protection*, *77*(9), 1612–1616. Available from https://doi.org/10.4315/0362-028X.JFP-13-527.

Sabry, M., Abd El-Moein, K., Hamza, E., & Abdel Kader, F. (2016). Occurrence of Clostridium perfringens types A, E, and C in fresh fish and its public health significance. *Journal of Food Protection*, *79*(6), 994–1000. Available from https://doi.org/10.4315/0362-028X.JFP-15-569.

Sadek, Z. I., Abdel-Rahman, M. A., Azab, M. S., Darwesh, O. M., & Hassan, M. S. (2018). Microbiological evaluation of infant foods quality and molecular detection of *Bacillus cereus* toxins relating genes. *Toxicology Reports*, *5*, 871–877. Available from https://doi.org/10.1016/j.toxrep.2018.08.013.

Saito, M. (1990). Production of enterotoxin by *Clostridium perfringens* derived from humans, animals, foods, and the natural environment in Japan. *Journal of Food Protection*, *53*, 115–118.

Saleh, I., Zouhairi, O., Alwan, N., Hawi, A., Barbour, E., & Harakeh, S. (2009). Antimicrobial resistance and pathogenicity of *Escherichia coli* isolated from common dairy products in the Lebanon. *Annals of Tropical Medicine and Parasitology*, *103*(1), 39–52. Available from https://doi.org/10.1179/136485909X384965.

Sallam, K. I., Mohammed, M. A., Ahdy, A. M., & Tamura, T. (2013). Prevalence, genetic characterization and virulence genes of sorbitol-fermenting *Escherichia coli O157:H-* and *E. coli O157:H7* isolated from retail beef. *International Journal of Food Microbiology*, *165*(3), 295–301. Available from https://doi.org/10.1016/j.ijfoodmicro.2013.05.024.

Scalfaro, C., Auricchio, B., De Medici, D., & Anniballi, F. (2019). Foodborne botulism: An evolving public health challenge. *Infectious Diseases (London)*, *51*(2), 97–101. Available from https://doi.org/10.1080/23744235.2018.1524584.

Scott, E., & Bloomfield, S. F. (1990). The survival and transfer of microbial contamination via cloths, hands and utensils. *The Journal of Applied Bacteriology*, *68*(3), 271–278. Available from https://doi.org/10.1111/j.1365-2672.1990.tb02574.x.

Shawish, R., & Tarabees, R. (2017). Prevalence and antimicrobial resistance of Bacillus cereus isolated from beef products in Egypt. *Open Veterinary Journal*, *7*(4), 337–341. Available from https://doi.org/10.4314/ovj.v7i4.9.

Shawish, R. R., & Al-Humam, N. A. (2016). Contamination of beef products with staphylococcal classical enterotoxins in Egypt and Saudi Arabia. *GMS Hygiene and Infection Control*, *11*, 1–6.

Shebib, Z. A., Abdul Ghani, Z. G., & Mahdi, L. K. H. (2003). First report of *Escherichia coli O157* among Iraqi children. *Eastern Mediterranean Health Journal = La Revue de Sante de la Mediterranee Orientale = al-Majallah al-sihhiyah li-sharq al-mutawassit*, *9*(1–2), 159–166.

Sperber, W. H. (1983). Influence of water activity on foodborne bacteria—A review. *Journal of Food Protection*, *46*, 142–150.

Stenfors Arnesen, L. P., Fagerlund, A., & Granum, P. E. (2008). From soil to gut: Bacillus cereus and its food poisoning toxins. *FEMS Microbiology Reviews*, *32*(4), 579–606.

Taha, S., Wilkins, S., Juusola, K., & Osaili, T. M. (2020). Food safety performance in food manufacturing facilities: The influence of management practices on food handler commitment. *Journal of Food Protection*, *83*(1), 60–67. Available from https://doi.org/10.4315/0362-028X.JFP-19-126.

Turnbull, P. C. B. (1996). Bacillus. In S. Baron (Ed.), *Medical microbiology* (4th ed.)). Galveston (TX): University of Texas Medical Branch at Galveston. Chapter 15. Available from https://www.ncbi.nlm.nih.gov/books/NBK7699/.

Udo, E. E., Al-Bustan, M. A., Jacob, L. E., & Chugh, T. D. (1999). Enterotoxin production by coagulase-negative staphylococci in restaurant workers from Kuwait City may be a potential cause of food poisoning. *Journal of Medical Microbiology*, *48*(9), 819–823. Available from https://doi.org/10.1099/00222615-48-9-819.

van der Vorst, M. M., Jamal, W., Rotimi, V. O., & Moosa, A. (2006). Infant botulism due to consumption of contaminated commercially prepared honey. First report from the Arabian Gulf States. *Medical Principles and Practice: International Journal of the Kuwait University, Health Science Centre*, *15*(6), 456–458. Available from https://doi.org/10.1159/000095494.

Weber, J. T., Hibbs, R. G., Jr, Darwish, A., Mishu, B., Corwin, A. L., Rakha, M., ... Tauxe, R. V. (1993). A massive outbreak of type E botulism associated with traditional salted fish in Cairo. *The Journal of Infectious Diseases*, *167*(2), 451–454. Available from https://doi.org/10.1093/infdis/167.2.451.

Wieckowski, E. U., Kokai-Kun, J. F., & McClane, B. A. (1998). Characterization of membrane-associated Clostridium perfringens enterotoxin following pronase treatment. *Infection and Immunity*, *66*, 5897–5905.

Yehia, H. M., Al-Masoud, A. H., Alarjani, K. M., & Alamri, M. S. (2020). Prevalence of methicillin-resistant (mecA gene) and heat-resistant *Staphylococcus aureus* strains in pasteurized camel milk. *Journal of Dairy Science*, *103*(7), 5947–5963. Available from https://doi.org/10.3168/jds.2019-17631.

Yehia, H. M., Ismail, E. A., Hassan, Z. K., Al-Masoud, A. H., & Al-Dagal, M. M. (2019). Heat resistance and presence of genes encoding staphylococcal enterotoxins evaluated by multiplex-PCR of Staphylococcus aureus isolated from pasteurized camel milk. *Bioscience Reports*, *39*(11). Available from https://doi.org/10.1042/BSR20191225, BSR20191225.

Zeinhom, M. M., Abdel-Latef, G. K., & Jordan, K. (2015). The use of multiplex PCR to determine the prevalence of enterotoxigenic *Staphylococcus aureus* isolated from raw milk, feta cheese, and hand swabs. *Journal of Food Science*, *80*(12), M2932–M2936. Available from https://doi.org/10.1111/1750-3841.13147.

Zouhairi, O., Saleh, I., Alwan, N., Toufeili, I., Barbour, E., & Harakeh, S. (2012). Antimicrobial resistance of Staphylococcus species isolated from Lebanese dairy-based products. *Eastern Mediterranean Health Journal = La Revue de Sante de la Mediterranee Orientale = al-Majallah al-sihhiyah li-sharq al-mutawassit*, *16*(12), 1221–1225. Available from https://doi.org/10.26719/2010.16.12.1221.

Chapter 5

Chemical residues: potential food safety hazards in the Middle East

Akram R. Alaboudi
Department of Pathology and Public Health, Faculty of Veterinary Medicine, Jordan University of Science and Technology, Irbid, Jordan

5.1 Introduction

A residue of a parent drug or chemical and its metabolites may accumulate and be deposited or stored within the plant or animal (meat) tissues and organs following:

- the use of drugs or chemicals to control diseases;
- the use of drugs or chemicals to treat diseases; and
- the use of feed additives to promote growth and improve feed efficiency.

Residues may be either Intentional or Unintentional.

A. Intentional residue (direct additive):
The drug or chemical substance is intentionally added to:
- control diseases
- promote growth
- preserve feed (antifungal)

B. Unintentional residue (indirect additive, or it is called "accidental") like, rodents' control drugs on pesticides, antibiotics to treat diseases related to infections of animals, growth hormones added on animal feed supplements, and so on.

The residue that occurs as an environmental contaminant or may be acquired at any phase in the production, processing, or storage of animal products are:

1. Antimicrobial agents: penicillin, streptomycin, polypeptides, tetracyclines, chloramphenicol (aplastic anemia), sulfonamides and quinolones.

Food Safety in the Middle East. DOI: https://doi.org/10.1016/B978-0-12-822417-5.00004-0

2. Antiparasitic agents including anthelmintic, antiprotozoal.
3. Insecticides: organophosphates, organochlorines, and so on.
4. Growth promoters and feed additives.
5. Naturally occurring toxins and environmental pollutants.
   - *Naturally occurring toxins* include mycotoxins, marine biotoxins, cyanogenic glycosides, and toxins occurring in poisonous mushrooms.
   - *Persistent organic pollutants*: chemicals that accumulate in the environment and human body, like dioxins and polychlorinated biphenyls, which are unwanted by-products of industrial processes and waste treatment. They find their way in the environment and accumulate in animal food chains. Dioxins are highly toxic and may cause health problems such as damaging the immune system, interfering with hormones and cause cancer.
6. Heavy metals such as lead, cadmium, and mercury that cause neurological and kidney damage. Contamination by heavy metal in food chain occurs mainly through pollution of air, water, or soil.
7. Dyes like Gentian Violet, Malachite Green, and Methylene Blue are used for numerous purposes, including animal husbandry and aquaculture. Food destined for human consumption could contain residues of these compounds and therefore unnecessary exposure to dye residues has the potential for human health hazards.
8. Hormones and antihormones: Estrogens, androgens, and corticoids.

5.2 Hormonal growth-promoting drugs

Of all the drugs used in food animal production, none has evoked greater emotional response among the public than the hormonal growth-promoting drugs. Several recent incidents involving precocious sexual development in infants and young children have been blamed on meat containing the residues of these substances. These production (as opposed to therapeutic) drugs are used to increase the rate of weight gain and/or improve feed efficiency in livestock.

5.3 Synthetic hormonal growth-promoting agents

Trenbolone acetate, a synthetic anabolic hormone with androgenic properties, and zeranol, a product with weak estrogenic activity formed by the reduction of the mycotoxin zearalenone (ZEN), are approved in some countries as growth-promoting implants for use in cattle. Unlike the naturally occurring hormones for which human food safety assessment is based (on a ratio of the amount of these substances consumed in food compared to the amount produced endogenously by the consumer), safety assessment for the synthetic hormones must be based on alternative strategies. The major impediment to establishing safe tissue concentrations of the synthetic hormones results primarily from their ability to produce tumors in laboratory animals, when these compounds are fed at high concentrations. These tumors occur only in endocrine-sensitive tissues and are similar to those produced by high doses of the naturally occurring hormones.

5.4 Somatotropic hormones

The newest member of the anabolic hormonal growth-promoting drugs is somatotropic hormone, also called growth hormone, somatotropin, bovine somatotropin or porcine somatotropin. Somatotropic hormone administered to livestock is reported to produce dramatic increases in animal growth, milk production, and altered body composition, favoring the development of lean muscle mass and a decrease in body fat. Residues of bovine somatotropic hormones in meat or milk are not a risk to the human consumer.

5.5 Chemical residues that constitute a real hazard to human health

1. Hypersensitivity or allergic reactions due to antibiotic residues

   Antibiotics (i.e., penicillin and streptomycin and, to a lesser extent, novobiocin and lindomycin) appear from clinical usage in human beings to be more inclined to produce hypersensitivity or allergies than others. A good example is that penicillin may enter food for human consumption from intramammary infusion to treat mastitis in dairy cows.
2. Carcinogenic effect

   This effect is produced by a substance having carcinogenic or cancer producing (substance) activity. There is good evidence that a large amount is required for a carcinogen to induce its effect. For example, 3×10^9 molecules/liver cell of aflatoxin (causes abortion in pregnant animals and humans) in a single dose produces hepato-carcinoma in rats.
3. Mutagenic effect

   Mutagen is used to describe those chemical agents that damage the genetic components of a cell (DNA) inducing gene mutations or chromosomal damages.
4. Teratogenic effect

   A teratogen applies to a drug or chemical agents that produce a toxic effect on the embryo or fetus during a critical phase of the gestation period. As a consequence, a congenital malformation that affects the structural and functional integrity of the organ is produced. Example: some anthelmintic feed additives.
5. Drug resistant and cross resistant

   The development of resistant strains of pathgenic bacteria, consequently finally leads to the failure of antimicrobial therapy in human beings.

5.6 Terminology used in residues

Most are derivatives from US Food and Drug Administration (FDA).

5.6.1 Permissible limits of drug residues

The quantity of the residue permitted for consumption. The assessment of this level is by the determination of the dose level showing no observable effect in at least two species of animals; one of them is nonrodent.

5.6.2 No effect (observable) level

The level of drug or chemical that produces no harmful effect (no change or effect on physiological activity, organ weight, body weight, and cellular structure and enzymatic activity of cells) when fed for 2 years to the most sensitive species.

5.6.3 Acceptable daily intake

It is the amount of drug (residue) that could be consumed by an adult person daily during his life span without any health disturbances.

5.6.4 Withdrawal time

It is clearly written in all veterinary drugs used and refers to the interval from the time an animal is removed from medication until the permitted time of consumption of animal products (meat, milk, eggs, etc.). This interval is not to safeguard the health of the animal but it is required to minimize or prevent high levels of drug residues in edible tissues for human consumptions.

Withdrawal time:

Vary from few hours to several days or months according to

- Drug type (synthesis)
- Route of administration
- Type of animal product (milk vs meat or spleen).

For example, 120 days are required, following the implantation of diethylstilbestrol before slaughtering for human consumption.

5.6.5 Tolerance level (maximum permissible residue level)

It is the maximum level or concentration of a drug or chemical that is permitted in or on food at a specified time of slaughter and processing, storage, and marketing of the feed up to the time of consumption by humans.

5.6.6 Maximum residue limit

It is the foremost consciousness of a chemical residue, counseled with the assist of the utilization of the Codex Alimentarius Commission (CAC) to be lawfully commissioned in or in food commodities and animal feeds (FAO/WHO, 2018).

5.6.7 Extraneous maximum residue limit

Pesticide residues coming from an environment. It is the most important contaminant that is stimulated by means of functionality of the CAC to be lawfully commissioned or diagnosed satisfactory on a food, agricultural goods, or animal nourishment (FAO/WHO, 2018).

5.6.8 Limit of determination

It is the minimal condensation of a residue that can be recognized and quantitatively measured in assurance in meal and feed commodity, which used to be 1.22 $\mu g\ kg^{-1}$ with a desirable degree of reliance by the way of a regulatory approach of analysis (FAO/WHO, 2018).

5.6.9 Acceptable daily intake

It is the everyday consumption which, at some stage in a complete lifetime, appears to be without good-sized danger to the health of the consumer (FAO/WHO, 2018).

5.6.10 Temporary acceptable daily intake

It is a proper each day consumption setup for a specified, restricted duration to allow additional biochemical, toxicological, or other records to be acquired as might also be required for estimating an applicable daily intake. (FAO/WHO, 2018).

5.7 General considerations in residues

Residues and chemical food contaminants come from different sources, like ingredients of natural toxins, industrial pollution, agrochemicals/veterinary drugs, food processing, and packaging. Residues can be deposited in plant or animal tissues. The main industrial or other contamination residue sources go to environment, air, food, water, and soil and then by inhalation, contact, or ingestion may reach human or livestock (Thompson & Darwish, 2019).

The major causes of drug residue in food-producing animals are no observation of withdrawal periods, no treatment records, overdose, or using prohibited drugs for animal treatment (Bobkov & Zbinden, 2018). The presence of unexpected residues in foods like meat, milk, and eggs may be due to unintentional or cross-contaminated feed and addition of antimicrobial to feed ingredients or water. Many drug-related factors like formulation type, site, route of administration, dose or animal-related factors such as breed, age, sex, and body condition play a major effect on drug residue levels in edible tissues. Drug residue concentration in tissues also depends on the physical or chemical characteristics of the drug. Highly lipid-soluble chemicals can easily enter tissues through passive diffusion, whereas drugs with poor lipid solubility may remain in the extracellular space.

Pesticide exposure can cause negative health effects like loss of coordination, reduced response to stimuli, reduced visual capacity, unusual general behavior, and reduced motor skills. Other health problems involve respiratory disease, hypersensitivity, and some chemicals might lead to cancer, fetal abnormalities, and disruption of hormones (Rather, Koh, Paek, & Lim, 2017).

5.8 Reduction of veterinary drug residues in animal products

The most useful scientifically based approach may depend on Risk Management for Animal Drug Residues (Risk Analysis and Risk Assessment) projects. To perform risk assessment of food safety problems, FDA uses Risk Analysis as suggested by the CAC, which involves risk management, risk assessment, and risk communication to monitor of chemical residues in foods.

Risk Analysis depends on using scientific knowledge combined with coordinated policy. It begins with managers to identify food safety problems that may pose risks and hazards to public health. The risk assessment team performs literature review and data collection, and thus plans a risk assessment case. If the plan is evaluated to be possibly implemented, the risk assessors develop a mathematical model that will answer the questions in concern. Then assessors review and comment on the questions for the ranking of the drug residues drafting a report that is also open for public judgment (inspection). A final report, in which comments are being considered, and upon fulfilling of all the requirements, is then approved.

Of the most important and common chemical residues in animal tissues that will be discussed are pesticides, antimicrobials, mycotoxins, and heavy metals.

5.9 Pesticides

5.9.1 Definition

Pesticides are natural or synthetic substances used by human beings to kill or deter organisms (pests) that threaten human health and well-being, pets and livestock health, or crops (Giliomee, 2008) and being used particularly in agriculture or in areas where human beings live.

It has been found that greater than 80% of the total intake of pesticide residues in human beings was through the food chain (Martinez, Angulo, Pozo, & Jo dral, 1997). Pesticide contamination of animal products results from feeding a diet containing low concentration of pesticides (Aulakh, et al., 2006; Noble, 1990).

Pesticides are used to increase crop yields, improve plant products and protection, and kill pests consisting of insects, rodents, and weeds. Pests consist of organisms that damage the vegetation, or compete with the vegetation for nutrients and water, a fungus that may cause plant illnesses, bacteria and viruses, nematodes, rodents, and bugs that may grow in animals' skin (Cooper & Dobson, 2007). Generally, they are unsafe to humans, both from direct contact or as residues in food. There are more than 1000 pesticides in use and each pesticide has different properties and toxicological effects (Pesticides & Water Pollution, 2017). Pesticides classified either by chemical characteristics like organophosphorus (OPs), organocarbamics (carbamates), organochlorine, hexachlorocyclohexane (HCH), aldrin, dieldrin, and malathion or by target pest (Table 5.1).

5.10 Food contamination by pesticides in the Middle East

5.10.1 Vegetables

Pesticides were heavily detected in fruits and vegetables (Guler, Cakmak, Dagli, Aktumsek, & Ozparlak, 1998), ground drinking water (Arya, 2005), soil (Khan, 1982), and in river water (Turgut, 2003). In a study on vegetables in Egypt, almost, 50% of the analyzed samples contained detectable residues with 32.5% of contaminated samples contain residues at levels lower than the MRLs and 17.5% (36 samples) had residues above the permissible limits. The most commonly detected pesticide groups were OPs

TABLE 5.1 Classification of various types of pesticides according to their action against various pests.

Pesticide	Pest controlled	Pesticide	Pest controlled
Algicide	Algae	Nematicide	Nematodes
Miticide	Mites	Fungicide	Fungi
Molluscicide	Snails, slugs	Herbicide	Weeds
Bactericide	Bacteria	Rodenticide	Rodents
Avicide	Birds	Insecticide	Insects

followed by pyrethroids then triazoles and carbamates, with frequencies percentages of 41.5%, 11.8%, 8.8%, and 8.0%, respectively (Gad Alla, Thabet, & Emil, 2013; Gad Alla, Almaz, Thabet, & Nabil, 2015).

A local Jordanian study conducted for detecting pesticides in a total of 73 samples showed that 46% were free from detectable residues, while 85 samples (54%) contained residues. Among the tested samples, 34 (22%) contained residues above MRLs and 51 (32%) contained residues at or below MRLs (Al Gharibeh & Al Fararjeh, 2019). In another Jordanian report on pesticides in fruits and vegetables (Al-Antary, Alawi, Shaderma, & Haddad, 2018) showed that chlorothalonil exceeded the MRL in all the citrus fruits and approached MRL as those in vegetables. Daminozide levels in citrus fruits were lower than for chlorothalonil but exceeded the MRL. Daminozide levels in cucumber, eggplant, and tomato exceeded the MRL. Several other pesticides, including bensulfuron-methyl and demeton-*S*-methyl-sulfoxide, exceeded the MRL in some of the fruits and vegetables. Chlorothalonil, daminozide, and other pesticides were present in relatively high levels in the irrigation water and soil at each cultivation site (Al-Nasir et al., 2020).

5.10.2 Animal products

In Egypt, Aboul-Enein, Nasr, Abou Elella, and Abdulla (2010) published a report about monitoring some organochlorines and OP residues in imported and locally raised chicken and bovine muscles. This study focused on the detection of pesticides (aldrin, endosulfan II, dieldrin, ppDDE, pirimiphos-methyl, diazinon, chlorpyrifos, and ethoprophos) in meat samples. Samples were prepared and extracts were analyzed using gas chromatography equipped with an electron capture detector and a flame photometric detector. The study demonstrated that high numbers of examined meat were contaminated with organochlorine pesticides (OCPs), especially locally produced products, while fewer samples were contaminated with OP pesticides. All of the imported chicken samples contained residues of aldrin, endosulfan II, dieldrin, and ppDDE, but none of these concentrations exceeded MRL given by the European Union (EU) and FAO/WHO-Codex Alimentarius (2020), whereas samples exceeding MRL values were two samples for diazinon, one sample for ethoprophos, and one sample for chlorpyrifos.

Milk and dairy products could be tainted by pesticides during its processing and handling. In the study in Giza, Palastine, raw milk samples of buffaloes and cows were analyzed for pesticide residues [malathion, profenofos, pirimiphos-methyl, dimethoate, HCB, lindane, aldrin, heptachlor epoxide, chlordane, endrin, and dichlorodiphenyltrichloroethane (DDT)] (Abou Donia, Abou-Arab, Enb, El-Senaity, & Abd-Rabou, 2010). In none of the raw milk samples examined, the presence of any OP pesticides was shown. However, OCPs were detected at values exceeding the MRL value of FAO/WHO for milk. Some residues of pesticides were removed from buttermilk and skimmed milk during the production of butter and cream. Yoghurt and butter were found to contain low levels of OCPs because of the impact of the thermal (heat) processing treatment.

A study aimed to detect some organochlorine, OP, pyrethroid, and carbamate pesticide residues in local fresh chicken meat and its viscera was conducted in Jordan using liquid chromatography−mass spectrophotometry (LC−Ms/MS) technique. A total of 260 samples from local fresh chicken meat and its products were collected. Results showed a prevalence of pesticides (25.16%) for all locally produced muscles, livers, and kidneys. Fenoxycarb, malathion, and diazinon being present in all of the examined samples with 100% prevalence and with 83%, 35.33%, and 0% above MRL for above three compounds, respectively. The profenofos and parathion-methyl from the OP group had 0% prevalence in all local samples (Alnatour, Alaboudi, & Al karasneh, 2019).

Another recent study aimed to determine the prevalence of hexachlorcyclohexane, aldrin, and malathion pesticides residues in home produced eggs in Jordan governorates and the distribution of pesticides in between egg yolk and egg white (Alaboudi, Osaili, & Alrwashdeh, 2019). High performance liquid chromatography was used to detect the pesticides residues. It was found that 66.5% of studied eggs were polluted within pesticides under study. The results indicated no residual level above the MRL for hexachlorcyclohexane, whereas 33% and 44% of samples were positive for aldrin and malathion, respectively. Malathion and aldrin are known for being rapidly distributed in the tissues that intricate and involve in egg development process. Both malathion and aldrin residues were detected in both yolk and white from all different Jordanian governorates' samples, whereas HCH was detected only in yolk. Samples from agricultural localities revealed the highest level of contamination in comparison to another Jordanian governorate. These findings may suggest that hen's body is exposed to pesticides directly through the ingestion of the chemical compounds (e.g., birds ingest seeds contaminated with pesticides) (Prosser & Hart, 2005) or through dermal exposure after a spray event, or by eating dead insects contaminated with pesticides (Mineau, 2011). Another study also in Jordan added new knowledge on pesticides contamination in home produced eggs, which reflect the misusage of pesticides and come on a parallel line to prior studies in the nearby areas on animal-origin products like meat, yogurt, milk, and cheese (Abdulkhaliq, Swaileh, Hussein, & Matani, 2012).

In other types of meat samples, a local Jordanian study conducted on 519 samples (lamb and poultry meat) including table eggs showed the presence of various pesticides. Aldrin, DDT and metabolites, dieldrin, endosulfan isomers, endrin, HCH isomers, heptachlor, heptachlor epoxide, and hexachlorobenzene (HCB) were present. The results showed that 28% (38/134), 20% (23/115), and 49% (131/270) of the eggs, chicken, and meat samples, respectively, were contaminated with OCP residues, prominently by HCHs and

DDTs. However, heptachlor, heptachlor epoxide, HCB, aldrin, and endrin compounds presented in less than 7% of the tested samples (Ahmad, Salem, & Estaitieh, 2010). Another study from Jordan was conducted on milk, table eggs, meat, and poultry. Results of milk products showed that there were only two samples contained residues but less than the MRL. Results of table eggs showed that there were 11 samples contained residues but less than the MRL. There were three samples of the table eggs contained residues more than the MRL. These contaminated samples contained p,p′-DDE. Results of meat and poultry showed that there were thirty-three meat samples contained residues, but less than the MRL. However, the contaminated samples were contained α-HCH, β-HCH, γ-HCH, heptachlor, aldrin, p,p′-DDE, p,p′-DDT, and p,p′-DDD (Al-Antary et al., 2018). Also, a study carried on chlorinated pesticides residues was done through 2013–14 (Alawi, Al-Antary, Estityah, & Haddad, 2016). All positive egg samples (11/35), milk products (2/30), and meat (21/55) contained HCH, DDT, heptachlor, and aldrin at a level below MRL level. A whole of 192 poultry eggs and chicken meat samples were assessed in an Iraqi province (Dyala). The residues evaluation confirmed that all poultry eggs and laying hens' meat samples were positive for delta-methrin residues and at value above the MRLs (Abbas, 2016).

Organophosphate insecticides, such as malathion, are strong acetylcholinesterase inhibitors used to control ticks and lice in poultry farms (Alawi, Ammari, & Al-Shuraiki, 1992). The routes of organophosphates transition in chickens are skin, eyes, inhalation, and digestion (Nasir, Bilto, & Al-Shuraiki, 1998). After absorption, organophosphates are widely processed and spread to surrounding tissues, muscle, fat, different organs, and skin and to the egg in poultry (Rafat, Salem, & Hussein, 2010). In chickens, the organophosphates residues can be detected in tissues and eggs after a few weeks (Le Doux, 2011). A study in Jordan on 500 samples of eggs, chicken, and meat, which were analyzed for OCP residues showed that 28% (38/134) of the examined eggs were contaminated with OCP residues with a high level of HCHs and DDTs (Rafat et al., 2010).

Pesticides are commonly recovered from marine environment. Pesticides enter the marine surroundings, streams, and rivers via leaching through waste and storm water systems, spray drift from agriculture, vapor, and as direct runoff. Also sometimes results in a rise of total suspended pesticides can enter the surface water as either water-dissolved or particle-associated chemicals (Maurya, Malik, & Sharma, 2019). Fishes are uncovered from pesticides contamination; these contaminants reach the aquatic animals via different routes such as inhalation by gills, through ingesting pesticides-contaminated water, or by consuming others influenced by chemicals (Helfrich, Weigmann, Hipkins, & Stinson, 2009).

Studies from in Egypt in fish collected from different locations (Delta Lakes) found that the OCPs were the foremost pesticides found in fish samples. DDTs was detected with mean concentrations of 0.59 ppm (Badawy and El Dib, 1984). Also, a hundred samples from five distinctive Egyptian fish collected from market were analyzed. Chemical analysis confirmed the presence of some OCs (DDTs), Gamma BHC, Delta BHC, methoxychlor, endrin, endosulfan sulfate, and heptachlor residues in the flesh of the examined fish. Endrin, or p,p-DDT, PP-DDD, and Delta BHC occurrence levels were above the MRL value (Marzouk, Shoukry, Ali, Naser, & Fayed, 2016).

In Saudi Arabia, a study conducted on cultured farm fish indicated that the pesticide residues detected in fish samples were five members of the organochlorine pesticides, namely p,p-DDT, p,p-DDE, p,p-DDD, γ-HCH, and heptachlor; and three members of OP pesticides, namely: α-endosulfan, diazinon, and chlorpyrifos with different concentrations levels. All detected pesticide residues were under the values set for MRLs (El-Saeid, 2010).

A recent Jordanian study was accomplished to determine the levels of 30 pesticide residues representing the organochlorines (DDTs and metabolites, endosulfan, chlordane, dieldrin, heptachlor, lindane, aldrin, heptachlor epoxide, methoxychlor, and HCB), OP (chlorpyrifos, malathion, fenitrothion, dichlorovos, diazinon, imidan, parathion, methyl parathion, azinphosmethyl, azamethiphos, and profenofos), pyrethroids (cypermethrin, delta-methrin, bifenthrin, and permethrin), and carbamates group (carbofuran, carbaryl, aldicarb, fenoxycarb, and methomy) in fishes (Alaboudi & Al Jarah, 2019). Various imported frozen fish samples (194) were collected from the most common fish type species (26) from different geographical location. Additionally, a total of 24 fish representing local 5 fresh species (Tilapia, Catfish, Gray Mullet, Tuna, and Shark) were also collected from the Al-Aghoar and Gulf of Aqaba districts. Samples were analyzed using LC−Ms/Ms and pesticides levels were compared with international and Jordanian acceptable standards (MRL). Results showed that all fish types (100%) were affected by a different percentage of 23 pesticides, and with no significant differences between local and imported types. In 15/23 pesticides detected residues were at concentrations >MRL (10 ppb). All 218 local (24 fresh samples) and imported (194 frozen) fish samples were contaminated with at least three different compounds. The contamination rate with four pesticides was 0.5%, whereas the percentage of fish contaminated with six pesticides was 55%. The highly contaminated species from all studied samples was Hake-Argentina (12 compounds) with a prevalence rate of 40%, whereas the lowest contaminated species was Mackerel-Iceland (three pesticides) with a prevalence rate of 10% The contamination prevalence rate for local fresh water fish species were: 13%, 17%, and 20% for the Tilapia, Gray Mullet, and Catfish species, respectively, whereas in 215 of the fish samples (98.6%) examined concentrations of pesticides were above the MRL values (Alaboudi & Al Jarah, 2019).

Other studies conducted in Jordan showed that the Gulf of Aqaba (water and biota) is exposed to the possibility of contamination with pesticides. A study conducted in 1995 showed that fish samples (50%) presented a high concentration of almost of all OCPs, with at least one OCP at a higher concentration than the maximum allowable concentration. Sediment samples collected in Gulf of Aqaba were free of OCP contamination and both heptachlor and HCB were detected in 58% of the samples at very low concentrations (Alawi, Hourani, & Abu Hilal, 1995). It is very interesting to notice that the concentration of α-HCH, HCB, o,p′-DDE, p,p′-DDE, o,p′-DDD, p,p′-DDD decreased from 1995 to 2006, whereas the concentration of p,p′-DDT and β-HCH increased significantly from 1995 to 2006 in the samples examined previously (Alawi, 2006).

5.10.3 Residue hazards

Most pesticides are toxic at animal or human in contact with. Toxicity defines as the characteristic poisonous potency of the compound under certain conditions. Hazards are defined as the risk of poisoning when a chemical is used or applied, while poison refers to a chemical substance that had harmful effect when in contact with living organisms during use (Pohanish, 2017). The relative hazard of a pesticide is dependent upon the toxicity of the pesticide, the dose, and the length of time exposed. The hazard in using a pesticide is related to the likelihood of exposure to harmful amounts of the pesticide. The toxicity of a pesticide can't be changed, but the risk of exposure can be reduced with the use of proper personal protective equipment, proper handling, and application procedures. Pesticides toxicity depends on the chemical and physical properties of a substance and can be defined as the ability of being poisonous or harmful to animals or plants. Pesticides have many different modes of action but in general cause biochemical changes that interfere with normal cell functions. This toxicity depends on its function and other factors like the route of exposure such as swallowing, inhaling, or direct contact with the skin. The same pesticide can have different effects at different doses. Generally, insecticides tend to be more toxic to humans than herbicides (Garvin, 2017; Kalyonova & El-Batawi, 2019).

In developing countries, such poisonings are associated strongly with excessive exposure to and inappropriate use of toxic chemicals (Goldman & Tran, 2002) and it comes among the leading causes of death by self-poisoning, particularly in low- and middle-income countries. As they are intrinsically toxic and deliberately spread in the environment, the production, distribution, and use of pesticides require strict regulation and control. Regular monitoring of residues in food and the environment is needed continuously. It has been found that greater than 80% of the total intake of pesticide residues in human beings was through the food chain (Martinez et al., 1997). Unintentional poisonings kill an estimated 355,000 people globally each year (WHO, 2003). The World Health Organization (WHO) report on pesticides in agriculture estimated 220,000 deaths due to pesticide poisoning in 1990; 99% of these were in the developing world and 20,000 were unintentional (WHO, 1990). The WHO estimates that there are 3,000,000 cases of pesticide poisoning each year and up to 220,000 deaths primarily in developing countries (Dixit, Srivastava, & Sharma, 2019).

Acute toxicity is the ability of a substance to cause harmful effects that develop rapidly following exposure, that is, a few hours or a day. Chronic toxicity is the ability of a substance to cause adverse health effects resulting from long-term exposure to a substance. Some pesticides are dangerous after one large dose (acute toxicity). Others can be dangerous after small, repeated doses (chronic toxicity) (Ministry of Agriculture, British Colombia, Canada, 2017). Acute or chronic pesticide poisoning symptoms are a headache, exhaustion, general weakness, dizziness, muscle weakness, anxiety, nausea and vomiting, excessive salivation, diarrhea, and anorexia. While in complicated cases, there is excessive saliva and perspiration, stomach cramps, trembling with poor muscle coordination, and twitching (Nimmo, Hamaker, Matthews, & Moore, 1981).

Each pesticide has different properties and toxicological effect (FAO, 2018). Unintentional poisonings kill an estimated 355,000 people globally each year (WHO, 2003). In developing countries, such poisonings are associated strongly with excessive exposure to, and inappropriate use of, toxic chemicals (Goldman & Tran, 2002).

The International Agency for Research on Cancer (IARC), a part of the WHO, and its monograph arrangement on the evaluation of carcinogenic risks to humans is broadly used to recognize environmental carcinogens and to help guide government policy in protecting people from the risk of cancer due to dietary, ecological, and occupational carcinogens. Right now, IARC classifies two pesticides as human cancer–causing agents specifically, the arsenical insecticides and 2,3,7,8 tetrachlorodibenzo-p-dioxin, a contaminant of the phenoxy herbicide (Tomatis, 2006).

People who face the greatest health risks from exposure to pesticides are those who come into contact with them at work or in their home. Global health agencies (WHO) are to ban pesticides that are most toxic to humans, as well as pesticides that remain for the longest time in the environment to protect public health. WHO, in collaboration with FAO, is responsible for assessing the risks to humans of pesticides—both through direct exposure and through residues in food. The ADIs are used by governments and international risk managers, such as the CAC, to establish MRLs for pesticides in food (USDA, 2019). FAO/WHO-Codex Alimentarius Commission (2020) has adopted MRLs for more than 30 different pesticides in various foods, including crops (barley, rye, and rice), vegetables (garlic, cucumber, and peas), fruits (banana, orange, and grape), and animal products (milk, eggs, and poultry). It has been a significant achievement to translate the results of the FAO/WHO expert meetings on pesticide residues into Codex MRLs.

5.10.4 Processing

Foods are invariably exposed to heat treatment during preparation and preservation; the heat treatment is given in many ways including boiling, pasteurization, frying, freezing, cooking, and so on, depending upon the nature of food and aim of processing, The loss of pesticide residue during heat processing may be due to evaporation, codistillation, thermal degradation, which vary with the chemical nature of the individual pesticide (Sharma, Satya, Kumar, & Tewary, 2005).

In recent study (Alnatour et al., 2019) boiling (90°C–100°C) treatment of pesticides of confirmed positive chicken meat samples (gamma-chlordane, malathion, fenoxcarb, and delta-methrin) for up to 20 min (at time intervals: (5, 10, 15, and 20 min)) caused reduction percentages of 8%, 14%, 25%, and 46%, respectively, for gamma-chlordane; 7%, 16%, 27%, and 48% for malathion; 6%, 13%, 25%, 50% for fenoxycarb; and 7%, 13%, 24%, and 49% for delta-methrin, respectively.

Similarly, to the previous data the effects of common cooking methods (boiling) on buffalo meat resulted in a 58.33% reduction on the levels of aldrin and total endosulfan (Muthukumar et al., 2010). Upon frying treatment, using olive oil at 160°C for 15 min, the percentage reductions were of 23%, 45%, 61%, and 73% after 3, 5, 10, and 15 min, respectively, for gamma-chlordane, whereas for malathion reduction percentages after frying treatment were at 26%, 42%, 59%, and 71%, respectively, after the aforementioned time intervals. Fenoxycarb reductions were at 28%, 45%, 62%, and 77% and finally, for delta-methrin, the percentages were at 23%, 39%, 58%, and 74% after 3, 5, 10, and 15 min, respectively. Frying also reduced organochlorine (lindane and DDT) pesticides residues in chicken meat by 75% (Street, 1969), which comes in parallel to the previous study. Frying is in general use in food industries due to its low cost. The process depends on the oil–food interaction at high temperatures, which cooks and dehydrates the food, leading to chemical and physical changes (protein denaturation, starch gelatinization, flavoring, and color production) via Maillard reaction (Bordin, Kunitake, Aracava, & Trindade, 2013). Therefore high temperature in frying treatment causes protein denaturation beside their effect on fat itself. Most pesticides being fat soluble and meats subjected to high temperatures may cause fat melting, consequently resulting in pesticides leaking out of the meat fat and into the frying oil. Various thermal processing treatments like pasteurization, blanching, boiling, cooking, steaming, canning, scrambling, and so on, have been found valuable in the degradation of various pesticides depending upon the type of pesticide and length of treatment (Bajwa and Sandhu, 2014). In Egypt, heat treatment of some selected muscles of chicken and bovine samples (boiling for 1.5 h) produced overall reductions of 40.4%, 55.0%, 32.4%, 33.5%, 29.2%, 42.7%, and 38.2% in DDTs, lindane, dieldrin, aldrin, endrin, toxaphene, and HCB contents, respectively (Aboul-Enein et al., 2010).

Although meat cooking is not the guarantee efficient way to destroy and remove pesticides from meat to acceptable level, that is, below MRL; high-temperature treatment like frying with oil is a better way to reduce the levels of pesticide residues in poultry meat compared to boiling. However, heat treatment is not the recommended way to substitute strict hygienic measures to avoid the presence of pesticides in poultry and efficient ways to limit the uncontrolled ways of using pesticides in agricultural industry.

In Egypt, organochlorine and OP pesticide residues were discovered to be degraded by boiling of milk samples of 5.48%, 24.49%, 6.06%, 22.38%, 100%, 45.1%, 16.67%, 2.63%, and 15.14% for HCB, β-HCH, Υ-HCH, heptachlor, H. epoxide, aldrin, endrin, p′p-DDT, and p′p-DDE, respectively, while, 100% degradation occurred to dimethoate, pirimiphos-methyl, phorate, and chlorpyrifos, respectively (Ismail & Elkassas, 2016). Also pasteurization with 4 mg of malathion and dimethioate spiked into 100 g buffalo milk samples, the result showed approximately 76% and 96%, respectively, of degradation (Abd-Rabo, Elsalamony, & Sakr, 2016). In contaminated eggs in Jordan (malathion, aldrin, and HCH) heat treatment (boiling at 100°C −15 min and frying at 160°C −5 min) significantly reduced contamination levels to values below maximum residual limit (0.02) ppm (Alaboudi et al., 2019).

A recent study in Jordan (Alaboudi & Al Jarrah, 2019) examined the effect of heat processing treatment by different cooking method (roasting and frying) applied to fish, contaminated with various pesticides (endosulfan, melathione, chlorpyrifos, bifenthrine, fenoxycarb). Generally, heat treatments applied by frying reduced the contamination levels by a range of 53%–95%, whereas roasting reduced the concentrations by 61%–90%. Therefore data of this study revealed that the frying process is more effective than roasting in removing pesticides from fish.

Generally frying greatly affects the organic process composition as a result of water loss, fat uptake, and changes within the profile of fatty acids caused by oxidization and isomerization, macromolecule oxidization, loss of amino acids, and variation within the contents of vitamins and minerals (Bouchon & Dueik, 2018).

Cooking time and temperature are the crucial factors influencing the reduction of residues. Most pesticides are reduced upon preparation (frying, roasting, and boiling). However, their reduction might lead to the formation of degradation products that vary little from original compounds (Bajwa & Sandhu, 2014). Cooking meat and fish containing pesticides residues might cause the formation of harmful compounds. Though reduction within the levels of chemical residues might occur by evaporation or thermal degradation throughout heat treatment, owing to their oleophilic behavior and affinity for fatty tissue, the removal of fat tissues in fish and meat, before preparation, might contribute to a reduced intake of those contaminants (Ali-Aberoumand, 2014). Frying resulted in higher water loss and macromolecule gain than the opposite preparation strategies principally because of the absorption of the fat by the fish throughout frying (García-Arias, Pontes, García-Linares, García-Fernández, & Sánchez-Muniz, 2003).

In Jordanian eggs, pesticides (malathion, aldrin, and HCH) levels were quite stable during refrigeration storage for up to 1 month (Alaboudi et al., 2019). Freezing treatment at −70°C for up to 4 weeks showed no significant reduction in the concentration of examined pesticides (gamma-chlordane, malathion, fenoxcarb, and delta-methrin) in Jordanian chicken meat. Reduction percentages ranged from 4%, 8%, 11%, and 15% after 1 week, 2 weeks, 3 weeks, and 4 weeks, respectively (Alaboudi et al., 2019). The same observations were noted on the effects of freezing for 1 month on pesticides (endosulfan, malathion, chlorpyrifos, bifenthrine, fenoxycarb) in contaminated fish purchased from various markets in Jordan. Reductions of only 6%−30% were recorded (Alaboudi & Al Jarah, 2019).

5.10.5 Conclusion

Therefore finally it may be concluded that food of plant or animal products surveyed in Middle East countries are highly contaminated with pesticides and heat treatment or freezing is not guarantee for pesticide clearance to reach acceptable level. Most pesticides are harmful to consumer and may be considerably toxic at high levels.

5.10.6 Recommended control measures

1. Additional efforts are needed to minimize the undesirable environmental consequences of the use of pesticides by the establishment of governmental routine pesticides residues monitoring.
2. Regular monitoring of food of animal or plant origin or their products for pesticides residues is strictly recommended.
3. Health education programs to raise the awareness and attitudes of using pesticides are highly supported.
4. Activation of legislations and laws to control the usage of pesticides in developing countries is highly recommended.

5.11 Antimicrobials

5.11.1 Introduction

Antibiotics are defined as the substances that are able to inhibit the growth of various microorganisms. They are produced naturally by living organisms or synthetically. Veterinary medicines, especially antibiotics, are among the most important compounds related to animal feed production. Approximately 80% of the animals used in food production are currently being treated with veterinary drugs in a certain part or all through their lives (Pavlov, Lashev, Vachin, & Rusev, 2008). Antibiotics are used for two main purposes: as preventive and curative drugs and as feed additives or growth promoters (Darwish et al., 2013). These drugs are quickly excreted from the animal; others are not readily metabolized or excreted and so, their residues will persist in the animal tissues and hence enter the human food chain constituting health risks to the consumers.

Antibiotics are administered to animals in different ways. It is known that residue levels occurring from injectable sources are more than those resulting from feeding (Katz & Brady, 2000). Improvement in growth due to antibiotics was first described in the middle of 1940s. Use of food additives may improve feed efficiency: 17% in beef cattle, 10% in lambs, 15% in poultry, and 15% in swine. But their indiscriminate use will produce toxicity in consumers (Nisha, 2008).

5.11.2 Sources and food contamination

In veterinary medicine, β-lactams (penicillin and cephalosporin), tetracyclines, chloramphenicol, macrolides, spectinomycin, lincosa-mide, sulfonamides, nitrofuranes, nitroimidazoles, trimethoprim, polymyxins, quinolones, and macrocyclines (ansamycins, glycopeptides, and aminoglycosides) are used for different purposes (Cháfer-Pericás, Maquieira, & Puchades, 2010). Antibiotics may enter to human body in different ways as directly or indirectly by using them as growth stimulants, disease prevention and treatment, and contamination in animals (Phillips et al., 2004).

Several studies confirmed the prevalence of antimicrobial residues in table eggs or chicken meat or large animals' products with levels exceeding permissible limits. In Jordan, a local screening study revealed that 84 out of 180 (46.6%) of the local fresh poultry samples contained antimicrobial residues, where 26.6%, 32.7%, and 38.3% of muscle, liver, and kidney tissues, respectively, showed positive results (Alaboudi & Al Hijazin, 2010). A 12.8% of 2500 table eggs (forming 500 composite samples) screened using Premi test were positive for the presence of antimicrobial residues. Antimicrobial residues were detected in either egg white, egg yolk, or both in Jordan (Alaboudi, Abu Basha, & Musallam, 2013). From all 64 antimicrobial positive samples, egg white had high prevalence (47 samples) of antimicrobial residues in comparison to that of yolk (17 samples) or the 9 samples that contain the residues in both yolk and white simultaneously. The distribution of antimicrobials in between white and yolk is mainly related to antimicrobial composition and egg compartments properties (Furusawa, 2001). These considerably high figure of residues in egg indicates an extensive abuse of veterinary drugs in local poultry industry. In Saudi Arabia, AL-Mustafa et al. (2000) designed a screening study in eastern province involving 32 broiler farms and 22 (69%) farms showed antibiotic residues.

In another Iraqi study, liver and breast muscle had the highest percentage of antibiotic detected in liver (56%), followed by (44%) for thigh muscle (Shareef, Jamel, & Yonis, 2009). In Saudi Arabia (El-Ghareeb et al., 2019), a study was conducted on antimicrobial residues in animal tissues. Results indicated the occurrence of antimicrobial residues in the examined samples at levels below the recommended MRL values, except for sulfamethazine that was detected at higher levels. Six antimicrobial residues were detected in samples collected from sheep; however, only three antimicrobials were detected in camel and cattle meat. Information on occurrence of residues of veterinary drugs varies considerably due to different veterinary practices and systems of veterinary drug residue control. An antibiotic residue at 10.8% was detected in raw beef or at 10.4%–13.2% in sheep meat in Erbil (Iraq) (Al Mashhadany, 2019, 2020).

Findings from another Middle East study of tetracycline residues in food products of animal origin in Kuwait showed that the level of antibiotic residues was higher than the maximum permissible limit (MPL) in 5% of poultry and 18% of milk samples examined (Al-Mazeedi et al., 2009). Another example of antibiotic residues in foods, consumed in the Middle East, involved a study of detection of antibiotics residues in chicken meat products in Al-Najaf, province of Iraq (Shamsa, 2013). In this study, both local and imported chicken products were examined and samples included liver, breast muscle, thigh muscle, and gizzard. Results showed that the prevalent antibiotic residues in imported products were 60% versus 42.5% in local products. The results also revealed that the most prevalent antibiotic was sulfadiazine (27.5%) followed by oxytetracycline and chloramphenicol, while the lowest neomycin was at 10%. In imported products the highest prevalent antibiotics were oxytetracycline (40%) followed by sulfadiazine, neomycin, and chloramphenicol in percentage rate of 27.5%, 15%, and 3%, respectively.

In many Middle Eastern countries, antibiotics can easily be obtained over the counter. Findings from a study done in 2010 in Riyadh, Saudi Arabia, showed that antibiotics could readily be obtained without a prescription in 244 (78%) of 327 pharmacies. In the same line a parallel survey of 405 community pharmacists in Jordan, 381 (94%) suspected that their staff dispensed drugs without prescription, mostly antibiotics, cough or cold preparations, and benzodiazepines (Habibzadeh, 2013).

5.11.3 Residues hazards

The assessment of the risk–benefit ratio for the use of the drug in living organisms should be made before using (Phillips et al., 2004). Prohibition of antibiotic use in the production of foodstuffs may not be a realistic approach. It is also important to ensure that antimicrobial agents in animal production are controlled by relevant authorities, and meat and internal organs should be investigated for drug residues before selling and consumption. The elimination half-life of antibiotics must be considered before the introduction of food products to the market. The WHO has urged a ban on growth-promoting antibiotics (GPAs) arguing that their use leads to various health problems in humans (Bacanlı & Başaran, 2019).

The misuse of antibiotics in Middle Eastern countries comes from an example study in Saudi Arabia. This study reported that 29 antimicrobial agents were identified as being available for poultry use, of which 22 (75.9%) were important for the treatment of human infections. Enrofloxacin, oxytetracycline, ampicillin, neomycin, sulfamethoxazole, colistin, doxycycline, and erythromycin were the most frequently used drugs. Food-borne hypersensitivity reactions and the emergence of microbial resistance, as well as cross-resistance to the various groups of antibiotics in animals and its transfer to human pathogens, are well documented. The study concluded that the misuse of antibiotics in the local poultry industry poses a serious health risk to the public and may complicate the treatment of human infections (Al-Mustafa and Al-Ghamdi, 2001). The most important pathological lesions produced by antibiotic residues in food are transfer of antibiotic-resistant bacteria to the human, Immunopathological effects, autoimmunity, carcinogenicity (sulfamethazine, oxytetracycline, furazolidone), mutagenicity, nephropathy (gentamicin), hepatotoxicity, reproductive disorders, bone marrow toxicity (chloramphenicol), and allergy (penicillin) (Nisha, 2008).

In many Middle East countries, authorities (EU) had banned the use of antibiotics as feed additives or growth promoters for livestock production (EU, 2010). In addition, WHO, EU, and other regulatory authorities had set MPLs for antimicrobial residues in food of animal origin; food products that contain higher levels of antimicrobials than MRLsare unsuitable for human consumption (European Center for Disease Prevention and Control, 2012). The maximum residue limits ($\mu g\ kg^{-1}$) may range from 0.0 level for novobiocin, chloramphenicol, fluoroquinolones or 20, 30, 40, and 50 for cefquinome, cloxacillin, erythromycin, and tyrosine, respectively, and may reach up to 100 for tetracycline, oxytetracycline, neomycin, and sulfonamides or 200 $\mu g\ kg^{-1}$ for streptomycin and apramycin (Nisha, 2008). In April, 2012, the FDA issued a promising voluntary plan to limit antibiotic use in agriculture and in turn limit the amount of antibiotics ingested by people.

In any way, the important questions to be asked is, how much effect on human therapy and is it enough to outweigh the benefits gained by the use of antibiotics in animal feed to maintain a cost-effective contact food supply. By all means, the safety levels of food must be strictly observed, drug products should be used in accordance with the labeled directions, and public awareness should be created on the public health significance of antibiotic residue using different media. There are few reports documenting adverse reactions in persons consuming drug residue–contaminated foods, and the overwhelming majority of these related to allergic (not toxic) reactions toward penicillin. Other harmful antibiotics residues effect in that it may cause various toxic effects such as transfer of antibiotic-resistant bacteria to humans, allergy, immunopathological effects, carcinogenicity mutagenicity, nephropathy (gentamicin), hepatotoxicity, reproductive disorders, bone marrow toxicity, and even anaphylactic shock in humans (Darwish et al., 2013; Nisha, 2008).

In the developing world including Middle East world, multiresistant bacteria to various antibiotics are becoming very big problem in the treatment of diseases (Willis, 2000). Several important factors can accelerate the evolution of drug resistance. These include the overuse and misuse of antimicrobials, inappropriate use of antimicrobials, subtherapeutic dosing, and patient noncompliance with the recommended course of treatment. Exposure of a pathogen to an antimicrobial compound can select for chromosomal mutations conferring resistance, which can be transferred vertically to subsequent microbial generations and eventually become predominant in a microbial population that is repeatedly exposed to the antimicrobial. The impact of transmissible drug resistance on public health has been controversial since the early days of antimicrobial use. The controversy is fueled by the amount of drug used in animal agriculture. The bulk of animal drugs are administered for growth-promoting purposes. Growth-promoting drugs are given to animals for much of their life at levels which are considered too low to inhibit the growth of most pathogens. When high concentrations of antibiotics were used, their residues have been found in the blood and the other tissues of the animals. Direct contamination of animal derived feed may occur from air and water during processing, storage, and transportation. Antibiotics in feed given to animals are the examples of indirect contamination (Nisha, 2008). The other problem is the contamination of feed with fecal recycling. The drug excreted in the feces of the treated animals. These feces can contaminate the feed of other untreated animals (Darwish et al., 2013). Vegetables may also be contaminated from feces especially in countries in where feces are generally used as a fertilizer (Phillips et al., 2004).

5.11.4 Effect of processing

Animal products are usually not consumed raw and are generally refrigerated and subjected to heat before being consumed. These treatments can cause protein denaturation, dehydration, and pH changes that can eventually result in chemical changes, concentration, or alter the solubility of the antimicrobial residues. Therefore some antimicrobial residues are chemically unstable and may undergo degradation during storage and heat treatment (Botsoglou & Fletouris, 2000).

Antimicrobials in egg components are sensitive to high temperatures. For example, boiling eggs at 100°C for 15 min or frying eggs at 160°C for 5 min resulted in an 87% and 93% reduction in the mean residual concentrations of ciprofloxacin and enrofloxacin, respectively. Also, it was shown that sulfanilamide content, in both egg albumen and yolk, was reduced by 66% (upon boiling) and by 89%–91% (upon frying) (Alaboudi and Al hijazin, 2010).

In other study in Egypt, in eggs subjected to thermal treatments, reduced enrofloxacin and tetracycline residues by 52% and 47%, and ciprofloxacin, enrofloxacin, and sulfanilamide residues by 87%, 93%, and 89%–91%, were obtained, respectively (Fath El-Bab, 2012). The heat stability of antimicrobial drug residues in poultry muscle tissues demonstrated a decrease in the concentration for oxytetracycline, tetracycline, and chlortetracycline. The decrease in the concentration was appreciable at 50°C, 70°C, and significant at 90°C with a percentage reduction of 3.2%, 3.1%, and 8.4%, respectively (Fath El-Bab, 2012).

However, such percentage reductions in antimicrobial-contaminated animal tissues will not make foods free of such residues or decrease them to safer levels for human consumption (lower than MRL) (Alaboudi & Al hijazin, 2010).

During meat thermal treatments, oxytetracycline, ampicillin, and chloramphenicol residues were decreased by 12%–50%, sulfonamide residues by 45%–61%. Milk sterilization helped degrading tetracycline by approximately 98%, and sulfonamides within a range of 0%–99%. Sterilization also reduced macrolides and aminoglycosides residues by 93%, and >95%, respectively. Lincomycin and tylosin are almost heat stable in milk treatment, whereas ampicillin is degraded by almost 25% in milk after boiling and penicillin-G by less than 40%. Quinolones are stable during thermal treatment and decreased by only 10% in milk, but ciprofloxacin and norfloxacin were degraded by almost 13% and 12% during thermal treatment of milk, respectively. In eggs, florfenicol is heat labile and degraded (by 78%) by frying and boiling. Oxytetracycline and tetracycline are reduced by 40% and 30%, respectively, but after milk pasteurization lincomycin and tylosin were almost heat stable in milk treatment (Rana Md, Lee, Kan, & Hur, 2019).

5.11.5 Storage effects on antimicrobials

In Jordan, it was found that the antimicrobials of enrofloxacin and ciprofloxacin in eggs under refrigeration conditions of 10°C were unstable. Instability of antimicrobials increased with refrigeration time where a 44%–50% reduction for enrofloxacin and ciprofloxacin after 4 weeks of storage. Ambient storage of eggs also reduced ciprofloxacin and enrofloxacin in eggs. After 2 weeks of storage at room temperature, a 34%–35% reduction in ciprofloxacin occurred in egg white and yolk whereas enrofloxacin concentrations were reduced to 54% in yolk and 69% in egg white after 2 weeks of storage (Alaboudi et al., 2013).

The mean concentration of tetracyclines residues decreased by 4% at the end of the 3-months freezing storage, which does not represent appreciable losses (oxytetracycline, tetracycline and chlortetracycline) in poultry muscle tissues. These findings suggest that freezing is not an effective treatment in treating high levels of these antimicrobials (Alaboudi & Al hijazin, 2010).

5.11.6 Conclusion

The misuse of antibiotics in the local animal industry poses a serious health risk to the public and may complicate the treatment of human infections. The veterinary use of antimicrobial agents, especially those with dual animal and human applications, should therefore be restricted. Food-borne hypersensitivity reactions and the emergence of microbial resistance, as well as cross-resistance to the various groups of antibiotics in animals and its transfer to human pathogens, are well documented. Therefore it can be concluded that the most common causes of drug residues in food products are:

1. the failure to meet the withdrawal times;
2. improper use of licensed substances; and
3. the improper health status of animals that may affect the drug pharmacokinetics.

5.11.7 Recommended control measures

Each country should regulate antimicrobial drugs as well as products containing them. A comprehensive approach suggested by the WHO (2013a, 2013b) and the EU (2010) should be adopted, and each country should establish a national monitoring program on antimicrobial use in food animals. Such an approach can be done by gathering data from veterinarians, animal producers, manufacturers, distributors, and pharmaceutical records. A number of countries have banned the use of certain antibiotics in agriculture (Castanon, 2007). Legislation regarding the control of antibiotic residues in animals and their products were given in EU Council Directive 96/23/EC (EU, 1996). Subtherapeutic doses of antibiotic usage in food animals have been banned in the EU countries. However, in spite of the prohibitions in these countries, most of the antibiotics are still being used in animals for the treatment and/or prevention of diseases and growth promotion in many countries (Muaz, Riaz, Akhtar, Park, & Ismail, 2018). Again, it is of interest to report on claiming by other authors that, the use of GPAs in poultry production is associated with economic losses to the producers. Collected data are of considerable importance in the ongoing national debate concerning the continued use of antibiotics for growth promotion of food animals. Based on one the industry study and the resulting economic impact, the use of GPAs in the United States poultry production should be reconsidered (Graham, Boland, & Silbergeld, 2007).

The development of simple and economic field test to identify drug residue in edible animal products and use of activated charcoal, resin, and UV irradiation also help in antibiotic inactivation. Increasing public awareness on the repercussions of overuse of antibiotics will place pressure on animal agriculture to incorporate good management practices so as to avoid the consumption of animal products that have illegal concentrations of antimicrobials residues exceeding MRL. The veterinary use of antimicrobial agents, especially those with dual animal and human applications, should therefore be restricted and finally, antimicrobial use in animal production should never substitute for poor farm management and veterinary practices.

5.12 Mycotoxins

5.12.1 Introduction

The term mycotoxin was used for the first time in 1961 in the aftermath of a veterinary crisis in England, during which thousands of animals died. The disease was linked to a peanut meal, incorporated in the diet, contaminated with a toxin produced by the filamentous fungus *Aspergillus flavus* (Bennett & Klich, 2003; Richard, 2007). Mycotoxin is a result of fungal growth or it may be defining as fungal metabolites when storage conditions are suitable for their growth. The ideal development condition for fungi are temperatures between 10°C and 40°C, pH extending from 4 to 8, and water activity of over 0.7 (Lacey, Smith, & Henderson, 1991). Dietary contaminants with high mycotoxins concentrations over the tolerable levels may cause injurious effects upon animal and human health. Mycotoxicoses mean the exposure through the ingestion of foods or feeds that were contaminated with mycotoxins (Nelson, Desjardins, & Plattner, 1993).

There are more than 400 known mycotoxins (Huffman, Gerber, & Du, 2010). However, only a few have public health impact according their effect on animal health, transmission, and human toxicity. There are six significant classes of mycotoxins: Aflatoxins, trichothecenes, fumonisins, ZEN, ochratoxin, and certain ergot alkaloids (Erber & Binder, 2004). *Aspergillus*, *Penicillium*, and *Fusarium* are different fungus types, which are the most important mycotoxin producers (Bhat, Sridhar, & Karim, 2010). Fungi species varied in the ability of growth, where Fusarium can grow at higher temperature and lower water activity than *Aspergillus* and *Penicillium* species (Reddy et al., 2010). Naturally we can find more than one toxin in one sample; this shows synergistic effects between mycotoxins, like aflatoxins with vomitoxin, ochratoxins and fumonisins, and fumonisins with vomitoxin. Aspergillus toxins can be categorized into four groups: nephrotoxins, neurotoxins, immunotoxins, and hepatotoxins (Binder, Tan, Chin, Handl, & Richard, 2007). The major mycotoxins are illustrated in Table 5.2 (D'Mello, Porter, Macdonald, & Placinta, 2019).

TABLE 5.2 Mycotoxins and their fungi producer.

Mycotoxin	Fungal species
Aflatoxins	*A. flavus; A. parasiticus; A. nomius*
Ochratoxin	*Penicillium viridicatum; P. cyclopium*
Patulin	*P. expansum*
Deoxynivalenol	*Fusarium culmorum; F. graminearum F. sporotrichioides*
T-2 toxin	*F. sporotrichioides; F. poae*
Diacetoxyscirpenol	*F. sporotrichioides; F. graminearum; F. poae*
Zearalenone	*F. culmorum; F. graminearum; F. sporotrichioides*
Fumonisins	*F. moniliforme*
Ergopeptine alkaloids	*Acremonium coenophialum*

5.12.2 Sources

Mycotoxins can attack the yields of crops at different phases of creation; preharvest, as harvests and in the field; like aflatoxins, deoxynivalenol (DON) (vomitoxin), and different species show up during transportation or during stock piling. Environmental conditions that favor fungus and molds growth are temperatures at 25°C − 40°C, while toxin production is enforced at temperatures ranging from 20°C to 30°C. That is why mycotoxins are considering a problem in Middle East countries where the optimal conditions prevail (Iqbal, Nisar, Asi, & Jinap, 2014).

Between February and October 2009, 324 grain, feed, and feed commodity samples were sourced from Middle East and Africa, tested for the presence of A- and B-trichothecenes, ZEN, fumonisins, aflatoxins, and ochratoxin A, or for selected groups of mycotoxins only. The percentage of positive samples of B-trichothecenes ranged from 0% to 87% of tested samples. The prevalence of fumonisins in the different countries was >50% in most cases. ZEN was present in tested commodities from all countries except three. The presence of aflatoxin in analyzed samples varied from 0% to 94%. Ochratoxin A was present in 67% of samples in two African countries. No A-trichothecenes were found in this survey (Rodrigues, Handl, & Binder, 2011).

The definition of carryover toxins is the ratio of toxin transfer from feed to food. Generally, it's below 1% and varied from skeletal musculature, meat, blood serum, and in fat tissue (Beaver, 1990). Based on their function in detoxification, higher carryover ratios can generally be seen in liver and kidney tissue compared to other tissues (Völkel, Schröer-Merker, & Czerny, 2011). Carryover ratios might be affected by animal species, breed, sex, age or production level, and general health status. Periods of toxin withdrawal certainly influence the accumulation of mycotoxins in tissues. A further problem linked to carryover is the enrichment of several mycotoxins due to food processing, as it can be seen for milk powder (AFM1, OTA) and in curd, whey, and cheese (aflatoxin M1) (Battacone, Nudda, Cannas, Cappio Borlino, & Bomboi, 2003).

5.12.3 Food contamination

Food and feed generally are widely exposed to mycotoxin contamination (Milicevica, Nesicb, & Jaksic, 2015).

In a local Jordanian study to detect aflatoxin B1, aflatoxin B2, aflatoxin G1, aflatoxin G2, aflatoxin M1, ochratoxin A, ZEN, fumonisin B1, and DON residues in 150 samples of local fresh chicken meat using LC−Ms/MS technique was reported. Except for ochratoxin all other above types were detected. The results show that 82.0% of local muscle tissue samples were contaminated with aflatoxin M1, exceeding MRL values. Aflatoxins, ZEN, and DON at above MRL values were found in 52.7%, 10.7%, and 8.7% of samples, respectively (Alaboudi & Otoum, 2019).

Another study conducted in Jordan was carried out to evaluate the prevalence of mycotoxins (fumonisin B, aflatoxin B1, DON, and ZEN) residues in local hen's table eggs. Randomly 250 fresh table eggs samples were collected locally from the markets of Jordan. A 67% of the tested samples were positive for mycotoxins presence. Out of 250 samples 168 investigated positive for the presence of one or more toxins, 105 samples revealed the presence of only one mycotoxin under study. A 42 of the samples contained more than one mycotoxin, while 21 of the samples showed the presence of three types of mycotoxins. Residues of aflatoxin B1 were detected in both eggs white and yolk at levels ranging from 0.19 to 1.06 ppb, with a mean of 0.54 ppb, fumonisin B, and zearalenon were detected with means of 0.5, 3.2 ppb, respectively, whereas DON was not detected in any samples (Alaboudi & AL Jbour, 2018). This local high percentage might be related to uncontrolled feed offer in poultry industry or due to poor and unhygienic storage of feed components and the absence of controlling measures to limit the presence of contaminated fungi (Amirkhizi, Arefhosseini, Ansarin, & Nemati, 2015).

In Egypt, aflatoxin mean values in eggs were reported by Salem, El-Kaseh, and El-Diasty (2009) in the range of 0.542 ± 0.226 ppb, which are almost equal to those reported previously in Jordan.

Herzallah (2013) in Jordan had documented an average value of 0.66 ppb in hen's eggs samples, which come from layer hen's fed AFB1 contaminated feed at 894.12 ppb and this value was decreased to 0.33 ppb for hen's fed contaminated with 190.02 ppb AFB1. This relationship between AFB1 in the feed and the residues level in hen's eggs was also reported by Hussain et al. (2010).

In local poultry products in Jordan, the following results on mycotoxin prevalence are being reported where no Ochratoxin are being detected (Table 5.3).

5.12.4 Hazardous prevalence

Low toxins residues detective values are not marked for safety; the accumulative factors for these residues give reasons to increase the public awareness of food safety. Good agricultural practices are very important in preventing fungal contamination, multiplication, and mycotoxin production in raw materials used in animal feed. According to the Food and Agriculture Organization (FAO), it has been estimated that mycotoxin contaminations affect up to 25% of the world's crop production (Binder et al., 2007). Mycotoxins can invade animals by inhalation, ingestion, or absorption by skin. By any route of invasion, mycotoxins can cause sickness, general weakness, or death in animals (Maresca & Fantini, 2010).

Mycotoxins are metabolized in the liver and in the kidney upon food consumption. Metabolizing results differ according to parent molecules, so there is a difficulty to follow or know all toxins metabolite derivation or its chemical structure or associated toxicity excreted by animals (Coppock, Margitta, & Dziwenka, 2014). Studying of mycotoxins and monitoring the toxins hazards in animal products are considered a worldwide trend for ensuring food safety (Marin, Ramos, Cano-Sancho, & Sanchis, 2013). Severity of mycotoxicosis depends on such factors as type and dose of mycotoxin, extent

TABLE 5.3 Comparison between local muscle, local liver, and local kidney samples for the prevalence of mycotoxin levels in local Jordanian chicken.

Sample	Positive sample above MRI (%)			*P*-value
	Local muscle	Local liver	Local kidney	
Aflatoxin B1	1 (0.7%)	0 (0.0%)	0 (0.0%)	.716
Aflatoxins	76 (52.7%)	31 (62.0%)	30 (60.0%)	.421
Aflatoxin M1	123 (82.0%)	38 (76.0%)	38 (76.0%)	.541
Ochratoxin A	ND	ND	ND	—
Fumonisins B1	0 (0.3%)	0 (0.0%)	4 (8.0%)	.000
Zearalenone	16 (14.7%)	15 (30.0%)	4 (8.0%)	.001
Deoxynivalenol	13 (8.7%)	0 (0.0%)	2 (4.0%)	.049

Source: Data from Alaboudi, A., & Otoum, G. (2019). *Determination and quantification of nine carried over mycotoxins' residues (aflatoxin b1, b2, g1, g2, m1 and ochratoxin A, zearalenone, fumonisins, deoxynivalenol) in poultry meat* (M.Sc. thesis). Jordan: Jordan University of Science and Technology.

of exposure, health condition, gender, and age of the individual (Binder et al., 2007). Depending on these factors, mycotoxin-contaminated foodstuffs can cause chronic and or acute health problems in humans and animals. Mycotoxins might reach human plate through animal products like meat, eggs, milk as the eventual outcome of the animal-eating spoiled feed. The limits of aflatoxins B1, B2, G2, and M1 in foods and feedstuffs vary from 0 to 40 ppb for foods and 0–1000 ppb in feed; for ochratoxin A (0–50 ppb in food and 0–1000 ppb in feed); for vomitoxin, also known as DON (500–2000 ppb in food and 5–10,000 ppb in feed); for ZEN (0–1000 ppb in food); for Patulin (0–50 ppb in foods) and for fumonisins (0–1000 ppb in food 5000–50,000 ppb in feedstuffs) (Mazumder & Sasmal, 2001).

Other suggested maximum values by European authority.

Mycotoxin	Food commodity	EU ($\mu g\ kg^{-1}$)
Aflatoxins B1, B2, G1, G2	Maize, rice, peanut, almond, groundnuts, figs, spices	2 for B1 4 for total
Aflatoxin M1	Milk products	0.05 in milk, 0.025 in infant formulae and infant milk
Ochratoxin A	Cereals, dried fruit, grapes, coffee, cheese	2–10
Fumonisins B1, B2, B3	Maize, asparagus	200–1000
Zearalenone	Cereals, maize, wheat or barley	20–100
Deoxynivalenol	Cereal products	500–750

Dietary contaminants with high mycotoxins concentrations over the tolerable levels may cause injurious effects upon animal and human health. According to WHO (2018a, 2018b), the effects of some food-borne mycotoxins are of acute nature with symptoms of severe illness, appearing fast after the consumption of food products contaminated with mycotoxins, whereas other mycotoxins have been associated with long-term effects on health, like including the induction of cancers and immune deficiency (Bosco & Mollea, 2012; Clark & Snedeker, 2006).

Aflatoxins are among the most poisonous mycotoxins and are produced by certain molds (*A. flavus* and *Aspergillus parasiticus*), which grow in soil or decaying plant. The toxins can also be found in the milk of animals. Large doses of aflatoxins can lead to acute poisoning (aflatoxicosis) and can be health threatening, through liver damaging. Aflatoxins also been shown to be genotoxic and cause cancer in animal species or liver cancer in humans (WHO, 2018a, 2018b).

Ochratoxin A is produced by the species of *Aspergillus* and *Penicillium* and is a common food-contaminating mycotoxin. Ochratoxin A is formed during the crops storage and is known with toxic effects in animal species. The most noticed effect is kidney damage, but the toxin may also have affected the immune system. Contrary to the clear evidence of kidney toxicity and kidney cancer due to ochratoxin A exposure in animals, this association in humans is unclear; however, effects on kidney have been demonstrated (Clark & Snedeker, 2006). Patulin is a mycotoxin produced by a variety of molds, particularly *Aspergillus*, *Penicillium*, and *Byssochlamys*, often found in rotting apples and apple products. The acute symptoms in animals include liver, spleen, and kidney damage, and toxicity to the immune system. For humans, nausea, gastrointestinal (GI) disturbances, and vomiting have been reported (WHO, 2018a, 2018b).

Fusarium fungi are common to the soil and produce a range of different toxins, including trichothecenes such as DON, nivalenol (NIV), and T-2 and HT-2 toxins, as well as ZEN and fumonisins. Trichothecenes can be acutely toxic to humans, causing rapid irritation to the skin or intestinal mucosa and lead to diarrhea. ZEN has been shown to have hormonal, estrogenic effects, and can cause infertility at high intake levels, whereas fumonisins have been related to esophageal cancer in humans, and to liver and kidney toxicity in animals (WHO, 2018a, 2018b).

5.12.5 Effect of processing

Most mycotoxins are relatively heat stable within the conventional food processing temperature range (80°C–121°C), therefore so little or no destruction occurs under normal cooking conditions, such as boiling and frying, or even following pasteurization (Bidhuri, 2018). The stability of mycotoxins during food processing has been reviewed in the work by Bullerman and Bianchini (2007). In general, the application of a food process reduces mycotoxin concentrations significantly but does not eliminate them completely. The food processes that have been examined include physical treatments (cleaning and milling) and thermal processing (e.g., cooking, baking, frying, roasting, and extrusion). The different treatments have various effects on mycotoxins, and those that utilize the highest temperatures have the greatest effects: Roasting or cooking at high temperatures (above 150°C) appear to reduce mycotoxin concentrations significantly (Bullerman & Bianchini, 2007).

In a Jordanian study, mycotoxins were almost stable during and after various ways of heat treatments of raw eggs like of refrigeration of raw eggs for 4 weeks; boiling (at 100°C for 15 min) and frying (at 160°C for 5 min). Thermal processing, as applied had no significant effect in detoxification aflatoxin B1, fumonisin B1, DON, and ZEN in eggs. In this study, the mean reduction of toxin concentrations was minimal and ranged from 0.2% to 1% (Alaboudi and AL Jbour, 2018). Almost similar findings were reported by authors outside Middle East like, Salwa and Anwer (2009) in Pakistan report on aflatoxins in eggs. Therefore it can be concluded that minimizing aflatoxin B transmission into eggs appears to be the only practical way to ensure their safety for human consumption.

5.12.6 Conclusion

Avoiding toxins to be transferred over to the food may appear to be the most effective practice to eliminate the contamination with mycotoxins and to ensure the food safety (Egmond, 2002). Therefore the implementation of a highly effective quality control systems and good surveillance to manage food and feed toxins residues are required. Mycotoxins are seriously injurious to animal or human health. Some of them are seriously carcinogenic. In recent years, a good control of mycotoxigenic fungi has been achieved using plant products (e.g., extracts and essential oils) as environmentally friendly fungicides (Musto, 2015; Reddy et al., 2010; Thembo, Vismer, Nyazema, Gelderblom, & Katerere, 2010). Moreover, biological control represents a new opportunity in control strategies: there is evidence that *Bacillus* sp., propionic acid bacteria and lactic acid bacteria are able to inhibit fungal growth and thus mycotoxin production (Bianchini and Bullerman, 2009).

5.12.7 Recommended control measures

1. Control aflatoxins contamination in rations to avoid the occurrence of aflatoxins in animal tissue intended for human consumption through many toxins detoxifications procedures.
2. Making good quality control system, started from feed storage, to feed processing to final ration then to check animal edible tissues residues, using highly compatible techniques.
3. Developing countries are encouraged to put more legislations which prevent import any feed contains mycotoxins residues. Therefore urgent steps should be taken to monitor and control these toxins in animal products. The strict permissible limits should be implemented to avoid fungal contamination.
4. Good agricultural practices are extremely important in preventing contamination, fungal multiplication, and mycotoxin production in raw materials used in feed.

5.13 Heavy metals

5.13.1 Introduction

In science, a heavy metal is a metallic element that is toxic and has a high density and specific gravity or atomic weight. However, the term means something slightly different in common usage, referring to any metal capable of causing health problems or environmental damage (Helmenstine, 2019). Examples of heavy metals include lead, mercury, and cadmium. Less commonly, any metal with a potential negative health effect or environmental impact may be termed a heavy metal, such as cobalt, chromium, lithium, and even iron. Heavy metals form one of the important contaminating agents in our food supply (Zaidi, Asrar, Mansour, & Farooqui, 2005). Food safety is a major concern at present and increasing demand of food safety has encouraged interest on the risk associated with food consumption contaminated by heavy metals (Mansour, Belal, Abou- Arab, & Gad, 2009).

5.13.2 Sources

Heavy metals exist naturally in the soil from the soil forming processes of disintegration of parent resources at rare levels ($<1000\,mg\,kg^{-1}$). Heavy metals come from manmade sources trying to be more moveable in the soil, hereafter biologically available than soil forming phenomena metal-containing solids at polluted places can originate from an extensive variation of manmade sources in terms of metal mine stakeouts, leaded gasoline and paints that are lead based, application of fertilizer, discarding high metal wastes in inappropriately protected landfills, animal manures, bio solids (sewage sludge), coal combustion remainders, compost, petrochemicals, pesticides, and deposition in atmosphere (Sardar et al., 2013).

The main safety risk to consumer health from heavy metals is tied to exposure to lead, cadmium, mercury, and arsenic. Although health effects due to heavy metals have been known for a long time, exposure to heavy metals continues to be a problem in developing countries. Serious health hazards can develop due to dietary accumulation of heavy metals such as Cr, Cd, Ni, and Pb (Oliver, 1997). Heavy metals usually accumulated in soils and from there can find its way to humans through various exposure pathways (Qishlaqi, Moore, & Forghani, 2008).

Wastewaters carry toxic heavy metals that get introduced into the soil, aquatic system, and plant root (Khan, Cao, Zheng, Huang, & Zhu, 2008). In case heavy metal accompanied aerosols, they mainly accumulated on the leaf surfaces. There is no efficient method to completely remove all heavy metals originating from the aerosol's deposition, as fine particulates may enter the leaves. The rate at which heavy metals are accumulated in the soil depends on the physiochemical properties of the soil and crops (Qishlaqi et al., 2008). Generally, heavy metals cannot be removed from wastewater and when they enter into the soil and interfere with the plant roots and enter into food chain when these contaminated plants eaten by animals or humans. Therefore heavy metals affect the quality and production of crop and these contamination of important and of concern because of increasing demand for food safety.

Cadmium emissions continued because its use in batteries and may often dumped together with household waste. Smoking may also be considered a source of cadmium. In nonsmokers, food is the most important source of cadmium exposure. Health effects of cadmium exposure may occur even at lower exposure levels, taking the forms of kidney damage or bone effects and fractures (WHO, 1992).

The primarily exposure to mercury is through food, where fish may form a major source of methyl mercury and high fish consumption may be associated with a risk of neurological damage to adults. Also, when pregnant women are exposed to high intake of fish from polluted waters, there would be a risk to the fetus (Government of Canada, 2013).

Population also can be exposed to lead from air and food. Lead emissions from petrol to air have created considerable pollution. Children are susceptible to lead exposure because of high GI uptake and the permeable blood–brain barrier. Blood levels in children should be below the levels that are considered acceptable as there may be neurotoxic effects at lower levels of exposure. Also the use of lead-based paints should be avoided, and lead should not be used in food containers (Järup, 2003).

Food or drinking water can also be exposed to arsenic. Long-term exposure to arsenic can be linked to the increased risks of skin cancer, so as exposure to arsenic, by inhalation, may also be associated with lung cancer (WHO, 2018a, 2018b). Therefore there are different sources for heavy metal like natural and manmade and air-borne sources (Duruibe, Ogwuegbu, & Egwurugwu, 2007). The maximum contamination levels for heavy metal concentration of Cd in air, soil, and water as suggested by US Environmental Protection Agency were 0.15, 85, and 0.005 mg/kg in air, soil, and drinking water, whereas for Zn the concentrations were 1.5, 7500, and 5.00, respectively. The figures for Pb were 420 and 0.01 $mg\,kg^{-1}$ and < 1 and 0.01 for Hg in soil and drinking water, respectively.

5.13.3 Food contamination

Heavy metals (As, Cd, Co, Cr, Cu, Mn, Ni, Pb, and Zn) in various vegetables from the market in Jordan were measured. Parsley, followed by spinach, contained the highest concentration of heavy metals and onion contained high levels of toxic heavy metals. The content of Cu in parsley and spinach and Pb in onion exceeded the Codex limits. However, the daily intake of heavy metals from the tested vegetables was lower than the maximum limits for allowable intake (Osaili, Al Jamali, Makhadmeh, Taha, & Jarrar, 2016).

Levels of heavy metals such as Cd, Cu, and Zn in three fish Species collected from the Northern Jordan Valley, Jordan, were examined. The levels of heavy metals (Cd, Cu, and Zn) in muscles of the three fish species were within acceptable limits by FAO standards, except for the Zn concentration in muscles of *Oreochromis aureus* ($70.76 \pm 31.21\ mg\,kg^{-1}$ dry weight), which might be due to the increase of agricultural influx and some other anthropogenic activity in that area (Al-Weher, 2008).

The concentrations of the heavy metals Cd, Co, Cr, Cu, Fe, Mn, Ni, Pb, and Zn were determined in the muscles, livers, gills, gonads, and the stomachs of three fish species collected from the Gulf of Aqaba, Jordan. In general, muscles contained lower metal concentrations than other organs. Comparing species, there was no significant difference in the mean concentration of metals except Zn in the muscles of the examined fish species. The concentration of metals in the muscle tissues was generally low and within the ranges expected for metals in the muscle of fish from relatively uncontaminated locations. The ranges are generally lower or within the ranges of the concentrations for these elements in fishes of the Red Sea (Hanna et al., 1997). Moreover, the values fall below the acceptable levels for human consumption recommended by FAO/WHO, which means that they do not pose a significant threat to the health of human consumers.

The muscles, livers, gills, gonads, and stomachs of 11 common fish species collected at three sites in the Northern Gulf of Aqaba were analyzed for the heavy metals Cd, Co, Cr, Cu, Fe, Mn, Ni, Pb, and Zn (Abu Hilal & Ismail, 2008). Large differences in trace metal concentrations (in $\mu g\ g^{-1}$ dry weight) were observed between different tissues or organ parts within each fish. In muscle tissue, Cd ranged from 0.5 to 2.0 $\mu g\ g^{-1}$ dry weight, while higher concentrations were found in liver, gill, and stomach. Cobalt concentrations were lowest in muscles and livers and highest in gills and stomachs. Similarly, Cr concentrations were highest in gills and stomachs, and lowest in livers. Copper was also low in muscles (0.5–2.0), but highest in liver tissue. Iron levels were highest in liver (30–1031) and lower in other organs (3.9–391.0). Muscle tissues contained lower concentrations of Mn than other organs, particularly the gills, which contained also higher concentrations of Ni and Pb compared to the livers and muscles. Gonads contained the highest concentration of Zn, while muscles contained the lowest (Abu Hilal & Ismail, 2008). Fishes of the families Carangidae, *Decapterus macarellus*, *Decapterus macrosoma*, and *Decapterus russelli* were collected from the Jordanian Aqaba coast for the determination of their metal concentrations in various organs (muscle, liver, kidney, gonads, gills, and stomach food contents). The results showed significant differences in metal concentration between species and significant differences of heavy metal elements among different organs of the same species. The results did not reveal any significant differences between male and female organs, and the only significant difference was found for Pb in *D. macorsoma* and for Cu in *D. russelli*. The low metal concentrations (below MRL) were found in muscle tissues of all the studied fishes (Khalaf et al., 2011). Another study from Egypt evaluated the concentrations of heavy metals (Cu, Zn, Pb, Cd, Fe, and Mn) were in the liver, gills, and muscles of 14 benthic and pelagic fish species collected from three main landing areas (Shalateen, Hurghada, and Suez) in the Egyptian Red Sea. The levels of heavy metals varied significantly among fish species and organs. As expected, muscle tissues possessed the lowest concentrations of all metals. In most studied fish, the liver was the target organ for Cu, Zn, and Fe accumulation. Pb and Mn, however, exhibited their highest concentrations in the gills. The concentration of metals in the present fish muscles were accepted by the international legislation limits and are safe for human consumption (El-Moselhy, Othman, Abd El-Azem, & El-Metwally, 2014).

The metal levels of arsenic, chromium, copper, lead, magnesium, manganese, selenium, vanadium, and zinc concentrations were determined in various fish body organs of sea, to assess the bioaccumulation of metals associated with petroleum input a decade after the 1991 Gulf War oil spillage (de Mora, Fowler, Wyse, & Azemard, 2004). High concentrations of Zn and Cu in the muscle and hepatopancreas tissues were a strong indicative of high exposure of blue crab (Portunus *pelagicus*) to these metals. However, muscle tissue had been found to accumulate the highest values for all metal speciation analyzed. The difference in patterns of metal occurrence and the significant increase in the Cu and Zn concentrations in various organs of the crab were largely associated with the 1991 Gulf War oil spill (Al-Mohanna and Subrahmanyam, 2001). The results clearly indicate the ability of decapods to accumulate metals to detectable levels. Metal bioaccumulation by crabs can be affected by the chemical composition of the sediment and interstitial seawater. Petroleum and petrochemical industry wastes contribute significantly to metal enrichment of the Arabian Gulf marine environment (de Mora et al., 2004).

Commercially important fresh (581) and frozen (292) marine fish samples of 10 species were collected from seafood factories in Oman. There were significant interspecific differences for all metals, and yellow-fin tuna had the highest level of cadmium and mercury; however, red seabream had maximum numbers above the standards. In general, fishes from these regions are within the safety levels recommended by various organizations and do not pose a health risk in terms of human diet (Al-Busaidi et al., 2011).

5.13.4 Heavy metal hazards

Heavy metals are toxic metals for living organisms. They get into body by different ways like ingestion, inhalation, or absorption. Heavy metals are one of the major contaminating agents in our food supply (Zaidi et al., 2005). They become harmful when their deposition rate is higher than their discharge. High concentration exposure is not a necessity to produce a state of toxicity in the body, as heavy metal accumulation occurs in body tissues gradually and, over time, can reach toxic concentration levels (Suruchi, 2011).

The excessive quantities of these metals in food is associated with a number of diseases, like cardiovascular, kidney, nervous, and so as bone diseases (Sanchez-Castillo et al., 1998; Steenland & Boffetta, 2000). Lead is known for its toxicity on public health. Absorption of ingested lead forms a serious risk to human health like colic, constipation, and anemia (Bolger et al., 1996). Serious systemic health risk may develop as a result of high dietary accumulation of heavy metals such as Cr, Cd, Ni, Pb, or Cu (Khair, 2009; Oliver, 1997). The bio-toxic effects of heavy metals refer to the harmful effects of heavy metals to the body when consumed above the bio-recommended limits. Although individual metals exhibit specific signs of their toxicity, the following have been reported as general signs associated with cadmium, lead, arsenic, mercury, zinc, copper, and aluminum poisoning: GI disorders, diarrhea, stomatitis, tremor, hemoglobin-urea causing a rust–red color to stool, ataxia, paralysis, vomiting and convulsion, depression, and pneumonia when volatile vapors and fumes are inhaled (McCluggage, 1991).

5.13.5 Effect of processing

Several worldwide studies have examined the effects of common food processing techniques on the levels of toxic elements in food. Some studies have reported negative effects of processing, whereas many others have shown that processing practices may have a positive effect on the reduction of toxic elements in foodstuffs (Hajeb, Sloth, Shakibazadeh, Mahyudin, & Afsah-Hejri, 2014). No specific studies are being reported in available literature on the effect of cooking processes on heavy metals in Middle East area and to quote some principles the following data will be cited.

To study the effects of food processing methods on the fate of heavy metals, heavy metals including cadmium (Cd), lead (Pb), arsenic (As), and aluminum (Al) were analyzed in oilseeds, noodles, tea leaves, and their processed or cooked products. Heavy metals in oilseeds, noodles, and teas were reduced by extracting oils, boiling noodles, and infusing teas. The movement of heavy metals into boiling water and infusion tea was increased as the boiling and infusion time is increased. Heavy metals in foods are water soluble, and heavy metals in foods would be decreased when foods are processed or cooked with water (Lee et al., 2019).

Cooking may reduce metal content although some foods can absorb metals if the cooking water is contaminated. Metals used in food processing equipment or food packaging material may contribute to food contamination. Contamination may also occur during kitchen preparation and storage (Morgan, 1999). Musaiger and O D'Souza (2008) also reported a reduction in arsenic, mercury, lead, and cadmium in fish and shrimp after different cooking processes (grilling, frying, and cooking both as a curry dish and in rice). Reduction ranged according to diet and cooking technique from 40% to 60%.

5.13.6 Conclusion

Heavy metals have bio-importance as trace elements but, the toxic effects of many of them in human are of great concern. Therefore there is a great need for understanding the conditions like the concentrations that make them harmful and how biotoxicity occurs. It is also of important to understand their sources, leaching or chemical conversions and ways of deposition to pollute foods or the environment. Usually they leach into underground waters and move along water pathways to be finally deposited in surface waters, thereby resulting in water and subsequently soil pollution. Poisoning and toxicity of humans or animals occur frequently through exchange and coordination mechanisms. When ingested, they combine with the body's biomolecules, like proteins and enzymes to form stable toxic compounds, affecting the physiological, biochemical, and normal body functions. Therefore studying toxic heavy metals, understanding their toxicity mechanisms, and understanding their biochemical activities are of importance. Effective mechanisms in reducing contamination in particularly of industrials sources and cleaning up of contamination sources and polluted foods are of seriously important.

5.13.7 Recommended control measures

The main sources of heavy metals in food are the contaminated wastewater beside industrial sources that may contaminate aerosols. Remediation of heavy metal-contaminated soils is necessary to reduce the associated risks. Thus attention has to be given to limit contamination sources. The concentration of toxic elements can also be reduced in a foodstuff by having a suitable method for preparation. Precooking treatments such as the peeling of plant products or certain cooking methods can remove some of the heavy metals. Cooking methods such as boiling and frying may alter the content of a toxic element through the loss of water and volatiles, the solubilization of the metal, and metal binding to macronutrients such as carbohydrates, lipids, and proteins. Since toxic elements are not evaporated or broken down to possible safer compounds, the elements that are removed from food during frying, boiling, or canning processes may also migrate from food to the frying oil or boiling water.

Heavy metals can be significantly reduced in food by using chelating agents. Chelating consists of the presence of a charged molecule (usually containing one or more − SH groups) to bind specific metal ions of opposite electrical charge and thus the removal of the consequent complex from the body via the urine (Risher & Amler, 2005). Chelators have also been applied to remove heavy metals through foods (Hajeb & Jinap, 2012). The metal chelation ability of organic compounds, such as ethylenediaminetetraacetic acid, nitrilotriacetic acid, acetic acid, citric acid, cysteine, HCl, or NaCl are commonly known; therefore they are often incorporated in food formulations (Hajeb et al., 2014).

Immobilization, soil washing, and phytoremediation techniques are frequently listed among the best demonstrated available technologies for cleaning up heavy metal–contaminated sites.

References

Abbas, O. S. (2016). Detection of deltamethrin residues in poultry egg and meat in Dyala province. *Al-Anbar Journal of Veterinary Sciences*, *9*(2), 41–46.

Abd-Rabo, F. H. R., Elsalamony, H., & Sakr, S. S. (2016). Reduction of pesticide residues in Egyptian buffalo milk by some processing treatments. *International Journal of Dairy Science, 11*(2), 75–78.

Abdulkhaliq, A., Swaileh, K., Hussein, R. M., & Matani, M. (2012). Levels of metals (Cd, Pb, Cu and Fe) in cow's milk, dairy products and hen's eggs from the West Bank, Palestine. *International Food Research Journal, 19*, 1089–1094.

Abou Donia, M. A., Abou-Arab, A. A. K., Enb, A., El-Senaity, M. H., & Abd-Rabou, N. S. (2010). Chemical composition of raw milk and the accumulation of pesticide residues in milk products. *Global Veterinaria, 4*, 6–14.

Aboul-Enein, A. M., Nasr, I. N., Abou Elella, F. M., & Abdulla, E. S. (2010). Monitoring of some organochlorines and organophosphorus residues in imported and locally raised chicken and bovine muscles in Egypt. *Journal of Applied Sciences Research, 6*(6), 600–608.

Abu Hilal, H., & Ismail, N. S. (2008). Heavy metals in eleven common species of fish from the Gulf of Aqaba, Red Sea. Jordan. *Journal of Biological Sciences., 1*, 13–18.

Ahmad, R., Salem, N. M., & Estaitieh, H. (2010). Occurrence of organochlorine pesticide residues in eggs, chicken and meat in Jordan. *Chemosphere, 78*(6), 667–671.

Alaboudi, A. R., Abu Basha, E., & Musallam, I. (2013). Chlortetracycline and sulfanilamide residues in table eggs: Prevalence, distribution between yolk and white and effect of refrigeration and heat treatment. *Food Control, 33*(1), 281–286.

Alaboudi, A. R., & Al hijazin, M. (2010). *Antibiotics residues in dressed poultry* (M.Sc. thesis). Jordan: Jordan University of Science and Technology.

Alaboudi, A. R., & Al Jarrah, B. S. (2019). *Determination and quantification of some of organochlorines, organophosphorus, carbamates and pyrethroids pesticide residues in local fresh fish and imported frozen fish in Jordan* (M.Sc. thesis). Jordan: Jordan University of Science and Technology.

Alaboudi, A. R. & AL Jbour, S. (2018). *Assessment of four well-known carried over toxin's residues (aflatoxin B1, fumonisin B1, deoxynivalenol, and zearalenone) in fresh and processed hen's eggs in Jordan market* (M.Sc. thesis). Jordan: Jordan University of Science and Technology.

Alaboudi, A. R., & Otoum, G. (2019). *Determination and quantification of nine carried over mycotoxins' residues (aflatoxin B1, B2, G1, G2, M1 and ochratoxin A, zearalenone, fumonisins, deoxynivalenol) in poultry meat* (M.Sc. thesis) Jordan: Jordan University of Science and Technology.

Alaboudi, A. R., Osaili, T. M., & Alrwashdeh, A. (2019). Pesticides hexachlorocyclohexane, aldrin, and malathion residues in home-grown eggs: prevalence, distribution, and effect of storage and heat treatments. *Journal of Food Science, 84*(12), 3383–3390.

Al-Antary, T. M., Alawi, M. A., Shaderma, A. M., & Haddad, N. A. (2018). Pesticides residues in agricultural crops in southern governorates of Jordan in 2016 and 2017. *Fresenius Environmental Bulletin, 27*(10), 6853–6857.

Alawi, M. A. (2006). Organochlorine pesticides in sea water and sediment samples from the Aqaba Gulf. *Fresenius Environmental Bulletin, 16*(9), 1131–1136.

Alawi, M. A., Al-Antary, T. M., Estityah, H., & Haddad, N. (2016). Evaluation of chlorinated pesticides residues in foodstuff of animal origin from middle districts of Jordan in 2013–2014. *Toxin Reviews, 36*(2), 94–100.

Alawi, M. A., Ammari, N., & Al-Shuraiki, Y. (1992). Organochlorine pesticide contaminations in human milk samples from women living in Amman, Jordan. *Archives of Environmental Contamination and Toxicology, 23*, 235–239.

Alawi, M. A., Hourani, M., & Abu Hilal, D. (1995). Levels of organochlorine pesticides in fish, algae, sediments and sea water samples in the Aqaba Gulf. *Toxicological & Environmental Chemistry*, *51*(1–4), 121–134.

Al-Busaidi, M., Yesudhason, P., Al-Mughairi, S., Al-Rahbi, W. A. K., Al-Harthy, K. S., Al-Mazrooei, N. A., & Al-Habsi, S. H. (2011). Toxic metals in commercial marine fish in Oman with reference to national and international standard. *Chemosphere*, *85*, 67–73.

Al Gharibeh, G. R., & Al Fararjeh, M. S. (2019). Pesticide residues in fruits and vegetables in Jordan using liquid chromatography/tandem mass spectrometry. *Food Additives & Contaminants: Part B*, *12*(1), 65–73.

Ali-Aberoumand, A. (2014). Nutrient composition analysis of Gish fish fillets affected by different cooking methods. *International Food Research Journal*, *21*(5), 1989–1991.

Al Mashhadany, D. A. (2019). Detection of antibiotic residues among raw beef in Erbil City (Iraq) and impact of temperature on antibiotic remains. *Italian Journal of Food Safety*, *8*, 7897.

Al Mashhadany, D. A. (2020). Monitoring of antibiotic residues among sheep meat in Erbil City and thermal processing effect on their remnants. *Iraqi Journal of Veterinary Sciences*, *34*(2), 217–222.

Al-Mazeedi, H. M., Abbas, A. B., Alomirah, H. F., Al-Jouhar, W. Y., Al-Mufty, S. A., Ezzelregal, M. M., … Al-Owaish, R. A. (2009). Screening for tetracycline residues in food products of animal origin in the State of Kuwait using Charm II radio- immunoassay and LC/MS/MS methods. *Food Additives & Contaminants: Part A*, *27*(3), 291–301.

Al-Mohanna, S. Y., & Subrahmanyam, M. N. V. (2001). Flux of heavy metal accumulation in various organs of the intertidal marine blue crab, *Portunus pelagicus* (L.) from the Kuwait coast after the Gulf War. *Environment International*, *27*(4), 321–326.

Al-Mustafa, Z. H., & Al-Ghamdi, M. R. (2001). Use of antibiotics in the poultry industry in Saudi Arabia: Implications for public health. *Annals of Saudi Medicine*, *22*(1–2), 4–7.

Al-Nasir, F. M., Jiries, A. G., Al-Rabadi, G. J., Alu'datt, M. H., Tranchant, C. C., Al-Dalain, S. A., … Al-Dmour, R. S. (2020). Determination of pesticide residues in selected citrus fruits and vegetables cultivated in the Jordan Valley. *LWT*, *123*, 109005.

Alnatour, M. K., Alaboudi, A. R., & Al karasneh, A. (2019). *Detection of some organochlorine, organophosphorus, pyrethroid and carbamate pesticide residues in imported frozen and local fresh chicken meat and its viscera in Jordan* (M.Sc. thesis). Jordan: Jordan University of Science and Technology.

Al-Weher, S. M. (2008). Levels of heavy metal Cd, Cu and Zn in three fish species collected from the Northern Jordan Valley, Jordan. *Jordan Journal of Biological Sciences*, *1*(1), 41–46.

Amirkhizi, B., Arefhosseini, S. R., Ansarin, M., & Nemati, M. (2015). Aflatoxin B1 in eggs and chicken livers by dispersive liquid–liquid microextraction and HPLC. *Food Additives & Contaminants: Part B*, *8*(4), 245–249.

Arya, N. (2005). Pesticides and human health: why public health officials should support a ban on nonessential residential use. *Canadian Journal of Public Health/Revue Canadienne de Sante'e Publique*, *96*, 89–92.

Aulakh, R. S., Gill, J. P., Bedi, J. S., Sharma, J. K., Joia, B. S., & Ockerman, H. W. (2006). Organochlorine pesticide residues in poultry feed, chicken muscle and eggs at a poultry farm in Punjab, India. *Journal of the Science of Food and Agriculture*, *86*, 741–744.

Bacanlı, M., & Başaran, N. (2019). Importance of antibiotic residues in animal food. *Food and Chemical Toxicology*, *125*, 462–466.

Badawy, M. I., & El Dib, M. A. (1984). Residues of organochlorine pesticides in fish from the Egyptian delta lakes. *Environment International*, *10*(1), 3–8.

Bajwa, U., & Sandhu, K. S. (2014). Effect of handling and processing on pesticide residues in food—A review. *Journal of Food Science and Technology*, *51*(2), 201–220.

Battacone, A., Nudda, A., Cannas, A., Cappio Borlino, G., & Bomboi, G. P. (2003). Excretion of aflatoxin M1 in milk of dairy ewes treated with different doses of aflatoxin B1. *Journal of Dairy Science*, *86*(8), 2667–2675.

Bennett, J. W., & Klich, M. (2003). Mycotoxins. *Clinical Microbiology Review*, *16*, 497–516.

Bhat, R., Sridhar, K., & Karim, A. (2010). Microbial quality evaluation and effective decontamination of nutraceutically valued lotus seeds by electron beams and gamma irradiation. *Radiation Physics and Chemistry*, *79*(9), 976–981.

Bianchini, A., & Bullerman, L. B. (2009). Biological control of molds and mycotoxins in foods. *ACS Symposium Series*, *1031*, 1–16.

Bidhuri, A. (2018). *Harmful effects of pesticides in fruits and vegetables.* https://www.onlymyhealth.com/harmful-effects-of-pesticides-in-fruits-and-vegetables-1.

Binder, E. M., Tan, L. M., Chin, L. J., Handl, J., & Richard, J. (2007). Worldwide occurrence of mycotoxins in commodities, feeds and feed ingredients. *Animal Feed Science and Technology*, *137*(3), 265–282.

Bobkov, M., & Zbinden, P. (2018). Occurrence of veterinary drug residues in poultry and products thereof. A review. *CHIMIA International Journal for Chemistry*, *72*(10), 707–712.

Bolger, P. M., Yess, N. J., Gunderson, E. L., Troxell, T. C., & Carrington, C. D. (1996). Identification and reduction of sources of dietary lead in the United States. *Food Additives & Contaminants*, *13*(1), 53–60.

Bordin, K., Kunitake, M. T., Aracava, K. K., & Trindade, C. S. F. (2013). Changes in food caused by deep fat frying—A review. *Archivos latinoamericanos de Nutrición*, *63*, 5–13.

Bosco, F., & Mollea, C. (2012). Mycotoxins in food. *The hidden danger in foods. Mycotoxins and food safety*. Available from https://www.intechopen.com/./mycotoxins-in-food.

Botsoglou, N. A., & Fletouris, D. J. (2000). Stability of residues during food processing. *Drug residues in foods: Pharmacology, food safety, and analysis*. Available from https://b-ok.org/book/818496/28d21a.

Bouchon, P., & Dueik, V. (2018). *Frying of foods* (Chapter 10), Biology 456, University of Santiago, Chile. https://www.coursehero.com/file/58076455/Control-5-Fryingpdf.

Bullerman, L. B., & Bianchini, A. (2007). Stability of mycotoxins during food processing. *International Journal of Food Microbiology*, *119*(1), 140–146.

Castanon, J. (2007). History of the use of antibiotic as growth promoters in European poultry feeds. *Poultry Science*, *86*, 2466–2471.

Cháfer-Pericás, C., Maquieira, A., & Puchades, R. (2010). Fast screening methods to detect antibiotic residues in food samples. *TrAc Trends in Analytical Chemistry*, *29*, 1038–1049.

Clark, H. A., & Snedeker, S. M. (2006). Ochratoxin A: Its cancer risk and potential for exposure. *Journal of Toxicology and Environmental Health, Part B: Critical Reviews*, *9*(3), 265–296.

Cooper, J., & Dobson, H. (2007). The benefits of pesticides to mankind and the environment. *Crop Protection*, *26*, 1337–1348.

Coppock, R. W., Margitta, M., & Dziwenka, M. M. (2014). *Mycotoxins. Biomarkers in toxicology* (pp. 549–562). Academic Press.

Darwish, W. S., Eldaly, E. A., El-abbasy, M. T., Ikenaka, Y., Naakyama, S., & Ishzuka, M. (2013). Antibiotics residues in food: The African scenario. *The Japanese Journal of Veterinary Research*, *61*, S13–S22.

de Mora, S., Fowler, S. W., Wyse, E., & Azemard, S. (2004). Distribution of heavy metals in marine bivalves, fish and coastal sediments in the Gulf and Gulf of Oman. *Marine Pollution Bulletin*, *49*(5–6), 410–424.

Dixit, S., Srivastava, M. P., & Sharma, Y. K. (2019). Pesticide and human health: A rising concern of the 21st century. In K. A. Wani, & Mamta (Eds.), *Handbook of research on the adverse effects of pesticide pollution in aquatic ecosystems* (pp. 85–104). IGI Global.

D'Mello, J. P. F., Porter, J. K., Macdonald, A. M. C., & Placinta, C. M. (2019). Fusarium mycotoxins. In D. Mello (Ed.), *Handbook of plant and fungal toxicants* (1st ed., p. 287). CRC Press.

Duruibe, J. O., Ogwuegbu, M. O. C., & Egwurugwu, J. N. (2007). Heavy metal pollution and human biotoxic effects. *International Journal of Physical Sciences*, *2*(5), 112–118.

Egmond, H. P. (2002). Worldwide regulations for mycotoxins FAO. *Advances in Experimental Medicine and Biology*, *504*, 257–269.

El-Ghareeb, W. R., Mulla, Z. S. H., Meligy, A. M. A., Darwish, W. S., & Edris, A. M. (2019). Antibiotic residue levels in camel, cattle and sheep tissues using LC-MS/MS. *The Journal of Animal & Plant Sciences*, *29*(4), 943–952.

El-Moselhy, K. M., Othman, A. I., Abd El-Azem, H., & El-Metwally, M. E. A. (2014). Bioaccumulation of heavy metals in some tissues of fish in the Red Sea, Egypt. *Egyptian Journal of Basic & Applied Sciences*, *1*(2), 97–105.

El-Saeid, M. H. (2010). Monitoring of pesticide residues in Riyadh cultured farm fish. *World Applied Sciences Journal*, *9*(9), 1075–1080.

Erber, E., & Binder, E. (2004). Managing the risk of mycotoxins in modern feed production. In *The 5th Korea Feed Ingredient Association international symposium, Korea Feed Ingredient Association* (pp. 21–45). Seoul, Korea.

EU. (1996). *Council Directive 96/23/EC on measures to monitor certain substances and residues thereof in live animals and animal products and repealing*. https://eur-lex.europa.eu/legal-content/EN/LSU/?uri=CELEX:31996L0023.

EU. (2010). *Directive 2010/63/EU is the European Union (EU) legislation "on the protection of animals used for scientific purposes."* https://en.wikipedia.org/wiki/Directive_2010/63/EU.

European Center for Disease Prevention and Control. (2012). *Summary of the latest data on antibiotic consumption in the European Union*. https://www.ecdc.europa.eu/./antibiotics-consumption-EU-data-2012.

FAO/WHO. (2018). *Pesticide residues in food, Rome, Italy*. Food and Agricultural Organization. http://www.who.int/mediacentre/factsheets/pesticide-residues-food/en/.

FAO/WHO-Codex Alimentarius. (2020). *International food standards*. http://www.fao.org/fao-who-codexalimentarius.

Fath El-Bab, G. F. A. (2012). Residues of some antibiotics in table eggs in some private farms. *The Journal of the Egyptian Medical Association*, *72*, 69–80.

Furusawa, N. (2001). Transference of dietary veterinary drugs into eggs. *Veterinary Research Communications*, *25*, 651–662.

Gad Alla, S. A., Almaz, M. M., Thabet, W. M., & Nabil, M. M. (2015). Evaluation of pesticide residues in some Egyptian fruits. *International Journal of Environment*, *4*(1), 87–97.

Gad Alla, S. A., Thabet, W. M., & Emil, Y. S. (2013). Monitoring and risk assessment of pesticide residues in some Egyptian vegetables. *Middle East Journal of Applied Science*, *3*(4), 216–230.

García-Arias, M. T. A., Pontes, E., García-Linares, M. C., García-Fernández, M. C., & Sánchez-Muniz, F. J. (2003). Cooking-freezing-reheating (CFR) of sardine (Sardinapichardus) fillets, effect of different cooking and reheating procedures on the proximate and fatty acid compositions. *Food Chemistry*, *83*(3), 349–356.

Garvin, K. S. (2017). *How herbicides affect people*. https://healthfully.com/199337-how-herbicides-affect-people.htm.

Giliomee, J. H. (2008). Pesticides. In H. A. Strydom, & N. D. King (Eds.), *Environmental management in South Africa*. Juta. Available from https://juta.co.za/catalogue/environmental-management-in-south-africa.

Goldman, L., & Tran, N. (2002). *Toxics and poverty: The impact of toxic substances on the poor in developing countries*. Washington, DC: World Bank. Available from http://documents.worldbank.org/curated/en/689811468315541722/Toxics-and-poverty-the-impact-of-toxic-substances-on-the-poor-in-developing-countries.

Government of Canada. (2013). *Mercury in the food chain. Guidelines for Canadian drinking water quality: Guideline technical document – Mercury*. https://www.canada.ca/en/health-canada/services/publications/healthy; https://www.canada.ca/./health-concerns/food-chain.html.

Graham, J. P., Boland, J. J., & Silbergeld, E. (2007). Growth promoting antibiotics in food animal production: An economic analysis. *Public Health Reports*, *122*, 79–87.

Guler, G. O., Cakmak, Y. S., Dagli, Z., Aktumsek, A., & Ozparlak, H. (1998). Organochlorine pesticide residues in wheat from Konya region, Turkey. *Food and Chemical Toxicology, 48*, 1218–1221.

Habibzadeh, F. (2013). Use and misuse of antibiotics in the Middle East. *The Lancet (Middle East Edition)*, *382*, 1175–1182.

Hajeb, P., & Jinap, S. (2012). Reduction of mercury from mackerel fillet using combined solution of cysteine, EDTA, and sodium chloride. *Journal of Agricultural and Food Chemistry*, *60*(23), 6069–6076.

Hajeb, P., Sloth, J. J., Shakibazadeh, S., Mahyudin, N. A., & Afsah-Hejri, L. (2014). Toxic elements in food: Occurrence, binding, and reduction approaches. *Comprehensive Reviews in Food Science and Food Safety*, *13*(4), 457–472.

Hanna, L. A., Peters, J. M., Wiley, L. M., Clegg, M. S., & Keen, C. L. (1997). Comparative effects of essential and nonessential metals on preimplantation mouse embryo development in vitro. *Toxicology*, *116*, 123–131.

Helfrich, L. A., Weigmann, D. L., Hipkins, P. A., & Stinson, E. R. (2009). Pesticides and aquatic animals: a guide to reducing impacts on aquatic systems. https://vtechworks.lib.vt.edu/bitstream/handle/10919/48060/420013_pdf.pdf?sequence=1&isAllowed=y.

Helmenstine, A. M., (2019) *Heavy metals in science – Definition and examples*. https://www.thoughtco.com/what-is-a-heavy-metal-608449.

Herzallah, S. M. (2013). Aflatoxin B1 residues in eggs and flesh of laying hens fed aflatoxin B1 contaminated diet. *American Journal of Agricultural & Biological Sciences*, *8*, 156–161.

Huffman, J., Gerber, R., & Du, L. (2010). Recent advancement in the biosynthetic mechanism for polyketide-derived mycotoxins. *Biopolymers*, *93*, 764–776.

Hussain, Z., Khan, M. Z., Khan, A., Javed, I., Saleemi, M. K., Mahmood, S., & Asi, M. R. (2010). Residues of aflatoxin B1 in broiler meat: Effect of age and dietary aflatoxin B1 levels. *Food and Chemical Toxicology*, *48*(12), 3304–3307.

Iqbal, S. Z., Nisar, S., Asi, M. R., & Jinap, S. (2014). Natural incidence of aflatoxins, ochratoxin A and zearalenone in chicken meat and eggs. *Food Control*, *43*, 98–103.

Ismail, T., & Elkassas, W. M. (2016). Prevalence of some pesticides residues in buffalo's milk with refer to impact of heating. *Alexandria Journal of Veterinary Science*, *48*(2), 113–123.

Järup, L. (2003). Hazards of heavy metal contamination. *British Medical Bulletin*, *68*(1), 167–182.

Kalyonova, F. K., & El-Batawi, M. A. (2019). *Human toxicology of pesticides (e-book)*. Hash file: 0fec3ae87169d558522dc58736391e98.pdf.

Katz, S. E., & Brady, M. S. (2000). Antibiotics residues in food and their significance. *Food Biotechnology*, *14*, 147–171.

Khair, M. H. (2009). Toxicity and accumulation of copper in Nannochloropsisoculata (Eustigmatophycea, Heterokonta). *World Applied Sciences Journal*, *6*(3), 378–384.

Khalaf, M., Al-Najjar, T., Alawi, M. A., & Disi, A. A. (2011). Levels of trace metals in three fish species *Decapterus macrellus, Decapterus macrosomos* and *Decapterus russelli* of the family Carangidae from the Gulf of Aqaba, Read Sea, Jordan. *Natural Science*, *4*(6), 362–367.

Khan, S., Cao, Q., Zheng, Y. M., Huang, Y. Z., & Zhu, Y. G. (2008). Health risks of heavy metals in contaminated soils and food crops irrigated with wastewater in Beijing, China. *Environmental Pollution*, *152*(3), 686–692.

Khan, S. U. (1982). Bound pesticide residues in soil and plants. In F. A. Gunther, & J. D. Gunther (Eds.), *Residue reviews* (pp. 1–25). New York: Springer.

Lacey, J. (1991). Natural occurrence of mycotoxins in growing and conserved forage crops. In J. E. Smith, & R. S. Henderson (Eds.), *Mycotoxins and animal foods* (pp. 363–397). CRC Press.

Le Doux, M. (2011). Analytical methods applied to the determination of pesticide residues in foods of animal origin. A review of the past two decades. *Journal of Chromatography A*, *1218*(8), 1021–1103.

Lee, J. G., Hwang, J. Y., Lee, H. E., Kim, T. H., Cho, J. D., & Gang, G. J. (2019). Effects of food processing methods on migration of heavy metals to food. *Applied Biological Chemistry*, *62*, 64.

Mansour, S., Belal, M., Abou- Arab, A. A. K., & Gad, M. F. (2009). Monitoring of pesticides and heavy metals in cucumber fruits produced from different farming systems. *Chemosphere*, *75*(5), 601–609.

Maresca, M., & Fantini, J. (2010). Some food-associated mycotoxins as potential risk factors in humans predisposed to chronic intestinal inflammatory diseases. *Toxicon: Official Journal of the International Society on Toxinology*, *56*(3), 282–294.

Marin, S., Ramos, A. J., Cano-Sancho, G., & Sanchis, V. (2013). Mycotoxins: Occurrence, toxicology, and exposure assessment. *Food and Chemical Toxicology*, *6*, 218–237.

Martinez, M. P., Angulo, R., Pozo, R., & Jo dral, M. (1997). Organochlorine pesticides in pasteurized milk and associated health risks. *Food and Chemical Toxicology: An International Journal Published for the British Industrial Biological Research Association*, *35*(6), 621–624.

Marzouk, N. M., Shoukry, H. M., Ali, H., Naser, G. A., & Fayed, A. M. S. (2016). Detection of harmful residues in some fish species. *Egyptian Journal of Chemistry and Environmental Health*, *2*(2), 363–381.

Maurya, P. K., Malik, D. S., & Sharma, A. (2019). Impacts of pesticide application on aquatic environments and fish diversity. In V. Kumar, R. Kumar, J. Singh, & P. Kumar (Eds.), *Contaminants in agriculture and environment: Health risks and remediation* (pp. 112–128). Agro Environ Media. Available from https://doi.org/10.26832/AESA-2019-CAE-0162-09.

Mazumder, P. M., & Sasmal, D. (2001). Mycotoxins – Limits and regulations. *Ancient Science of Life*, *20*(3), 1–19.

McCluggage, D. (1991). *Heavy metal poisoning*. Columbus, OH: The Bird Hospital. Available from http://www.cocktatiels.org/articles/Diseases/Metals.html.

Milicevica, D., Nesicb, K., & Jaksic, S. (2015). Mycotoxin contamination of the food supply chain – Implications for One Health programme. *Food Science*, *5*, 187–190.

Mineau, P. (2011). Barking up the wrong perch: Why we should stop ignoring nondietary routes of pesticide exposure in birds. *Integrated Environmental Assessment and Management*, *7*, 297–299.

Ministry of Agriculture, British Colombia, Canada. (2017). *Pesticide toxicity and hazard*. https://www2.gov.bc.ca/./ministries-organizations/ministries/agriculture.

Morgan, J. N. (1999). Effects of processing on heavy metal content of foods. In L. S. Jackson, M. G. Knize, & J. N. Morgan (Eds.), *Impact of processing on food safety* (pp. 195–211). Kluwer Academic/Plenum Publishers. Available from https://doi.org/10.1007/978-1-4615-3-4859.

Muaz, K., Riaz, M., Akhtar, S., Park, S., & Ismail, A. (2018). Antibiotic residues in chicken meat: Global prevalence, threats, and decontamination strategies: A review. *Journal of Food Protection*, *81*, 619–627.

Musaiger, A., & O D'Souza, R. (2008). The effects of different methods of cooking on proximate, mineral and heavy metal composition of fish and shrimps consumed in the Arabian Gulf. *Archivos Latinoamericanos de Nutricion*, *58*(1), 103–109.

Musto, M. (2015). Preliminary report on antifungal activity of a Solanum nigrum extract against five mycotoxin-producing fungi. *Emirates Journal of Food and Agriculture*, *27*(11), 1–6.

Muthukumar, M., Reddy, K. S., Reddy, K. K., Reddy, A. G., Reddy, D. J., Kondaiah, N., & Reddy, C. N. (2010). Organochlorine pesticides residues in chicken muscle and organs. *Indian Journal of Poultry Science*, *45*, 372–375.

Nasir, K., Bilto, Y. Y., & Al-Shuraiki, Y. (1998). Residues of chlorinated hydrocarbon insecticides in human milk of Jordanian women. *Environmental Pollution*, *99*, 141–148.

Nelson, P. E., Desjardins, A. E., & Plattner, R. D. (1993). Fumonisins, mycotoxins produced by Fusarium species: Biology, chemistry, and significance. *Annual Review of Phytopathology*, *31*(1), 233–252.

Nimmo, D. R., Hamaker, T. L., Matthews, E., & Moore, J. C. (1981). An overview of the acute and chronic effects of first- and second-generation pesticides on an estuarine mysid. In F. J. Vernberg, A. Calabrese, F. P. Thurberg, & W. B. Vernberg (Eds.), *Biological monitoring of marine pollutants* (pp. 3–20). New York: Academic Press.

Nisha, A. (2008). Antibiotics residues – A global health hazard. *Veterinary World*, *1*, 375–377.

Noble, A. (1990). The relation between organochlorine residues in animal feeds and residues in tissues, milk and egg: A review. *Australian Journal of Experimental Agriculture.*, *30*, 145–154.

Oliver, M. A. (1997). Soil and human health: A review. *European Journal of Soil Science*, *48*, 573–592.

Osaili, T. M., Al Jamali, A. F., Makhadmeh, I. M., Taha, M., & Jarrar, S. K. (2016). Heavy metals in vegetables sold in the local market in Jordan. *Food Additives & Contaminants: Part B*, *3*, 223–229.

Pavlov, A., Lashev, L., Vachin, I., & Rusev, V. (2008). Residues of antimicrobial drugs in chicken meat and offals. *Trakia Journal of Sciences*, *6*, 23–25.

Pesticides and Water Pollution - Safe Drinking Water. (2017). *Pesticides and water pollution fact sheet*. https://www.safewater.org/fact-sheets-1/2017/1/23/pesticides.

Phillips, I., Casewell, M., Cox, T., De Groot, B., Friis, C., Jones, R., ... Waddell, J. (2004). Does the use of antibiotics in food animals pose a risk to human health? A critical review of published data. *Journal of Antimicrobial Chemotherapy*, *53*(1), 28–52.

Pohanish, R. P. (2017). *Sittig's handbook of toxic and hazardous chemicals and carcinogens* (7th ed.). Oxford: William Andrew Publishing.

Prosser, P., & Hart, A. D. M. (2005). Assessing potential exposure of birds to pesticide-treated seeds. *Ecotoxicology*, *14*, 679–691.

Qishlaqi, A., Moore, F., & Forghani, G. (2008). Impact of untreated wastewater irrigation on soils and crops in Shiraz suburban area, Iran. *Environmental Monitoring and Assessment*, *141*, 257–273.

Rafat, A., Salem, N., & Hussein, E. (2010). Occurrence of organochlorine pesticide residues in eggs, chicken and meat in Jordan. *Chemosphere*, *78*, 667–671.

Rana Md, S., Lee, S. Y., Kan, H. J., & Hur, S. J. (2019). Reducing veterinary drug residues in animal products: A review. *Food Science of Animal Resources*, *39*(5), 687–703.

Rather, I. A., Koh, W. Y., Paek, W. K., & Lim, J. (2017). The sources of chemical contaminants in food and their health implications. *Frontiers in Pharmacology*, *8*, 830.

Reddy, K. R. N., Salleh, B., Saad, B., Abbas, H. K., Abel, C. A., & Shier, W. T. (2010). Overview of mycotoxin contamination in foods and its implications for human health. *Toxin Reviews*, *29*(1), 3–26.

Richard, J. L. (2007). Some major mycotoxins and their mycotoxicoses - An overview. *International Journal of Food Microbiology*, *119*(1–2), 3–10.

Risher, J. F., & Amler, S. N. (2005). Mercury exposure: Evaluation and intervention, the inappropriate use of chelating agents in diagnosis and treatment of putative mercury poisoning. *Neurotoxicology*, *26*(4), 691–699.

Rodrigues, I., Handl, J., & Binder, E. M. (2011). Mycotoxin occurrence in commodities, feeds and feed ingredients sourced in the Middle East and Africa. *Food Additives & Contaminants: Part B*, *4*(3), 168–179.

Salem, R. M., El-Kaseh, R. M., & El-Diasty, E. M. (2009). A study on the fungal contamination and prevalence of aflatoxins and some antibiotic residues in table eggs. *Arab Journal of Biotechnology*, *12*(1), 65–71.

Salwa, A. A., & Anwer, W. (2009). Effect of naturally contaminated feed with aflatoxins on performance of laying hens and the carryover of aflatoxin B residues in table eggs. *Pakistan Journal of Nutrition*, *8*(2), 181–186.

Sanchez-Castillo, C. P., Dewey, P. J. S., Aguirre, A., Lara, J. S., Vaca, R., & de la Barra, P. L. (1998). The mineral content of Mexican fruits and vegetables. *Journal of Food Composition and Analysis*, *11*, 340–356.

Sardar, K., Ali, S., Hameed, S., Afzal, S., Fatima, S., Shakor, M. B., ... Tauqeer, H. M. (2013). Heavy metals contamination and what are the impacts on living organisms. *Greener Journal of Environmental Management and Public Safety*, *2*(4), 172–179.

Shamsa, M. T. (2013). Detection of antibiotics residue in chicken meat products in Al-Najaf province. *Al-Qadisiyah Journal of Veterinary Medicine Sciences*, *12*(2), 11–15.

Shareef, A. M., Jamel, Z. T., & Yonis, K. M. (2009). Detection of antibiotic residues in stored poultry products. *Iraqi Journal of Veterinary Sciences*, *23*, 45–48.

Sharma, I., Satya, S., Kumar, V., & Tewary, D. K. (2005). Dissipation of pesticides during bread-making. *Chemical Health and Safety*, *12*(1), 17–22.

Steenland, K., & Boffetta, P. (2000). Lead and cancer in humans: Where are we now? *American Journal of Industrial Medicine*, *38*(3), 295–299.

Street, J. C. (1969). Methods of removal of pesticide residues. *Canadian Medical Association Journal*, *100*(4), 154.

Suruchi, P. K. (2011). Assessment of heavy metal contamination in different vegetables grown in and around urban areas. *Research Journal of Environmental Toxicology*, *5*(3), 162–179.

Thembo, K. M., Vismer, H. F., Nyazema, N. Z., Gelderblom, W. C. A., & Katerere, D. R. (2010). Antifungal activity of four weedy plant extracts against selected mycotoxigenic fungi. *Journal of Applied Microbiology*, *109*, 1479–1486.

Thompson, L. A., & Darwish, W. S. (2019). Environmental chemical contaminants in food: Review of a global problem. *Journal of Toxicology*, *2019*(6), 1–14, Article ID 2345283.

Tomatis, L. (2006). Identification of carcinogenic agents and primary prevention of cancer. *Annals of the New York Academy of Sciences*, *1076*(1), 1–14. Available from https://suraclux.bestbuddieskentucky.org/131bf2/human-toxicology-o.

Turgut, C. (2003). The contamination with organochlorine pesticides and heavy metals in surface water in KUCUK Menderes River in Turkey, 2000–2002. *Environment International*, *29*, 29–32.

United States Department of Agriculture (USDA). (2019). *Maximum residue limits (MRL) database*. Foreign Agricultural Services. https://www.fas.usda.gov/data/china-china-releases-standard-maximum.

Völkel, I., Schröer-Merker, E., & Czerny, C. P. (2011). The carry-over of mycotoxins in products of animal origin with special regard to its implications for the European food safety legislation. *Food and Nutrition Sciences*, *2*, 852–867.

World Health Organization (WHO). (1992) *Cadmium. Environmental health criteria. Cadmium exposure and human health.* https://www.scirp.org/reference/ReferencesPapers.aspx?ReferenceID=1790319.

World Health Organization (WHO). (2003). *The health and environment linkages initiative - HELI*. Geneva, Switzerland: World Health Organization. Available from https://www.who.int/heli/risks/toxics/chemicals/en/.

World Health Organization (WHO). (2013a). *Evaluations of the Joint FAO/WHO Expert Committee on Food Additives (JECFA)*. https://apps.who.int/food-additives-contaminants-jecfa-database/.

World Health Organization (WHO). (2013b). *Integrated surveillance of antimicrobial resistance: Guidance from a WHO Advisory Group*. http://www.who.int.

World Health Organization (WHO). (2018a). *Mycotoxins*. https://www.who.int/news-room/fact-sheets/detail/mycotoxins.

World Health Organization (WHO). (2018b). *Pesticide residues in food*. http://www.who.int/news-https://www.who.int/news-room/fact-sheets/detail/pesticide-residues-in-foodroom/fact-sheets/detail/pesticide-residues-in-food.

World Health Organization and United Nations Environment Programme. (1990). *Public health impact of pesticides used in agriculture*. Geneva, Switzerland. http://www.who.int/iris/handle/10665/39772.

Willis, C. (2000). Antibiotics in the food chain: their impact on the consumer. *Reviews in Medical Microbiology*, *11*, 153–160.

Zaidi, M. I., Asrar, A., Mansour, A., & Farooqui, M. A. (2005). The heavy metal concentrations along roadsides trees of Quetta and its effects on public health. *Journal of Applied Sciences*, *5*(4), 708–711.

Chapter 6

Control of foodborne pathogens in common foods in the Middle East

Amin N. Olaimat[1], Anas A. Al-Nabulsi[2] and Tareq M. Osaili[2,3]
[1]Department of Clinical Nutrition and Dietetics, Faculty of Applied Medical Sciences, The Hashemite University, Zarqa, Jordan, [2]Department of Nutrition and Food Technology, Jordan University of Science and Technology, Irbid, Jordan, [3]Department of Clinical Nutrition and Dietetics, University of Sharjah, Sharjah, United Arab Emirates

6.1 Introduction

Food safety is a health and socioeconomic concern worldwide. The consumption of unsafe food is associated with various illnesses which could have major repercussions especially for the vulnerable segments of society like immunocompromised patients, pregnant women, and children. Foodborne outbreaks could be prevented and controlled. Prevention strategies include government-imposed food safety regulations, implementation of frequent and successful food safety associated programs, research development which identify gaps in practice, and lastly the adaptation of new advanced technologies which help in improving food safety. Controlling or limiting an outbreak solely rests on one concrete factor, which is an efficient surveillance and epidemiological information system. A platform integrates all the entities of concern such as the healthcare system, municipal organization, and food catering services (Faour-Klingbeil & Todd, 2020; Todd, 2017).

Barring a few exceptions, countries in the Middle East still have some major voids in the system which hamper their management/prevention of foodborne outbreaks; the predicament being even more obvious in traditional food products. Maintaining checks and balances to control pathogenic microorganisms (especially in traditional products) is not a common phenomenon, be it at the processing plant level or at retail (Faour-Klingbeil & Todd, 2020; Todd, 2017). The entire regulatory system pertaining to food safety usually comes into play in the event of an outbreak, later leading to product recalls.

Food Safety in the Middle East. DOI: https://doi.org/10.1016/B978-0-12-822417-5.00003-9

Although a gap exists in practice at the retail level, an effort to combat this issue has been made by academia. Multiple research studies have been conducted which identify various biological, chemical, and physical interventions to control foodborne pathogens in traditional food products usually consumed in the Middle East including dips (Table 6.1), salads (Table 6.2), dairy products (Table 6.3), meat products (Table 6.4), and miscellaneous items (Table 6.5). This chapter reviews these approaches in detail.

6.2 Chemical and natural preservation treatments

The use of natural and chemical antimicrobials for food preservation purposes has been passed down by generations. One such set of natural compounds used for this purpose are organic acids. Acetic, lactic, malic, citric, formic, sorbic, propionic, and benzoic acids are the most common examples (Anyasi, Jideani, Edokpayi, & Anokwuru, 2017). Organic acids are low-molecular-weight compounds containing one or more carboxyl groups. They posess the ability to penetrate the pathogenic cell membrane and dissociate inside it. This leads to a decrease in intracellular pH which disrupts the synthesis of adenosine triphosphate (ATP), RNA, DNA, and other proteins all eventually retarding cell growth.

Al-Nabulsi et al. (2014) incorporated $\leq 0.5\%$ citric acid/acetic acid in commercial tahini ($a_w = 0.3$). They observed a reduction in *Salmonella* Typhimurium numbers by 2.5–3.8 log CFU mL^{-1} and 2.7–4.8 log CFU mL^{-1}, respectively, upon storage for 28 days at 10°C–37°C. The same authors hydrated the tahini and observed that *S.* Typhimurium cells reduced to undetectable levels upon the addition of 0.5% citric acid or acetic acid after 21 and 7 days of storage, respectively. In another study, *Staphylococcus aureus* numbers in commercial tahini incorporated with 0.5% citric or acetic acid were reduced by 2.3 log CFU mL^{-1} after 28 days of storage. In comparison, *Staph. aureus* cells were not detected in hydrated tahini to which 0.3% or 0.5% acetic acid was added after 14, 7 days of storage (at 21°C and 37°C) and after 28, 14 days (at 10°C), respectively. A lower concentration, that is, 0.1% acetic acid was also capable of reducing bacterial numbers to undetectable levels within 14, 28 days of storage at 21°C and 37°C, respectively. *Staph. aureus* cells were also reduced in rehydrated tahini to undetectable levels within 21–28 days by adding 0.1%–0.5% citric acid, respectively (Olaimat, Al-Nabulsi, et al., 2017).

In tabbouleh salad, stored at 21°C, 0.4% acetic acid reduced the numbers of *S.* Typhimurium and *Escherichia coli* O157:H7 to below detectable levels by 5 and 7 days, respectively. It also reduced the *Staph. aureus* population by 2.8 log CFU g^{-1} within 7 days. However, upon storing the tabbouleh at 4°C and 10°C, citric acid (compared to acetic acid) was more inhibitory against the tested pathogens. A citric acid concentration of 1.4% reduced *E. coli* O157:H7, *S.* Typhimurium, and *Staph. aureus* by 2.2, 3.9, and 3.6 log

TABLE 6.1 Control methods of different foodborne pathogens in common dips in the Middle East.

Antimicrobial treatment	Concentration or dose	Foodborne pathogen	Food product	Storage duration	Temperature	Log reduction	References
Citric acid	$\leq$0.5%	*Salmonella* Typhimurium	Tahini	28 days	10, 21, 37	2.5–3.8 log CFU mL^{-1}	Al-Nabulsi et al. (2014)
Acetic acid	$\leq$0.5%	*Salmonella* Typhimurium	Tahini	28 days	10, 21, 37	2.7–4.8 log CFU mL^{-1}	
Citric acid	0.50%	*Salmonella* Typhimurium	Hydrated tahini	21 days	10, 21, 37	Not detected	
Acetic acid	0.50%	*Salmonella* Typhimurium	Hydrated tahini	7 days	10, 21, 37	Not detected	
Citric or acetic acid	0.1%–0.5%	*Staphylococcus aureus*	Tahini	28 days	10, 21, 37	$\leq$2.3 log CFU mL^{-1}	Olaimat, Al-Nabulsi, et al. (2017)
Acetic acid	0.30%	*Staphylococcus aureus*	Hydrated tahini	14 days	21, 37	Not detected	
Acetic acid	0.50%	*Staphylococcus aureus*	Hydrated tahini	7 days	21, 37	Not detected	
Acetic acid	0.30%	*Staphylococcus aureus*	Hydrated tahini	28 days	10	Not detected	
Acetic acid	0.50%	*Staphylococcus aureus*	Hydrated tahini	14 days	10	Not detected	

(*Continued*)

TABLE 6.1 (Continued)

Antimicrobial treatment	Concentration or dose	Foodborne pathogen	Food product	Storage duration	Temperature	Log reduction	References
Acetic acid	0.10%	*Staphylococcus aureus*	Hydrated tahini	14 days	21	Not detected	
Acetic acid	0.10%	*Staphylococcus aureus*	Hydrated tahini	28 days	37	Not detected	
Citric acid	0.50%	*Staphylococcus aureus*	Hydrated tahini	21 days	10, 21, 37	Not detected	
Citric acid	0.10%	*Staphylococcus aureus*	Hydrated tahini	28 days	21	Not detected	
Citric acid	0.30%	*Staphylococcus aureus*	Hydrated tahini	21 days	21	Not detected	
Cinnamon EO	2.00%	*Salmonella*	Tahini	28 days	10–37	2.4–2.9 log CFU mL^{-1}	Al-Nabulsi, Osaili, Olaimat, Almasri, Ayyash, et al. (2020)
Thyme EO	2.00%	*Salmonella*	Tahini	28 days	10–37	2.2–3.3 log CFU mL^{-1}	
Cinnamon EO	2.00%	*Salmonella*	Hydrated tahini	7 days	10, 25, 37	Not detected	
Thyme EO	2.00%	*Salmonella*	Hydrated tahini	28 days	25, 37	Not detected	

Cinnamon EO	2.00%	*E. coli* O157:H7	Tahini	28 days	10, 25, 37	1.38–2.20 log CFU mL^{-1}	Al-Nabulsi, Osaili, Olaimat, Almasri, Al-Holy, et al. (2020)
Thyme EO	2.00%	*E. coli* O157:H7	Tahini	28 days	10, 25, 37	1.65–2.01 log CFU mL^{-1}	
Thyme EO	0.5% or 1.0%	*E. coli* O157:H7	Hydrated tahini	28 days	25, 37	Not detected	
Gamma irradiation	2.0 kGy	*Salmonella*	Tahini			4.5–4.7 log CFU g^{-1}	Osaili, Al-Nabulsi, Abubakar, Alaboudi, & Al-Holy (2016)
Gamma irradiation	1.0 kGy	*E. coli* O157:H7	Tahini			2.6–3.2 log CFU g^{-1}	Osaili & Al-Nabulsi (2016)
Citric acid	0.1%–0.3%	*L. innocua*	Hummus	6 days	4	No effect	Al-Holy, Al-Qadiri, Lin, & Rasco (2006)
Nisin and citric acid	1000 IU g^{-1}, 0.3%	*L. innocua*	Hummus	6 days	4	2.1 log CFU g^{-1}	
Citric acid	1.0%	*Sh. sonnei*	Hummus	10 days	10	2.0 log CFU g^{-1}	Olaimat, Al-Holy, et al. (2017)
Citric acid	2.0%	*Sh. sonnei*	Hummus	10 days	10	4.0 log CFU g^{-1}	
Citric acid	2.0%	*Sh. sonnei*	Hummus	7 days	4	Not detected	
Citric acid	2.0%	*Sh. flexneri*	Hummus	10 days	4	1.4 log CFU g^{-1}	
Citric acid	2.0%	*Sh. flexneri*	Hummus	10 days	10	1.0 log CFU g^{-1}	

(*Continued*)

TABLE 6.1 (Continued)

Antimicrobial treatment	Concentration or dose	Foodborne pathogen	Food product	Storage duration	Temperature	Log reduction	References
Garlic extract	3.00%	*Sh. sonnei*	Hummus	10 days	4	4.0 log CFU g^{-1}	
Garlic extract	3.00%	*Sh. sonnei*	Hummus	10 days	10	3.0 log CFU g^{-1}	
Garlic extract	3.00%	*Sh. flexneri*	Hummus	10 days	10	Inhibited growth	
Citric acid and garlic extract	1.0%, 2.0%	*Sh. flexneri*	Hummus	10 days	4	2.7 log CFU g^{-1}	
Citric acid and garlic extract	1.0%, 2.0%	*Sh. flexneri*	Hummus	10 days	10	2.1 log CFU g^{-1}	
Thiamine dilaurylsulfate and malic acid	2.0%, 1.0%	G − and G + bacteria	Hummus	30 days	4	Inhibited growth	Shaheen, Nsaif, & Borjac (2019)
Cinnamon EO	0.50%	*Salmonella*	Hummus	7 days	4, 10	Not detected	Olaimat et al. (2019)
Cinnamon EO	1.00%	*Salmonella*	Hummus	1 day	4, 10	Not detected	
Thyme EO	0.5%–1.5%	*Salmonella*	Hummus	10 days	4	1.0–2.9 log CFU g^{-1}	
Thyme EO	0.5%–1.5%	*Salmonella*	Hummus	10 days	10	<1 log CFU g^{-1}	
Allyl isothiocyanate	0.1%–0.25%	*S. enterica*	Hummus	10 days	4	3.0–5.7 log CFU g^{-1}	Olaimat et al. (2018)

Allyl isothiocyanate	0.10%	*S. enterica*	Hummus	10 days	10	6.7 log CFU g^{-1}	
Allyl isothiocyanate	0.25%	*S. enterica*	Hummus	10 days	10	Not detected	
Allyl isothiocyanate	≥0.5%	*S. enterica*	Hummus	3 days	4, 10	Not detected	
Allyl isothiocyanate	≥0.5%	*L. monocytogenes*	Hummus	3 days	10	Not detected	
Allyl isothiocyanate	≥0.5%	*L. monocytogenes*	Hummus	7 days	4	Not detected	
Allyl isothiocyanate	0.1%–0.25%	*L. monocytogenes*	Hummus	10 days	10	4.8–6.4 log CFU g^{-1}	
Allyl isothiocyanate	0.1%–0.25%	*L. monocytogenes*	Hummus	10 days	4	2.7–3.9 log CFU g^{-1}	
Hydrostatic pressure	500 MPa for 10 min	*Salmonella*, *L. monocytogenes*, *E. coli*	Hummus		Room temperature	> 5 log CFU g^{-1}	Sokołowska, Nasiłowska, Rutkowska, Fonberg-Broczek, & Rzoska (2019)

TABLE 6.2 Control methods of different foodborne pathogens in common salads in the Middle East.

Antimicrobial treatment	Concentration or dose	Foodborne pathogen	Food product	Storage duration	Temperature	Log reduction	References
Acetic acid	0.40%	*Salmonella* Typhimurium	Tabbouleh	5 days	21	Not detected	Al-Rousan et al. (2018)
Acetic acid	0.40%	*E. coli* O157:H7	Tabbouleh	7 days	21	Not detected	
Acetic acid	0.40%	*Staphylococcus aureus*	Tabbouleh	7 days	21	2.8 log CFU g^{-1}	
Citric acid	1.40%	*E. coli* O157:H7	Tabbouleh	7 days	10	2.2	
Citric acid	1.40%	*Salmonella* Typhimurium	Tabbouleh	7 days	10	3.9	
Citric acid	1.40%	*Staphylococcus aureus*	Tabbouleh	7 days	10	3.6	
Citric acid	1.40%	*E. coli* O157:H7	Tabbouleh	7 days	4	2	
Citric acid	1.40%	*Salmonella* Typhimurium	Tabbouleh	7 days	4	4.4	
Citric acid	1.40%	*Staphylococcus aureus*	Tabbouleh	7 days	4	4.3	
Citric and acetic acid	1.4, 0.3%	*Salmonella* Typhimurium/ *E. coli* O157:H7	Tabbouleh	2 days	21	Not detected	

Citric and acetic acid	1.0, 0.4%	*Salmonella* Typhimurium/ *E. coli* O157:H7	Tabbouleh	3 days	21	Not detected	
Citric and acetic acid	1.4, 0.3%	*Salmonella* Typhimurium	Tabbouleh	2 days	4	Not detected	
Citric and acetic acid	1.0, 0.4%	*Salmonella* Typhimurium	Tabbouleh	6 days	4	Not detected	
Citric and acetic acid	1.4, 0.3%	*Salmonella* Typhimurium	Tabbouleh	4 days	10	Not detected	
Citric and acetic acid	1.0, 0.4%	*Salmonella* Typhimurium	Tabbouleh	4 days	10	Not detected	
Citrus extract	1 and 2 mL kg^{-1}	*E. coli* O157:H7	Tzatziki	70, 35, 15 days	4, 10, 21	2.8–4.8 log CFU g^{-1}	Tsiraki et al. (2018)
Citrus extract	1 and 2 mL kg^{-1}	*L. monocytogenes*	Tzatziki	70, 35, 15 days	4, 10, 21	1.5–3.0 log CFU g^{-1}	
Lemon juice and NaCl	1%, 0.5%	*Salmonella*	Tomato-cucumber salad	5 days	4, 10	0.7–1.0 log CFU g^{-1}	Olaimat, Al-Holy, et al. (2020), Olaimat, Osaili, et al. (2020)
Lemon juice and NaCl	1%, 0.5%	*Shigella*	Tomato-cucumber salad	5 days	4, 10	0.6–1.4 log CFU g^{-1}	
Lemon juice and NaCl	1%, 0.5%	*Salmonella*	Tomato-cucumber salad	4 days	24	Not detected	

(*Continued*)

TABLE 6.2 (Continued)

Antimicrobial treatment	Concentration or dose	Foodborne pathogen	Food product	Storage duration	Temperature	Log reduction	References
Lemon juice and NaCl	1%, 0.5%	*Shigella*	Tomato-cucumber salad	5 days	24	1.9 log CFU g^{-1}	
Pomegranate molasses (PG) vinaigrette salad dressing	70 mL PG 30 mL extra virgin olive oil 15 mL white wine vinegar (6% acetic acid) 1.5 tsp salt	*Salmonella* Typhimurium	Mixed salad vegetables	1 h	5, 21	2.0–3.1 log CFU g^{-1}	Faour-Klingbeil and Todd (2018)

TABLE 6.3 Control methods of different foodborne pathogens in common dairy products in the Middle East.

Antimicrobial treatment	Concentration or dose	Foodborne pathogen	Food product	Storage duration	Temperature	Log reduction	References
Binium persicum essential oil	1.0%–2.0%	*E. coli* O157:H7	White-brined cheese	45 days	Ripening at 14°C for 15 days and storage at 4°C for 30 days	<0.7 log CFU g^{-1}	Ehsani, Hashemi, Naghibi, Mohammadi, & Khalili Sadaghiani (2016)
Binium persicum essential oil	1.0%–2.0%	*L. monocytogenes*	White-brined cheese	45 days	Ripening at 14°C for 15 days and storage at 4°C for 30 days	<0.7 log CFU g^{-1}	
Zataria multiflora essential oil	150 ppm	*E. coli* O157	White-brined cheese	60 days	4	2.0 log CFU g^{-1}	Mehdizadeh, Narimani, Mojaddar Langroodi, Moghaddas Kia, & Neyriz-Naghadehi (2018)
Dill essential oil	150 ppm	*E. coli* O157:H7	White-brined cheese	60 days	4	1.1 log CFU g^{-1}	Mojaddar Langroodi, Mehdizadeh, Majidi, & Neyriz-Naghadehi (2020)

(*Continued*)

TABLE 6.3 (Continued)

Antimicrobial treatment	Concentration or dose	Foodborne pathogen	Food product	Storage duration	Temperature	Log reduction	References
Cayenne and green pepper extract	6%–9%	*Staphylococcus aureus*	Egyptian Kareish cheese	2 days	4	Not detected	Wahba et al. (2010)
Dill and parsley extracts	6%–9%	*Staphylococcus aureus*	Egyptian Kareish cheese	2 days	4	3–4 log CFU g^{-1}	
Nisin	10 ppm	*Staphylococcus aureus*	Kareish cheese	1 month	4	1.6 log CFU g^{-1}	Meshref, Hassan, Riad, & Ashour (2019)
Nisin	12.5 ppm	*Staphylococcus aureus*	Kareish cheese	1 month	4	2.6 log CFU g^{-1}	
Starter LAB		*E. coli* O157:H7	White-brined cheese	28 days	10	2.6–3.4 log CFU g^{-1}	Osaili et al. (2014)
Starter LAB		*E. coli* O157:H7	White-brined cheese	28 days	21	1.0–1.6 log CFU g^{-1}	
Lb. reuteri		*E. coli* O157:H7	White-brined cheese stored in 10% NaCl brine	28 days	25	2.6 log CFU g^{-1}	Al-Nabulsi et al. (2021)
Lb. reuteri		*E. coli* O157:H7	White-brined cheese stored in 15% NaCl brine	28 days	10	2.2 log CFU g^{-1}	

Zataria Multiflora EO and *Lb. acidophilus* PTCC 1643	150 ppm	*E. coli* O157:H7	White-brined cheese in sterile 11% brine solution	60 days	4	2 log CFU g^{-1}	Mehdizadeh, Narimani, Mojaddar Langroodi, Moghaddas Kia, & Neyriz-Naghadehi (2018)
Lb. acidophilus PTCC 1643 along with dill EO	150 ppm	*E. coli* O157:H7	White-brined cheese in sterile 11% brine solution	60 days	4	1.6 log CFU g^{-1}	Mojaddar Langroodi, Mehdizadeh, Majidi, & Neyriz-Naghadehi (2020)
Lb. acidophilus ATCC 4356		*L. monocytogenes*	White-brined cheese in sterile 11% brine solution	15 / 45 days	14/4	3.16 log CFU g^{-1}	Mahmoudi, Tajik, Ehsani, & Zare (2012)
Active packaging (chitosan coating consisting of Mentha aquatica *L. essence*)	1.5%	*E. coli* O157:H7	White-brined cheese	10 days	4	Not detected	Hani Tabaie Zavareh & Ardestani (2020)
Active packaging (chitosan	1.5%	*L. monocytogenes*	White cheese	15 days	4	5.4 log CFU g^{-1}	

(*Continued*)

TABLE 6.3 (Continued)

Antimicrobial treatment	Concentration or dose	Foodborne pathogen	Food product	Storage duration	Temperature	Log reduction	References
coating consisting of Mentha aquatica *L. essence*)							
Active packaging (chitosan coating consisting of Mentha aquatica *L. essence*)	1.5%	*Staphylococcus aureus*	White cheese	15 days	4	4.9 log CFU g^{-1}	
Chitosan coating 1% (wt./vol.) ZnO nanoparticles		*E. coli* O157:H7	White-brined cheese	28 days	4	2.8 log CFU g^{-1}	Al-Nabulsi, Osaili, Sawalha, et al. (2020)
Chitosan coating 1% (wt./vol.) ZnO nanoparticles		*E. coli* O157:H7	White-brined cheese	28 days	10	2.1 log CFU g^{-1}	
Electron beam radiation	5 kGy	*Brucella abortus*	Tradiitional ice cream	21 days		Not detected	Ganjaroudi, Raeisi, Hajimohammadi, & Zandi (2016)

Electron beam radiation	5 kGy	*Brucella melitensis*	Tradiitional ice cream	21 days		>4 CFU g^{-1}	
Electron beam radiation	1 kGy	*Brucella abortus*	Tradiitional ice cream	21 days		>4 CFU g^{-1}	
Electron beam radiation	1 kGy	*Brucella melitensis*	Tradiitional ice cream	21 days		>4 CFU g^{-1}	
Starter LAB		*L. monocytogenes*	Camel yoghurt	14 days	4	2.0 log CFU mL^{-1}	Al-Nabulsi et al. (2016)
Starter LAB		*L. monocytogenes*	Camel yoghurt	14 days	10	2.9 log CFU mL^{-1}	
Starter LAB		*E. coli* O157:H7	Camel yoghurt	5 h	43	1.1 log CFU mL^{-1}	
Starter LAB		*E. coli* O157:H7	Camel yoghurt	7 days	4, 10	6.3 log CFU mL^{-1}	
Green tea and ginger	1.0% (wt./vol.)	*E. coli* O157:H7	Ayran	5 days	4	< 0.6 log CFU g^{-1}	Belal et al. (2019)

TABLE 6.4 Control methods of different foodborne pathogens in common meat products in the Middle East.

Antimicrobial treatment	Concentration or dose	Foodborne pathogen	Food product	Storage duration	Temperature	Log reduction	Reference
Marinade	1.5 g salt, 1.5 g white pepper, 3.6 mL corn oil, 0.6 mL vinegar, 2.0 g red chili paste, 2.4 g mixed fruit/vegetables	*E. coli* O157:H7	Chicken tawook	7 days	4	1.2 log CFU g^{-1}	Osaili, Hasan, Dhanasekaran, Obaid, Al-Nabulsi, Ayyash, et al. (2021)
Marinade	1.5 g salt, 1.5 g white pepper, 3.6 mL corn oil, 0.6 mL vinegar, 2.0 g red chili paste, 2.4 g mixed fruit/vegetables	*E. coli* O157:H7	Chicken tawook	7 days	10	3.8 log CFU g^{-1}	
Marinade	1.5 g salt, 1.5 g white pepper, 3.6 mL corn oil, 0.6 mL vinegar, 2.0 g red chili paste, 2.4 g mixed fruit/vegetables	*Salmonella* spp.	Chicken tawook	7 days	4	2.2 log CFU g^{-1}	
Marinade	1.5 g salt, 1.5 g white pepper, 3.6 mL corn oil, 0.6 mL vinegar, 2.0 g red chili paste, 2.4 g mixed fruit/vegetables	*Salmonella* spp.	Chicken tawook	7 days	10	5.1 log CFU g^{-1}	
Marinade	1.5 g salt, 1.5 g white pepper, 3.6 mL corn oil, 0.6 mL vinegar, 2.0 g red chili paste, 2.4 g mixed fruit/vegetables	*L. monocytogenes*	Chicken tawook	7 days	4	No effect	

Marinade	1.5 g salt, 1.5 g white pepper, 3.6 mL corn oil, 0.6 mL vinegar, 2.0 g red chili paste, 2.4 g mixed fruit/vegetables	*L. monocytogenes*	Chicken tawook	7 days	10	2.2 log CFU g^{-1}	
Marinade with carvacol or cinnamaldehyde or thymol	2.00%	*E. coli* O157:H7	Chicken tawook	7 days	4	1.7–2.3 log CFU g^{-1}	Osaili, Hasan, Dhanasekaran, Obaid, Al-Nabulsi, Karam, et al. (2021)
Marinade with carvacol or cinnamaldehyde or thymol	2.00%	*E. coli* O157:H7	Chicken tawook	7 days	10	3.8–4.8 log CFU g^{-1}	
Marinade with carvacol or cinnamaldehyde or thymol	2.00%	*Salmonella* spp.	Chicken tawook	7 days	4	2.7 log CFU g^{-1}	
Marinade with carvacol or cinnamaldehyde or thymol	2.00%	*Salmonella* spp.	Chicken tawook	7 days	10	5.1–5.6 log CFU g^{-1}	
Marinade with carvacol or cinnamaldehyde or thymol	2.00%	*L. monocytogenes*	Chicken tawook	7 days	4	No effect	

(*Continued*)

TABLE 6.4 (Continued)

Antimicrobial treatment	Concentration or dose	Foodborne pathogen	Food product	Storage duration	Temperature	Log reduction	Reference
Marinade with carvacol or cinnamaldehyde or thymol	2.00%	*L. monocytogenes*	Chicken tawook	7 days	10	2.4–2.7 log CFU g^{-1}	
Fermnted ginger paste	10 g for 10 g chicken	Aerobic bacteria	Chicken	2 days	8	2.8 log CFU mL^{-1}	Muhialdin, Kadum, Fathallah, & Meor Hussin (2020)
Fresh ginger paste	10 g for 10 g chicken	Aerobic bacteria	Chicken	2 days	8	No effect	
CoNShP-3 Phage	8 log	Coagulase negative staphylococci	Chicken breast samples	7 days	4	>6.0 CFU cm^{-2}	Sofy, El Haliem, Refaey, & Hmed (2020)
CoNShP-3 Phage	8 log	Coagulase negative staphylococci	Chicken breast samples	30 days	−20	>6.0 CFU cm^{-2}	
Thermal treatment		*Salmonella* Typhimurium	Chicken for sahwarma		54	*D* value: 9.15–12.44	Osaili et al. (2013)
Thermal treatment		*Salmonella* Typhimurium	Chicken for sahwarma		56	*D* value: 2.89–3.92 min	
Thermal treatment		*Salmonella* Typhimurium	Chicken for sahwarma		58	*D* value: 1.06–1.30 min	

Thermal treatment		*Salmonella* Typhimurium	Chicken for sahwarma		60	*D* value: 0.32–0.52 min	
Gamma irradiation	4.5 kGy	*Salmonella*	Cooked chicken samples	15 days		Not detected	Fallah et al. (2010)
Gamma irradiation	4.5 kGy	*E. coli* O157:H7	Cooked chicken samples	15 days		Not detected	
Gamma irradiation	4.5 kGy	*L. monocytogenes*	Cooked chicken samples	15 days		Not detected	
Ginger and citric acid incorporated in cellulose nanofibres		Total viable counts	Chicken barbeque meat	10 days	4	4.94–5.12 log CFU g^{-1}	Khaledian et al. (2019)
Ginger and citric acid incorporated in cellulose nanofibres		Psychrotrophic bacteria	Chicken barbeque meat	10 days	4	4.64–4.97 log CFU g^{-1}	
Ginger and citric acid incorporated in cellulose nanofibres		*Enterobacteriaceae*	Chicken barbeque meat	10 days	4	2.91–4.64 log CFU g^{-1}	
Thermal treatment		*E. coli* O157:H7	Ground camel meat		57.5–65	*D* value: 1.8–0.07 min;	Osaili, Al-Nabulsi, et al. (2020)

(Continued)

TABLE 6.4 (Continued)

Antimicrobial treatment	Concentration or dose	Foodborne pathogen	Food product	Storage duration	Temperature	Log reduction	Reference
						z value 4.6–5.0 C	
Thermal treatment		*Salmonella*	Ground camel meat		55–62.5	*D* value: 2.2–0.06 min; *z* value 5.1–5.5 C	
Thermal treatment		*E. coli* O157:H7	Marinated camel meat with hump fat		60–67.5	*D* value: 76.0–4.1 s	Osaili, Hasan, et al. (2020)
Thermal treatment		*Salmonella*	Marinated camel meat with hump fat		55–62.5	*D* value: 512.1–8.4 s	
Thermal treatment		*E. coli* O157:H7	Marinated camel meat		60–67.5	*D* value: 53.5–3.0 s	
Thermal treatment		*Salmonella*	Marinated camel meat		55–62.5	*D* value: 349.2–6.7 s	
Carvacrol	2%	*Salmonella*	Marinated camel meat	7 days	4	3.2 log CFU g^{-1}	Osaili, Hasan, Dhanasekaran, Obaid, Al-Nabulsi, Karam, et al. (2021)

Cinnamldehyde	2%	*Salmonella*	Marinated camel meat	7 days	4	3.4 log CFU g^{-1}	
Thymol	2%	*Salmonella*	Marinated camel meat	7 days	4	3.4 log CFU g^{-1}	
Carvacrol	2%	*E. coli* O157:H7	Marinated camel meat	7 days	4	2.5 log CFU g^{-1}	
Cinnamldehyde	2%	*E. coli* O157:H7	Marinated camel meat	7 days	4	2.6 log CFU g^{-1}	
Thymol	2%	*E. coli* O157:H7	Marinated camel meat	7 days	4	3 log CFU g^{-1}	
ZnO nanoparticles containing acetic acid	1%	*L. monocytogenes*	Sheep meat	12 days	4	4.7 log CFU g^{-1}	Mirhosseini & Arjmand (2014)
ZnO nanoparticles containing acetic acid	1%	*E. coli*	Sheep meat	12 days	4	1.2 log CFU g^{-1}	
ZnO nanoparticles containing acetic acid	1%	*Staphylococcus aureus*	Sheep meat	12 days	4	2.8 log CFU g^{-1}	

TABLE 6.5 Control methods of different foodborne pathogens in common miscellaneous items in the Middle East.

Antimicrobial treatment	Concentration or dose	Foodborne pathogen	Food product	Storage duration	Temperature	Log reduction	References
Phage ZCSE 1	7 log	*S. enterica*	Chicken skin	2 days	4	3.3 log CFU g^{-1}	El-Shibiny et al. (2017)
Phage ZCSE 1	7 log	*S. enterica*	Eggs	2 days	4	Not detected	
Phage ZCEC1	7 log	*E. coli*	Meat, tomatoes	1 day	4	Not detected	
Thermal treatment		*Salmonella*	Sesame seeds		150 C, 30 min; 130 C, 50 min; 110 C, 60 min	5.9 log CFU g^{-1}	Torlak, Sert, & Serin (2013)
Ultrasound	50%	*E. coli*	Pomegranate juice			<1.5 log	Alighourchi, Barzegar, Sahari, & Abbasi (2014)
Ultrasound	75%	*Saccharomyces cerevisiae*	Pomegranate juice			<1.5 log	
Ultrasound	100%	*E. coli*	Pomegranate juice			3.47 log CFU mL^{-1}	
Ultrasound	100%	*Saccharomyces cerevisiae*	Pomegranate juice			1.86 log CFU mL^{-1}	
Gamma irradiation	1 kGy	*E. coli*	Pomegranate juice			6.66 log CFU mL^{-1}	
Gamma irradiation	3 kGy	*Saccharomyces cerevisiae*	Pomegranate juice			5.08 log CFU mL^{-1}	

CFU g^{-1}, respectively, at 10°C and by 2.0, 4.4, and 4.3 log CFU g^{-1}, respectively, at 4°C. The combination of acetic and citric acids showed a synergistic effect against *E. coli* O157:H7 and *S.* Typhimurium, but not against *Staph. aureus*. Both *S.* Typhimurium and *E. coli* O157:H7 were not detected in tabbouleh salad after 2–3 days of storage at 21°C when the salad received a combination treatment of 1.4% citric acid and 0.3% acetic acid or 1% citric acid and 0.4% acetic acid, respectively. However, the two combination treatments reduced the numbers of *S.* Typhimurium below the detection levels after 2 and 6 days when the salad was stored at 4°C, and after 4 days (for both treatments) at 10°C (Al-Rousan et al., 2018). In another study, Tsiraki et al. (2018) investigated the antimicrobial activity of 1 and 2 mL kg^{-1} citrus extract against *E. coli* O157:H7 and *Listeria monocytogenes* in Tzatziki (yogurt-based salad) stored for 70, 35, and 15 days at 4°C, 10°C, or 21°C, respectively. Citrus extract showed a significant antimicrobial activity against *E. coli* O157:H7, with reductions of 2.8–4.8 log CFU g^{-1} in the treated salad samples at the tested temperatures by the end of the storage period. However, the citrus extract showed lower activity against *L. monocytogenes* and reduced its numbers only by 1.5–3.0 log CFU g^{-1} by the end of storage period at all the above-mentioned storage temperatures. Faour-Klingbeil and Todd (2018) found that pomegranate molasses (PG) vinaigrette salad dressing containing 70 mL PG, 30 mL extra virgin olive oil, 15 mL white wine vinegar (6% acetic acid), 1.5 tsp salt reduced numbers of low (3 log CFU g^{-1}) or high (6 log CFU g^{-1}) inoculated *S.* Typhimurium in mixed vegetable salad (parsley, radish, cucumber, tomato, lettuce, and onion) by 2.0–3.1 log CFU g^{-1} after 1 h at 5°C and 21°C. A study conducted on tomato-cucumber salad showed that an addition of 1.0% lemon juice and 0.5% NaCl reduced numbers of *Salmonella* spp. and *Shigella* sp. by 0.7–1.0 and 0.6–1.4 log CFU g^{-1} at 4°C and 10°C after 5 days, respectively. Surprisingly, *Salmonella* cells were not detected at 24°C after the addition by 4 days (Olaimat, Al-Holy, et al., 2020). This observation should be of great interest to the general public/food safety authorities as these salads are traditionally consumed at room temperatures and are not chilled.

Some studies have combined organic acids with other natural antimicrobials such as nisin and plant extracts to inhibit foodborne pathogens. Al-Holy, Al-Qadiri, Lin, & Rasco (2006) studied the antimicrobial effect of nisin (500 or 1000 IU g^{-1}), citric acid (0.1%, 0.2%, or 0.3%), or their combinations against *Listeria innocua* in hummus stored at 4°C. Citric acid displayed no antimicrobial activity against *L. innocua* in hummus. However, a combination of 1000 IU g^{-1} nisin and 0.3% citric acid was effective in reducing *L. innocua* by approximately 1.5 log CFU g^{-1} after 6 days. Olaimat, Al-Holy, et al. (2017) observed that 1.0% and 2.0% citric acid reduced numbers of *Shigella sonnei* by 2.0 and 4.0 log CFU g^{-1} at 10°C within 10 days. However, when the hummus treated with 2.0% citric acid was stored at 4°C for 7 days, *Sh. sonnei* cells reached undetectable levels.

Furthermore, 2% citric acid reduced numbers of *Sh. flexneri* in hummus by 1.4 and 1.0 log CFU g^{-1} at 4°C and 10°C, respectively, by 10 days. Garlic extract with a concentration of 3% reduced the numbers of *Sh. sonnei* by 4.0 and 3.0 log CFU g^{-1}, respectively, at 4°C and 10°C within 10 days in hummus. The garlic extract also inhibited the growth of *S. flexneri* in hummus at 10°C compared to the control. The combination of 1.0% citric acid and 2.0% garlic extract showed an increase in the inhibitory effect compared to the use of single agents; *S. flexneri* numbers were reduced by 2.7 and 2.1 log CFU g^{-1}, respectively, at 4°C and 10°C by 10 days. Shaheen, Nsaif, & Borjac (2019) reported that the addition of 2.0% thiamine dilaurylsulfate with 1% malic acid completely inhibited the growth of Gram-negative and Gram-positive bacteria in hummus at 4°C up to 30 days.

Essential oils are derived from different parts (flowers, leaves, seeds, fruits, roots, rhizomes, and bark) of the plant besides spices and herbs. They contain mixtures of volatile and aromatic compounds. Essential oils have largely been employed in food products as preservatives due to their antimicrobial action against pathogenic microorganisms. The Middle Eastern traditional foods are usually blended with spices and herbs such as cardamom, coriander, thyme, oregano, cumin, nutmeg, cloves, paprika, pepper, and cinnamon. They are commonly used to enhance flavor. Incorporating essential oils extracted from these spices into the Middle Eastern dishes is hence expected to have a dual effect; antimicrobial and organoleptic enhancement.

Essential oils can be incorporated into food products via different methods, direct liquid mixing, direct vapor phase exposure, or incorporation in active edible or biodegradable coatings and films. The antimicrobial activity of essential oils is exerted by damaging the structure and eventually the function of the bacterial cell membrane. The phospholipid bilayer of the cell membrane is attacked which leads to loss of vital intracellular contents like proteins, reducing sugars, inhibition of the ATP generation, disruption of enzyme systems and functions, and damage of bacterial genetic material (Chouhan, Sharma, & Guleria, 2017). Several factors effect the antimicrobial activity of essential oils including the presence of functional groups, their composition, and synergistic interactions (Dorman & Deans, 2000). Furthermore, the mechanism of antimicrobial action may vary with the type of essential oil based on its stereochemistry and lipophilicity. Terpenoids and phenylpropenes are the major antimicrobial compounds present in essential oils which show fairly good activity against foodborne pathogens. Some aldehydes and nonphenolic ingredients present in these essential oils also show antimicrobial effect (Hyldgaard, Mygind, & Meyer, 2012).

Furthermore, the species and strain of the microorganism may also affect the activity of essential oils. Generally, Gram-negative bacteria are more resistant to plant-origin antimicrobials than Gram-positive bacteria. The outer membrane of Gram-negative bacteria composed of lipopolysaccharides which prevent the diffusion of hydrophobic compounds (Chouhan, Sharma, & Guleria, 2017).

Ehsani, Hashemi, Naghibi, Mohammadi, & Khalili Sadaghiani (2016) observed that 1% and 2% essential oil of *Bunium persicum* (Black Cumin) significantly reduced the growth of *E. coli* O157:H7 and *L. monocytogenes* in white-brined cheese compared to the control throughout the storage period of 45 days. The cheese samples treated with tested concentrations of essential oils showed significantly higher scores of color, odor, flavor, texture, and general acceptability than the control when evaluated by panelists. Mehdizadeh, Narimani, Mojaddar Langroodi, Moghaddas Kia, & Neyriz-Naghadehi (2018) found that addition of 150 ppm *Zataria multiflora* essential oil inhibited growth of *E. coli* O157 in white-brined cheese by 2 log CFU g^{-1} after 60 days of storage at 4°C. Treatment of white-brined cheese with 150 ppm dill essential oil decreased numbers of *E. coli* O157:H7 by 1.1 log CFU g^{-1} compared to control samples after 60 days of storage at 4°C (Mojaddar Langroodi, Mehdizadeh, Majidi, & Neyriz-Naghadehi, 2020).

Osaili, Hasan, Dhanasekaran, Obaid, Al-Nabulsi, Ayyash, et al. (2021) investigated the antimicrobial activity of 1% and 2% (vol./vol.) carvacrol, cinnamaldehyde, and thymol against *L. monocytogenes*, *Salmonella* spp., and *E. coli* O157:H7 in marinated chicken tawook stored at 4°C or 10°C for 7 days. Addition of these compounds reduced numbers of *Salmonella* spp. and *E. coli* O157:H7 by 0.5−1.5 log CFU g^{-1}, whereas no antimicrobial activity against *L. monocytogenes* was observed at both 4°C and 10°C. The same authors also studied the effect of these active essential oil components (i.e., carvacrol, cinnamaldehyde, and thymol) on inoculated marinated camel meat chunks (Osaili, Hasan, Dhanasekaran, Obaid, Al-Nabulsi, Karam, et al., 2021). Adding these essential oils resulted in a decrease by 2.5−3.0, 3.2−3.4 log CFU g^{-1} for *E. coli* O157:H7 and *Salmonella* sp, respectively, when the meat chunks were stored at 4°C for 7 days. It was observed that elevating the essential oil concentration impacted *E. coli* O157:H7 and *Salmonella* spp. counts significantly with both the microorganisms experiencing a greater reduction by 3.6−4.4 and 1.0−2.7 log CFU g^{-1}, respectively. It was reported that 2% thymol and cinnamaldehyde were the most effective against *E. coli* O157:H7 and *Salmonella* spp. among all the tested types/concentrations of essential oils. Incorporating cinnamaldehyde onto the camel meat chunks was associated with positive sensory score values. Olaimat et al. (2019) investigated the antimicrobial effect of essential oils of cinnamon (*Cinnamomum zeylanicum*) and thyme (*Thymus vulgaris*) to control *Salmonella* spp. in hummus stored at 4°C or 10°C. Cinnamon essential oil at 0.5%−1.0% concentration reduced numbers of *Salmonella* in hummus to undetectable levels by 7 or 1 day, respectively, at both 4°C and 10°C. However, thyme essential oil at 0.5%−1.5% concentration reduced *Salmonella* in hummus by 1.0−2.9 log CFU g^{-1}, at 4°C by 10 days. Essential oils of thyme and cinnamon exhibited the highest in vitro antimicrobial activity from the 10 essential oils tested against five *Salmonella* spp. at 37°C and 10°C. In another study, incorporating tahini with 2.0%

cinnamon or thyme essential oil reduced *Salmonella* numbers by 2.4–2.9 and 2.2–3.3 log CFU mL^{-1}, respectively, at 10°C–37°C, by 28 days. However, their antimicrobial activity was more noticeable in hydrated tahini, and *Salmonella* cells were not detected by 7 days when 2.0% of cinnamon oil was added at all storage temperatures (10°C, 25°C, 37°C) or by 28 days when 2.0% thyme oil was added at 37°C or 25°C (Al-Nabulsi, Osaili, Olaimat, Almasri, Ayyash, et al., 2020).

Al-Nabulsi, Osaili, Olaimat, Almasri, Al-Holy, et al. (2020) performed a storage study (10°C, 25°C, 37°C) on tahini treated with essential oils for 28 days. The authors reported a decrease in *E. coli* O157:H7 counts by 1.4–2.24 and by 1.7–2.0 log CFU mL^{-1} (depending on storage temperature) in the samples treated with cinnamon and thyme essential oils, respectively. Upon diluting the tahini and storing it at 25°C or 37°C, thyme essential oil decreased the *E. coli* O157:H7 counts to undetectable levels after the 28-day storage period. An interesting observation in this study was the superior action of essential oils upon temperature increase. This could be a very beneficial finding as foods placed at ambient temperatures are usually associated with a higher risk of microbial growth. The essential oils incorporated into the tahini seem to play a role in overcoming this risk.

Abdel-Khalek (2008) reported that the essential oils of Caraway, Cumin, and a mixed spice powder were more effective against Gram-positive bacteria as compared to their Gram-negative counterparts and the bacteria in general as compared to molds. The antimicrobial effect of the mixed spice essential oil varied greatly depending on the type of microorganism.

Muhialdin, Kadum, Fathallah, & Meor Hussin, 2020 reported that the use of fermented ginger paste to marinate chicken significantly reduced the numbers of aerobic bacteria by 2.8 log CFU g^{-1} at 8°C after 2 days of storage. However, fresh ginger paste had no antimicrobial activity in the same condition tested. The antimicrobial effect of 0.1%–1.5% (vol./wt.) allyl isothiocyanate (AITC) against *S. enterica* and *L. monocytogenes* in hummus was investigated. AITC at $\leq$0.25% reduced *S. enterica* by 2.5–5.1 log CFU g^{-1} at 4°C and by 4.7–6.0 log CFU g^{-1} at 10°C by 10 days of storage. However, AITC at $\geq$0.5% reduced numbers of *S. enterica* by >6 log CFU g^{-1} after 3 days of storage at both 4°C and 10°C. *Listeria monocytogenes* numbers were also reduced by >6 log CFU g^{-1} in hummus treated with $\geq$0.5% AITC at 4°C or with $\geq$1.0% AITC at 10°C after 3 days of storage. Furthermore, 0.25% AITC reduced the numbers of *L. monocytogenes* by 4.3 and 2.7 log CFU g^{-1} in hummus stored at 10°C and 4°C, respectively. A 0.1% AITC concentration decreased *L. monocytogenes* numbers by 1.8 log CFU g^{-1} in hummus stored at 10°C, and this concentration inhibited the *L. monocytogenes* growth for up to 10 days of storage at 4°C (Olaimat, Al-Holy, Abu Ghoush, Al-Nabulsi, & Holley, 2018).

Belal et al. (2019) reported that addition of 1% (wt./vol.) green tea and ginger slightly but not significantly reduced the numbers of *E. coli* O157:H7 in Ayran compared to control (without spices). Wahba, Ahmed, and Ebraheim (2010) reported that addition of 6%–9% cayenne and green pepper extracts to Egyptian Kareish cheese reduced *Staph. aureus* numbers to undetectable levels within 2 days of storage. The addition of 6%–9% dill or parsley extract also significantly reduced the *Staph. aureus* numbers within the cheese. In another study, Meshref, Hassan, Riad, & Ashour, 2019 found that incorporating 10 and 12.5 ppm nisin into Kareish cheese reduced numbers of *Staph. aureus* by 1.6 and 2.6 log CFU g^{-1} compared to control samples (without nisin) after 1 month of storage at 4°C.

From the above-mentioned studies, it is evident that natural compounds have some antimicrobial potential against foodborne pathogens in the Middle Eastern foods. However, further studies are needed to evaluate the antimicrobial potency of other naturally occurring compounds, the most appropriate combinations/concentrations as well as the effect of these antimicrobials on the organoleptic characteristics and overall acceptability of the food products.

6.3 Biological preservation treatments

In the Middle Eastern cuisine, multiple traditional fermented foods such as white-brined cheese and vegetable pickles exist. To enhance the microbial safety and quality of these products, lactic acid bacteria (LAB) has been extensively added. Osaili et al. (2014) observed that the presence of starter LAB (*Streptococcus thermophilus* and *Lactobacillus bulgaricus*) reduced *E. coli* O157:H7 numbers in white-brined cheese stored for 28 days at 10°C and 21°C by 2.6–3.4; 1.0–1.6 log CFU g^{-1}, respectively. Al-Nabulsi et al. (2016) investigated the effect of starter LAB inoculation (*St. thermophilus* and *Lb. bulgaricus*) against *L. monocytogenes* and *E. coli* O157:H7 during manufacture and storage of camel yogurt. The presence of LAB reduced the growth of *E. coli* O157:H7 by 1.1 log CFU mL^{-1} during fermentation compared to yogurt samples without LAB. The presence of LAB also reduced *L. monocytogenes* growth by 2.0 and 2.9 log CFU mL^{-1} after 14 days of storage at 4°C or 10°C, respectively. Furthermore, about 6.3 log CFU mL^{-1} reduction in *E. coli* O157:H7 was observed in camel yogurt prepared with LAB compared to 3.5 log CFU mL^{-1} without LAB upon storage for 7 days. Recently, Al-Nabulsi et al. (2021) reported that addition of *Lactobacillus reuteri* enhanced the inhibition of *E. coli* O157:H7 in white-brined cheese stored at both 10°C and 25°C. In the presence of *Lb. reuteri*, numbers of *E. coli* O157:H7 in cheese stored in 10% NaCl brine at 25°C were reduced by 2.6 log CFU g^{-1} compared to 1.0 log CFU g^{-1} in the absence of *Lb. reuteri* and by 2.2 log CFU g^{-1} in 15% NaCl brine at 10°C compared to 1.9 log CFU g^{-1} in the absence of *Lb. reuteri*. It was reported that *Lb. reuteri* grew in all white-brine cheese samples up to 28 days. Mehdizadeh, Narimani, Mojaddar Langroodi, Moghaddas Kia, & Neyriz-Naghadehi (2018) observed that the combination of 150 ppm *Zataria multiflora* essential oil with probiotic

Lactobacillus acidophilus PTCC 1643 inhibited growth of *E. coli* O157:H7 in white-brined cheese by 2.0 log CFU g^{-1} after 60 days of storage in 11% sterile brined solution at 4°C. In another study, inoculation of white-brined cheese in brine solution (11%) with 8 log CFU mL^{-1} probiotic *Lb. acidophilus* PTCC 1643 in combination with 150 ppm dill essential oil decreased growth of *E. coli* O157:H7 by 1.6 log CFU g^{-1} after 2 months at 4°C compared to control cheese samples (Mojaddar Langroodi, Mehdizadeh, Majidi, & Neyriz-Naghadehi, 2020). Inoculation of white-brined cheese with 8–9 log CFU mL^{-1} probiotic *Lb. acidophilus* ATCC 4356 decreased the growth of *L. monocytogenes* by 3.2 log CFU g^{-1} compared with untreated cheese samples after both ripening in a sterile salt brine (8%) at 14°C for 15 days and storage at 4°C for 45 days (Mahmoudi, Tajik, Ehsani, & Zare, 2012).

Hence, probiotics and LAB could be used as an effective biological preservation method to inhibit foodborne pathogens, particularly when combined with other natural or chemical preservatives under appropriate storage conditions. Further studies are required to examine the antagonistic effect of LAB against foodborne pathogens in other types of the Middle Eastern foods.

Bacteriophages are viruses that infect bacteria during exponential and stationary phases, and they are considered as smart antimicrobials due to their ability to bind only to the target pathogenic bacteria without affecting the natural flora (Moye, Woolston, & Sulakvelidze, 2018). During the last two decades, bacteriophages have gained interest as a method to inhibit pathogens in food products. Although bacteriophages have been extensively studied due to their ability to mitigate pathogenic and spoilage bacteria (Moye, Woolston, & Sulakvelidze, 2018; Sillankorva, Oliveira, & Azeredo, 2012), there are very few studies pertaining to their use in traditional food products of the Middle East. It has been observed that the addition of phage ZCSE1 at a concentration of 7 log reduced the number of *S. enterica* on the surface of chicken skin and eggs by 3.3 log and to undetectable levels (<2 log), respectively, after 2 days of storage at 4°C. While another phage ZCEC1 reduced numbers of *E. coli* on both meat and tomatoes to undetectable levels (<2 log) after 1 day of storage at 4°C (El-Shibiny, El-Sahhar, & Adel, 2017). In another study, coagulase-negative staphylococci (*S. haemolyticus* and *S. epidermidis*) on the surfaces of chicken breast samples treated with 8 log CoNShP-3 Phage were reduced by >6.0 CFU cm^{-2} after 7 days at 4°C or 30 days at −20°C (Sofy, El Haliem, Refaey, & Hmed, 2020).

6.4 Physical preservation treatments

Multiple physical techniques such as heat treatment, ionizing or ultraviolet radiation, and high hydrostatic pressure (HHP) have been used to preserve the Middle Eastern food products. For example, in the processing of halva and tahini, roasting of sesame seeds is the first step. It is carried out mainly to enhance the microbial quality besides for an improvement to the texture, color, flavor, and overall palatability. The foodborne pathogen of utmost concern to regulatory agencies and food processors especially in tahini is *Salmonella*. Several researchers reported different roasting time–temperature combinations to help manage this dreadful pathogen (Kahyaoglu & Kaya, 2006; Torlak, Sert, & Serin, 2013). A 5.9 log CFU g^{-1} reduction in inoculated *Salmonella* (*S.* Montevideo, *S.* Typhimurium, and *S.* Newport) levels was observed when sesame seeds were roasted at a time–temperature combination of 150°C for 30 min; 130°C for 50 min, and 110°C for 60 min (Torlak, Sert, & Serin, 2013). Although, roasting of sesame seeds is a satisfactory method to eradicate foodborne pathogens like *Salmonella* spp. from tahini; numerous outbreaks have been linked to its consumption (Olaimat, Osaili, et al., 2020). This is mainly because of its contamination after this stage of processing (Al-Nabulsi et al., 2014). This is a classic example explaining the dire need for practical methods which maintain antimicrobial efficacy till the product reaches the costumer.

Osaili, Al-Nabulsi, et al. (2020) studied the effect of thermal treatment (55°C–65°C) on ground camel meat inoculated with two strains of *E. coli* O157:H7 and *Salmonella*. The *D* values for the two pathogens ranged from 1.8 to 0.07 min (57.5°C–65°C) and 2.2 to 0.06 min (55°C–62.5°C), respectively. While the *z* values for both pathogens spanned from 4.6°C to 5.0°C and 5.1°C to 5.5°C, respectively. The same authors (Osaili, Hasan, et al., 2020) in a later study marinated the meat and incorporated camel hump fat into the formulation. The *D* values upon thermal treatment (55°C–67.5°C) for both *E. coli* O157:H7 and *Salmonella* were significantly consistently higher in the formulation which contained hump fat (76.0–4.1 s; 512.1–8.4 s) compared to the control (53.5–3.0 s; 349.2–6.7 s). The *z* values spanned from 5.0°C to 6.0°C and 4.1°C to 4.4°C for the two pathogens, respectively. *Salmonella* was reported to be more resistant to the heat treatment than *E. coli* O157:H7. These findings are a tad bit concerning. This is because camel meat recipes are expected to incorporate different amounts of fat. A specific time–temperature combination may not be adequate to destroy pathogenic microorganisms found in high fat recipe products. Perhaps, the presence of a quick, sensitive, and portable pathogen detection tool would help people involved in food preparation to gauge microbial risk and consequently aid in preventing outbreaks.

Osaili et al. (2013) investigated the *D*- and *z* values of two strains of *S.* Typhimurium in ground marinated and nonmarinated chicken breast prepared for shawarma. The *D* values of *S.* Typhimurium strains inoculated on ground nonmarinated chicken, chicken marinated for 30 min, and marinated chicken stored for 15 h ranged from 9.15 to 12.44, 2.89 to 3.92, 1.06 to 1.30, and 0.32 to 0.52 min at 54°C, 56°C, 58°C, and 60°C, respectively. No significant difference in the *D* values based on the tested treatments was reported by the authors. The *z* values of *S.* Typhimurium in the same study ranged from 3.78°C to 4.58°C.

Recently, there has been an increased consumer demand/interest to use nonthermal preservation methods that enhance safety level and maintain the nutritional and organoleptic quality of food. HHP is a nonthermal preservation method that involves applying pressures in the ranges of 100–600 MPa to food so as to inactivate foodborne pathogens (Cheftel, 1995; Hendrickx & Knorr, 2001). It revolves around the following basic principles (Farkas & Hoover, 2000; Yousef & Balasubramaniam, 2013).

1. Le Chatelier's principle: A phenomena disrupting a system in equilibrium will result in a new equilibrium which diminishes the disrupting phenomena. The application of pressure during HHP may result in a phase change, molecular reconfiguration, and/or a chemical reaction besides a decrease in volume.
2. Isostatic principle: The transmission of pressure is uniform and quasiinstantaneous in an entire sample and can be considered independent of the sample's geometry and volume (unlike thermal processing). However, some researchers caution that pressure nonhomogeneity can occur, especially during the treatment of large solid foods.
3. Microscopic ordering principle: The order degree of molecules increases with increasing pressure in a given substance if kept under constant temperature. However, the possibility of synergistic or antagonistic reactions should be kept into account.

With regards to its application in food substances, it was observed that this technique had limited efficacy in destroying pathogenic microorganisms in high fat foods. The viability of *L. monocytogenes* was not significantly reduced in tahini (a high fat food) treated either for 4 min at 350 MPa or 10 min at 600 MPa (Salazar et al., 2019). In contrast, in hummus, a hydrostatic pressure of 500 MPa for 10 min at room temperature inhibited individual cocktails of *Salmonella*, *L. monocytogenes*, and *E. coli* strains by >5 log CFU g^{-1}. As a matter of fact, the bacterial cells were not detected in the product despite storing it for about 2 months (Sokołowska, Nasiłowska, Rutkowska, Fonberg-Broczek, & Rzoska, 2019).

Ionizing radiations are those radiations which have a wavelength less than 200 nm and include alpha particles, beta rays, gamma rays, and X rays. Gamma irradiation and electron beams have been investigated as an alternative preservation method to thermal treatment. When ionizing radiation penetrates a food or a microorganism, all or part of the radiation energy is absorbed which leads to the conversion of atoms and molecules to ions via removal of electrons. The antimicrobial effects of ionizing radiations could be via two pathways as stated below (Munir & Federighi, 2020).

1. Direct effect: When radiation is absorbed directly by the microorganism, there is a possibility that critical targets will be hit. Nucleic acid molecules may be ionized or excited which initiate a chain of events leading to cell death

2. Indirect effect: Alternatively, the radiation may interact with other atoms or molecules in the cell, particularly water (cytoplasm consists of about 90% water), to produce free radicals which can diffuse and damage the DNA.

These methods have been approved by the US Food and Drug Administration for the inactivation of undesirable bacteria in poultry, meat, vegetables, fresh fruits, and spices (Ban & Kang, 2014). Microorganisms which have been stressed through some means are usually expected to show higher resistance; gamma irradiation has been recorded to have the ability to destroy such pathogens too. Osaili, Al-Nabulsi, Abubakar, Alaboudi, & Al-Holy (2016) observed that the viability of a stressed *Salmonella* cocktail (*S.* Cubana, *S.* Aberdeen, *S.* Typhimurium, and *S.* Paratyphi) inoculated onto tahini was reduced by 4.5–4.7 log CFU g^{-1} upon being gamma irradiated (2.0 kGy). Similarly, Osaili & Al-Nabulsi (2016) reported *E. coli* O157:H7 unstressed cells and cold, heat, starvation, ethanol, alkaline, or acid stressed cells reduced by 2.6–3.2 log CFU g^{-1} when 1 kGy of gamma radiation was applied to tahini. The sensitivity of *Salmonella* and *L. monocytogenes* to gamma radiation was reported to increase when cells were exposed to desiccation stress; however, the scenario was the opposite in heat stressed *E. coli* O157:H7 and *L. monocytogenes* (sensitivity decrease was recorded) (Osaili, Al-Nabulsi, & Aljaafreh, 2018). Radiation is capable of not only destroying the bacteria but even their genes (Umar, Roddick, & Fan, 2019) and spores. It was observed that gamma radiating (4 kGy) raw milk, carrot juice, and water decreased the *D* values of *Bacillus cereus* spores found in these products in a multifold manner (2.8–3.4 times). The *D* and *z* values of the bacterial spores for the above-mentioned food products spanned from 7.6 to 11.6 min and 9.81°C–11.24°C, respectively (El-Nour & Hammad, 2013).

Abdel-Khalek (2008) irradiated (10 kGy) cumin, caraway, and mixed spice powder and reported that irradiation reduced moisture content of the products and decreased yeast and molds, mesophilic and thermophilic bacterial counts to acceptable levels. Al-Qadiri, Amr, Al-Holy, & Shahein (2020) irradiated hummus using gamma rays ranging from 0.1 to 2.5 kGy and stored it at refrigeration temperatures. It was reported that an irradiation of 2.5 kGy reduced LAB to undetectable levels up to 10 days. Post this period, although the counts increased, they fell within the acceptable range. Towards the end of the 35-day storage period, mesophilic bacteria in the hummus increased significantly from 4.1 to 6.7 log CFU g^{-1} in samples irradiated at 0.1 kGy, whereas in those samples irradiated at 1.5 kGy, the numbers significantly increased from 2.3 to 3.9 log CFU g^{-1}. As for yeasts and molds, the mean counts in hummus significantly increased from 2.9 to 5.8 log CFU g^{-1} in samples irradiated at 0.1 kGy, whereas they increased from 2.1 to 3.8 log CFU g^{-1} in samples irradiated at 1.5 kGy. A significant decrease in numbers of mesophilic bacteria, LAB, and yeast and molds was observed as the radiation dose increased in majority of the cases.

Gamma (γ) irradiation was also used to reduce microbial contamination on bee pollen (Hosny, Sabbah, & El-Bazza, 2018). Various strains belonging to *Bacillus* sp. were reported to be resistant to radiation of up to 5 kGy. The resistant fungi reported include *Penicillium chrysogenum*, *P. expansum*, and *P. corylophilum*. A point to observe from the above studies is the resistance exhibited by microorganisms despite receiving a fair dose of irradiation. This sheds light on their rather excellent adaptation responses which are indeed a challenge to the food industry.

Gamma irradiating ready to cook chicken samples at 4.5 kGy resulted in a total destruction of pathogenic microorganisms namely *Salmonella*, *E. coli* O157: H7, and *L. monocytogenes* (Fallah, Saei-Dehkordi, & Rahnama, 2010). They were not detected in the samples up to 15 days of storage. *Enterobacteriaceae*, yeasts, and molds inherent to the chicken were reported to be less resistant to irradiation when compared to LAB and aerobic mesophilic bacteria.

Ganjaroudi, Raeisi, Hajimohammadi, & Zandi (2016) inoculated a traditional ice cream with *Brucella abortus* and *Brucella melitensis* and performed an electron beam radiation (1–5 kGy) prior to storage for 21 days. The authors reported a decrease in counts from 5.5×10^4 to 1.6×10^3 CFU g^{-1} and from 6.5×10^4 to 1.3×10^3 CFU g^{-1}, respectively, at an irradiation dose of 1 kGy post the storage period. Irradiating the ice cream at 5 kGy completely eliminated the bacterial growth.

Using ultrasounds/sonication for microbial destruction has been attempted previously in pomegranate juice (Alighourchi, Barzegar, Sahari, & Abbasi, 2014). The juice treated at 50%–75% ultrasound amplitude levels decreased *E. coli* and *Saccharomyces cerevisiae* counts by less than 1.5 log. However, upon increasing the amplitude to 100%, the reduction was reported to be 3.5 and 1.9 log CFU mL^{-1}, respectively. On a comparative note, gamma irradiation decreased the counts of *E. coli* and *S. cerevisiae* in the juice by 6.7 (1 kGy) and 5.1 (3 kGy) log CFU mL^{-1}, respectively.

6.5 Use of active packaging for the preservation of the Middle Eastern food products

Active packaging is a ground-breaking technique which aims to preserve or extend the shelf-life of food products without compromising on their quality, safety, and integrity. Active packaging incorporates substances such as antimicrobials and antioxidants within the packaging layer. The active substances are either released into or absorbed from the environment surrounding the enclosed product. This decreases the need to directly add these substances to food during production and hence reduces their overall quantity in food products (Yildirim et al., 2018).

The antimicrobial effect of chitosan coating containing *Mentha aquatica L.* (water mint) essence against *E. coli* O157:H, *L. monocytogenes*, and *Staph. aureus* in white-brined cheese was investigated by Hani Tabaie

Zavareh & Ardestani (2020). Chitosan coating with 1.5% *Mentha aquatica L.* essence reduced numbers of *E. coli* O157:H to undetectable levels by 10 days of storage at 4°C. It also reduced numbers of *L. monocytogenes* and *Staph. aureus* by 5.4 and 4.9 log CFU g^{-1}, respectively, after 15 days of storage at 4°C. Al-Nabulsi, Osaili, Sawalha, et al. (2020) reported that chitosan coating without or with 1% (wt./vol.) ZnO nanoparticles reduced the numbers of inoculated *E. coli* O157:H7 in white-brined cheese by 2.5 and 2.8 log CFU g^{-1}, respectively, at 4°C or by 1.9 and 2.1 log CFU g^{-1}, respectively, at 10°C. The addition of starter LAB significantly inhibited the growth of *Staph. aureus* in white-brined cheese where its numbers decreased by 0.5 and 2.5 log CFU g^{-1} in cheese stored in 10% and 15% NaCl brine, respectively, compared to cheese samples without starter LAB (at 10°C). Furthermore, the presence of a starter culture may partially prevent production of enterotoxins by *Staph. aureus* in white-brined cheese (Al-Nabulsi, Osaili, AbuNaser, et al., 2020). Spray washing of sheep meat for 2–4 min with ZnO nanoparticles containing 1% acetic acid reduced numbers of *L. monocytogenes*, *E. coli*, and *Staph. aureus* by 4.7, 1.2, and 2.8 log CFU g^{-1}, respectively compared with the control after 12 days of storage at 4°C (Mirhosseini & Arjmand, 2014). Alizadeh Sani, Ehsani, and Hashemi (2017) observed that whey protein isolate/cellulose nanofiber nanocomposite films containing 1.0% (wt./wt.) titanium dioxide and 2.0% (wt./vol.) rosemary essential oil significantly inhibited the growth of inoculated *Staph. aureus*, *L. monocytogenes*, and *E. coli* O157:H7 in lamb meat stored at 4°C.

In another study, ginger essential oil and citric acid were incorporated in cellulose nanofibers; the antimicrobial effect of the resultant coating on chicken barbeque meat was studied (Khaledian, Pajohi-Alamoti, & Bazargani-Gilani, 2019). It was reported that the oil and citric acid although displayed significant antimicrobial effect, it was lower when compared to the antimicrobial activity upon cellulose coating integration. This finding was explained by the phenomenon of continuous, gradual, and long-term release of the antimicrobials from the packaging resulting in higher antimicrobial activity. Upon a 10-day storage period, the authors reported total viable counts and pyschrotrophic bacteria were 10.0 and 8.1 log CFU g^{-1}, respectively, in the uncoated control samples. The active agents (depending on concentration) incorporated onto the cellulose nanofibers decreased the total viable counts and pyschrotrophic bacteria to 4.9–5.1 and 4.6–5.0 log CFU g^{-1}, respectively. The *Enterobacteriaceae* counts post the storage period were reported to be 9.1 log CFU g^{-1}, the fusion of the cellulose coating along with the essential oil and acid decreased it to between 2.9 and 4.6 log CFU g^{-1}.

6.6 Conclusions and future work

Although, a fair amount of literature concerning the microbiological safety of traditional Middle Eastern food products exists, a great deal is yet to be explored. Appropriate time–temperature combinations for food products, their microbiological safety upon long storage periods, and practices during production which compromise microbial quality need to be worked upon on different types of traditional foods.

As the Middle East area, and mostly the Gulf region, suffers from a dry climate, especially during the summer period (July to September) where high temperatures prevail, it is imperative to use a multihurdle approach (i.e., added preservatives, ideally natural combined with packaging, or physical treatments) so as to retain both freshness and safety of perishable food products in mostly the Gulf region.

Despite the fact that industry which manufactures these food products at a large scale does exist, these products are generally prepared at the home/retail level. Identifying feasible antimicrobial methods which could be applied at this stage without compromising on organoleptic properties would contribute a great deal towards enhancing overall food safety.

Natural antimicrobials, including organic acids, essential oils, and plant extracts, have a potential to inhibit growth of major foodborne pathogens in traditional foods in the Middle East; further strategies should be developed and explored to enhance their antimicrobial activity perhaps by synergistic combinations, controlling antimicrobial delivery during food storage, as well as the incorporation of antimicrobial compounds into packaging tools such as coating and films.

Novel nonthermal techniques including HHP, ionizing radiation, and pulsed electric fields have the ability to inactivate pathogens in several foods, hence extending their shelf life. Furthermore, these methods compromise less on nutritional content compared to thermal treatments. However, these strategies have not been extensively studied and applied in the Middle Eastern foods. Combined effects of the above-mentioned physical treatments with natural antimicrobials may prove to be successful in controlling foodborne pathogens in the Middle Eastern foods.

Good packaging methods play a vital role in preservation of food products because they maintain the food under good hygienic and safe conditions until it reaches the consumer. The usage of protective coatings and films in the food industry can certainly extend the shelf life of food products and enhance their safety. Recent advances in technology have resulted in intelligent active food packaging systems which incorporate nano-antimicrobial ingredients. They are released throughout the storage period and reduce the required concentrations for antimicrobial activity. Further studies in this context are needed for commonly consumed foods in the Middle East. Probiotics and bacteriophages can perhaps be explored to be used potentially by the food industry, as preservation methods at the pre or postharvest stage. However, the nature and safety of these biocontrol techniques are considered a critical future challenge in their application in food products of the Middle East.

References

Abdel-Khalek, H.H., 2008. Effect of gamma irradiation on the microbial, chemical quality and the biological activity of some spices and herbs.

Al-Holy, M., Al-Qadiri, H., Lin, M., & Rasco, B. (2006). Inhibition of *Listeria innocua* in hummus by a combination of nisin and citric acid. *Journal of Food Protection*, *69*(6), 1322–1327. Available from http://www.ncbi.nlm.nih.gov/pubmed/16786852.

Alighourchi, H., Barzegar, M., Sahari, M. A., & Abbasi, S. (2014). The effects of sonication and gamma irradiation on the inactivation of *Escherichia coli* and *Saccharomyces cerevisiae* in pomegranate juice. *Iranian Journal of Microbiology*, *6*(1), 51.

Alizadeh Sani, M., Ehsani, A., & Hashemi, M. (2017). Whey protein isolate/cellulose nanofibre/TiO2 nanoparticle/rosemary essential oil nanocomposite film: Its effect on microbial and sensory quality of lamb meat and growth of common foodborne pathogenic bacteria during refrigeration. *International Journal of Food Microbiology*, *251*, 8–14. Available from https://doi.org/10.1016/j.ijfoodmicro.2017.03.018.

Al-Nabulsi, A., Osaili, T., Olaimat, A., Almasri, W., Al-Holy, M., Jaradat, Z., Ayyash, M., Awaisheh, S., & Holley, R. (2020). Inhibitory effect of thyme and cinnamon essential oils against E. coli O157: H7 in Tahini. *Food Science and Technology*, *40*(4), 885–893. Available from https://doi.org/10.1590/fst.21619.

Al-Nabulsi, A., Osaili, T., Sawalha, A., Olaimat, A. N., Albiss, B. A., Mehyar, G., Ayyash, M., & Holley, R. (2020). Antimicrobial activity of chitosan coating containing ZnO nanoparticles against E. coli O157:H7 on the surface of white brined cheese. *International Journal of Food Microbiology*, *334*, 108838. Available from https://doi.org/10.1016/j.ijfoodmicro.2020.108838.

Al-Nabulsi, A. A., Olaimat, A. N., Osaili, T. M., Ayyash, M. M., Abushelaibi, A., Jaradat, Z. W., Shaker, R., Al-Taani, M., & Holley, R. A. (2016). Behavior of Escherichia coli O157: H7 and Listeria monocytogenes during fermentation and storage of camel yogurt. *Journal of Dairy Science*, *99*(3), 1802–1811. Available from https://doi.org/10.3168/jds.2015-9872.

Al-Nabulsi, A. A., Olaimat, A. N., Osaili, T. M., Shaker, R. R., Zein Elabedeen, N., Jaradat, Z. W., Abushelaibi, A., & Holley, R. A. (2014). Use of acetic and citric acids to control Salmonella Typhimurium in tahini (sesame paste). *Food Microbiology*, *42*, 102–108. Available from https://doi.org/10.1016/j.fm.2014.02.020.

Al-Nabulsi, A. A., Osaili, T. M., AbuNaser, R. A., Olaimat, A. N., Ayyash, M., Al-Holy, M. A., Kadora, K. M., & Holley, R. A. (2020). Factors affecting the viability of Staphylococcus aureus and production of enterotoxin during processing and storage of white-brined cheese. *Journal of Dairy Science*, *103*(8), 6869–6881. Available from https://doi.org/10.3168/jds.2020-18158.

Al-Nabulsi, A. A., Osaili, T. M., Olaimat, A. N., Almasri, W. E., Ayyash, M., Al-Holy, M. A., Jaradat, Z. W., Obaid, R. S., & Holley, R. A. (2020). Inactivation of Salmonella spp. in tahini using plant essential oil extracts. *Food Microbiology*, *86*, 103338. Available from https://doi.org/10.1016/j.fm.2019.103338.

Al-Nabulsi, A. A., Osaili, T. M., Oqdeh, S. B., Olaimat, A. N., Jaradat, Z. W., Ayyash, M., & Holley, R. A. (2021). Antagonistic effects of *Lactobacillus reuteri* against *Escherichia coli* O157:H7 in white-brined cheese under different storage conditions. *Journal of Dairy Science*, *104*, 2719–2734. Available from https://doi.org/10.3168/jds.2020-19308.

Al-Qadiri, H., Amr, A., Al-Holy, M. A., & Shahein, M. (2020). Effect of gamma irradiation against microbial spoilage of hummus preserved under refrigerated storage. *Food Science and Technology International*. https://doi.org/10.1177/1082013220975891. In press.

Al-Rousan, W. M., Olaimat, A. N., Osaili, T. M., Al-Nabulsi, A. A., Ajo, R. Y., & Holley, R. A. (2018). Use of acetic and citric acids to inhibit *Escherichia coli* O157:H7, *Salmonella* Typhimurium and Staphylococcus aureus in tabbouleh salad. *Food Microbiology*, *73*, 61–66. Available from https://doi.org/10.1016/j.fm.2018.01.001.

Anyasi, T. A., Jideani, A. I. O., Edokpayi, J. N., & Anokwuru, C. P. (2017). *Application of organic acids in food preservation. Organic acids: Characteristics, properties and synthesis.* Nova Science. Available from https://doi.org/10.1201/9781420078435-4.

Ban, G. H., & Kang, D. H. (2014). Effects of gamma irradiation for inactivating *Salmonella* Typhimurium in peanut butter product during storage. *International Journal of Food Microbiology*, *171*, 48–53. Available from https://doi.org/10.1016/j.ijfoodmicro.2013.11.016.

Belal, M., Abulola, H., Olaimat, A. N., Odeh, R. A, Attlee, A., Al-Nabulsi, A. A., Osaili, T. M., Al-Shami, I., Ayyash, M. M., & Obaid, R. S. (2019). Viability of *Escherichia coli* O157:H7 during fermentation and storage of plain and spiced ayran. *Journal of Hygienic Engineering and Design*, *29*, 21–25.

Cheftel, J. C. (1995). Review: High pressure, microbial inactivation and food preservation. *Food Science and Technology International*, *1*, 75–90.

Chouhan, S., Sharma, K., & Guleria, S. (2017). Antimicrobial activity of some essential oils-present status and future perspectives. *Medicines (Basel, Switzerland)*, *4*(3)58. Available from https://doi.org/10.3390/medicines4030058.

Dorman, H. J. D., & Deans, S. G. (2000). Antimicrobial agents from plants: Antibacterial activity of plant volatile oils. *Journal of Applied Microbiology*, *88*, 308–316. Available from https://doi.org/10.1046/j.1365-2672.2000.00969.x.

Ehsani, A., Hashemi, M., Naghibi, S. S., Mohammadi, S., & Khalili Sadaghiani, S. (2016). Properties of *Bunium Persicum* essential oil and its application in Iranian white cheese against *Listeria Monocytogenes* and *Escherichia coli* O157:H7. *Journal of Food Safety*, *36* (4), 563–570. Available from https://doi.org/10.1111/jfs.12277.

El-Nour, S. A., & Hammad, A. (2013). Inactivation of *Bacillus cereus* spores in liquid food by combination treatments of heat and irradiation. *Food Science and Quality Management*, *19*, 31–40.

El-Shibiny, A., El-Sahhar, S., & Adel, M. (2017). Phage applications for improving food safety and infection control in Egypt. *Journal of Applied Microbiology*, *123*(2), 556–567. Available from https://doi.org/10.1111/jam.13500.

Fallah, A. A., Saei-Dehkordi, S. S., & Rahnama, M. (2010). Enhancement of microbial quality and inactivation of pathogenic bacteria by gamma irradiation of ready-to-cook Iranian barbecued chicken. *Radiation Physics and Chemistry*, *79*(10), 1073–1078.

Faour-Klingbeil, D., & Todd, E. C. D. (2018). The inhibitory effect of traditional pomegranate molasses on *S. typhimurium* growth on parsley leaves and in mixed salad vegetables. *Journal of Food Safety*, e12469. Available from https://doi.org/10.1111/jfs.12469.

Faour-Klingbeil, D., & Todd, E. C. D. (2020). Prevention and control of foodborne diseases in middle-east north african countries: Review of national control systems. *International Journal of Environmental Research and Public Health*, *17*(1), 1–23. Available from https://doi.org/10.3390/ijerph17010070.

Farkas, D. F., & Hoover, D. G. (2000). High pressure processing. *Journal of Food Science*, *65* (Suppl), 47S–64S.

Ganjaroudi, F. H., Raeisi, M., Hajimohammadi, B., & Zandi, H. (2016). Effect of electron beam irradiation on survival of *Brucella* spp. In traditional ice cream. *Journal of Food Processing and Preservation*, *40*(3), 567–571.

Hani Tabaie Zavareh, S. A., & Ardestani, F. (2020). Antibacterial effects of chitosan coating containing *Mentha aquatica L.* essence against *Escherichia coli*, *Staphylococcus aureus* and *Listeria monocytogenes* in Iranian white cheese. *International Journal of Dairy Technology*, *73*(3), 585–593. Available from https://doi.org/10.1111/1471-0307.12678.

Hendrickx, M. E. G., & Knorr, D. (2001). *Ultra high pressure treatments of food.* New York, NY: Kluwer Academic/Plenum Publishers.

Hosny, A. S., Sabbah, F. M., & El-Bazza, Z. E. (2018). Studies on the microbial decontamination of Egyptian bee pollen by γ radiation. *Egyptian Pharmaceutical Journal*, *17*(3), 190.

Hyldgaard, M., Mygind, T., & Meyer, R. L. (2012). Essential oils in food preservation: mode of action, synergies, and interactions with food matrix components. *Frontiers in Microbiology*, *3*, 12. Available from https://doi.org/10.3389/fmicb.2012.00012.

Kahyaoglu, T., & Kaya, S. (2006). Determination of optimum processing conditions for hot-air roasting of hulled sesame seeds using response surface methodology. *Journal of the Science of Food and Agriculture*, *86*(10), 1452–1459. Available from https://doi.org/10.1002/jsfa.2509.

Khaledian, Y., Pajohi-Alamoti, M., & Bazargani-Gilani, B. (2019). Development of cellulose nanofibers coating incorporated with ginger essential oil and citric acid to extend the shelf life of ready-to-cook barbecue chicken. *Journal of Food Processing and Preservation*, *43* (10), e14114.

Mahmoudi, R., Tajik, H., Ehsani, A., & Zare, P. (2012). Physicochemical and hygienic effects of *Lactobacillus acidophilus* in Iranian white cheese. *Veterinary Research Forum: An International Quarterly Journal*, *3*(3), 193–197. Available from http://www.ncbi.nlm.nih.gov/pubmed/25610568%0Ahttp://www.pubmedcentral.nih.gov/articlerender.fcgi?artid = PMC4299982.

Mehdizadeh, T., Narimani, R., Mojaddar Langroodi, A., Moghaddas Kia, E., & Neyriz-Naghadehi, M. (2018). Antimicrobial effects of *Zataria multiflora* essential oil and *Lactobacillus acidophilus* on *Escherichia coli* O157 stability in the Iranian probiotic white-brined cheese. *Journal of Food Safety*, *38*(4), 1–8. Available from https://doi.org/10.1111/jfs.12476.

Meshref, M. S. A., Hassan, M. G., Riad, M. E., & Ashour, A. W. (2019). Effect of nisin on the viability of *Staphylococcus aureus* in kareish cheese. *Journal of Veterinary Medical Research*, *26*(2), 174–185. Available from https://doi.org/10.21608/jvmr.2019.66100.

Mirhosseini, M., & Arjmand, V. (2014). Reducing pathogens by using zinc oxide nanoparticles and acetic acid in sheep meat. *Journal of Food Protection*, *77*, 1599–1604. Available from https://doi.org/10.4315/0362-028X.JFP-13-210.

Mojaddar Langroodi, A., Mehdizadeh, T., Majidi, L., & Neyriz-Naghadehi, M. (2020). *Lactobacillus acidophilus* and *Anethum graveolens* essential oil in Iranian cheese against *Escherichia coli* O157:H7. *Flavour and Fragrance Journal*, *36*, 1–7. Available from https://doi.org/10.1002/ffj.3629, August.

Moye, Z. D., Woolston, J., & Sulakvelidze, A. (2018). Bacteriophage applications for food production and processing. *Viruses*, *10*(4), 1–22. Available from https://doi.org/10.3390/v10040205.

Muhialdin, B. J., Kadum, H., Fathallah, S., & Meor Hussin, A. S. (2020). Metabolomics profiling and antibacterial activity of fermented ginger paste extends the shelf life of chicken meat. *LWT-Food Science and Technology*, *132*, 109897. Available from https://doi.org/10.1016/j.lwt.2020.109897.

Munir, M. T., & Federighi, M. (2020). Control of foodborne biological hazards by ionizing radiations. *Foods*, *9*, 878. Available from https://doi.org/10.3390/foods9070878.

Olaimat, A. N., Al-Holy, M. A., Abu Ghoush, M., Al-Nabulsi, A. A., & Holley, R. A. (2018). Control of Salmonella enterica and Listeria monocytogenes in hummus using allyl isothiocyanate. *International Journal of Food Microbiology*, *278*. Available from https://doi.org/10.1016/j.ijfoodmicro.2018.04.033.

Olaimat, A. N., Al-Holy, M. A., Abu Ghoush, M. H., Abu Hilal, H. M., Al-Nabulsi, A. A., Osaili, T. M., & Rasco, B. A. (2020). Population dynamics of Salmonella spp. and Shigella spp. in ready-to-eat Mediterranean vegetable salads. *Journal of Food Safety*, *40*. Available from https://doi.org/10.1111/jfs.12734.

Olaimat, A. N., Al-Holy, M. A., Abu Ghoush, M. H., Al-Nabulsi, A. A., Osaili, T. M., & Holley, R. A. (2019). Inhibitory effects of cinnamon and thyme essential oils against Salmonella spp. in hummus (chickpea dip). *Journal of Food Processing and Preservation*, *43*. Available from https://doi.org/10.1111/jfpp.13925.

Olaimat, A. N., Al-Holy, M. A., Abu-Ghoush, M. H., Osaili, T. M., Al-Nabulsi, A. A., & Rasco, B. A. (2017). Inhibition of *Shigella sonnei* and *Shigella flexneri* in hummus using citric acid and garlic extract. *Journal of Food Science*, *82*(8), 1908–1915. Available from https://doi.org/10.1111/1750-3841.13803.

Olaimat, A. N., Al-Nabulsi, A. A., Osaili, T. M., Al-Holy, M., Ayyash, M. M., Mehyar, G. F., Jaradat, Z. W., & Abu Ghoush, M. (2017). Survival and inhibition of Staphylococcus aureus in commercial and hydrated tahini using acetic and citric acids. *Food Control*, *77*, 179–186. Available from https://doi.org/10.1016/j.foodcont.2017.02.022.

Olaimat, A. N., Osaili, T. M., Al-Holy, M. A., Al-Nabulsi, A. A., Obaid, R. S., Alaboudi, A. R., Ayyash, M., & Holley, R. (2020). Microbial safety of oily, low water activity food products: A review. *Food Microbiology*, *92*, 103571. Available from https://doi.org/10.1016/j.fm.2020.103571.

Osaili, T. M., & Al-Nabulsi, A. (2016). Inactivation of stressed *Escherichia coli* O157:H7 in tahini (sesame seeds paste) by gamma irradiation. *Food Control*, *69*, 221–226. Available from https://doi.org/10.1016/J.FOODCONT.2016.05.009.

Osaili, T. M., Al-Nabulsi, A. A., Abubakar, S. A., Alaboudi, A. R., & Al-Holy, M. A. (2016). Feasibility of using gamma irradiation for inactivation of starvation-, heat-, and cold-stressed *Salmonella* in tahini. *Journal of Food Protection*, *79*(6), 963–969. Available from https://doi.org/10.4315/0362-028X.JFP-15-495.

Osaili, T. M., Al-Nabulsi, A. A., & Aljaafreh, T. F. (2018). Use of gamma radiation for inactivating *Salmonella* spp., *Escherichia coli* O157:H7 and *Listeria monocytogenes* in tahini halva. *International Journal of Food Microbiology*, *278*, 20–25. Available from https://doi.org/10.1016/j.ijfoodmicro.2018.04.029.

Osaili, T. M., Al-Nabulsi, A. A., Dhanasekaran, D. K., Hasan, F., Rao, S., Fatima, H., Ayyash, M., Holley, R., & Obaid, R. S. (2020). Growth behaviour and thermal inactivation of E. coli O157: H7 and Salmonella spp. in ground lean camel meat. *International Journal of Food Microbiology*, *316*, 108423. Available from https://doi.org/10.1016/j.ijfoodmicro.2019.108423.

Osaili, T. M., Al-Nabulsi, A. A., Olaimat, A. N., Shaker, R. R., Taha, M., & Holley, R. A. (2014). Survival of *Escherichia coli* O157:H7 during manufacture and storage of white brined cheese. *Journal of Food Science*, *79*(9), M1750–M1755. Available from https://doi.org/10.1111/1750-3841.12547.

Osaili, T. M., Al-Nabulsi, A. A., Shaker, R. R., Olaimat, A. N., Jaradat, Z. W., & Holley, R. A. (2013). Thermal inactivation of *Salmonella* Typhimurium in chicken shawirma (gyro).

International Journal of Food Microbiology, 166. Available from https://doi.org/10.1016/j.ijfoodmicro.2013.06.009.

Osaili, T. M., Hasan, F., Dhanasekaran, D. K., Obaid, R. S., Al-Nabulsi, A. A., Ayyash, M., Karam, L., Savvaidis, I. N., & Holley, R. (2021). Effect of active essential oils added to chicken tawook on the behaviour of Listeria monocytogenes, Salmonella spp. and Escherichia coli O157:H7 during storage. *International Journal of Food Microbiology, 337*, 108947. Available from https://doi.org/10.1016/j.ijfoodmicro.2020.108947.

Osaili, T. M., Hasan, F., Dhanasekaran, D. K., Obaid, R. S., Al-Nabulsi, A. A., Karam, L., Savvaidis, I. N., Olaimat, A. N., Ayyash, M., Al-Holy, M., & Holley, R. (2021). Effect of yogurt-based marinade combined with essential oils on the behavior of Listeria monocytogenes, Escherichia coli O157:H7 and Salmonella spp. in camel meat chunks during storage. *International Journal of Food Microbiology, 343*, 109106. Available from https://doi.org/10.1016/j.ijfoodmicro.2021.109106.

Osaili, T. M., Hasan, F., Dhanasekaran, D. K., Obaid, R. S., Al-Nabulsi, A. A., Rao, S., Fatima, H., Ayyash, M., Savvaidis, i., & Holley, R. (2020). Thermal inactivation of Escherichia coli O157: H7 strains and Salmonella spp. in camel meat burgers. *LWT, 120*, 108914. Available from https://doi.org/10.1016/j.lwt.2019.108914.

Salazar, J. K., Natarajan, V., Stewart, D., Warren, J., Gonsalves, L. J., Mhetras, T., & Tortorello, M. L. (2019). Fate of *Listeria monocytogenes* in ready-to-eat refrigerated dips treated with high pressure processing. *Journal of Food Protection, 82*, 1320–1325. Available from https://doi.org/10.4315/0362-028X.JFP-18-550.

Shaheen, M., Nsaif, M., & Borjac, J. (2019). Effect of TDS on bacterial growth in Lebanese hummus dip. *BAU Journal—Health and Wellbeing, 15*. Available from https://digitalcommons.bau.edu.lb/hwbjournal/vol1/iss2/5.

Sillankorva, S. M., Oliveira, H., & Azeredo, J. (2012). Bacteriophages and their role in food safety. *International Journal of Microbiology, 2012,* 863945. Available from https://doi.org/10.1155/2012/863945.

Sofy, A. R., El Haliem, N. F. A., Refaey, E. E., & Hmed, A. A. (2020). Polyvalent phage CoNShP-3 as a natural antimicrobial agent showing lytic and antibiofilm activities against antibiotic-resistant coagulase-negative Staphylococci strains. *Foods, 9,* 673. Available from https://doi.org/10.3390/foods9050673.

Sokołowska, B., Nasiłowska, J., Rutkowska, M., Fonberg-Broczek, M., & Rzoska, S. J. (2019). The usage of high hydrostatic pressure (HHP) to control food-borne pathogens in hummus. *High Pressure Research, 39*, 525–532. Available from https://doi.org/10.1080/08957959.2019.1630402.

Todd, E. C. D. (2017). *Foodborne disease in the middle east. Water, energy and food sustainability in the Middle East: The sustainability triangle*. Available from https://doi.org/10.1007/978-3-319-48920-9_17.

Torlak, E., Sert, D., & Serin, P. (2013). Fate of *Salmonella* during sesame seeds roasting and storage of tahini. *International Journal of Food Microbiology, 163*(2–3), 214–217. Available from https://doi.org/10.1016/j.ijfoodmicro.2013.03.010.

Tsiraki, M. I., Yehia, H. M., Elobeid, T., Osaili, T., Sakkas, H., & Savvaidis, I. N. (2018). Viability of and *Escherichia coli* O157:H7 and *Listeria monocytogenes* in a delicatessen appetizer (yogurt-based) salad as affected by citrus extract (Citrox©) and storage temperature. *Food Microbiology, 69*. Available from https://doi.org/10.1016/j.fm.2017.07.014.

Umar, M., Roddick, F., & Fan, L. (2019). Moving from the traditional paradigm of pathogen inactivation to controlling antibiotic resistance in water-Role of ultraviolet irradiation. *Science of the Total Environment, 662*, 923–939.

Wahba, N. M., Ahmed, A. S., & Ebraheim, Z. Z. (2010). Antimicrobial effects of pepper, parsley, and dill and their roles in the microbiological quality enhancement of traditional Egyptian Kareish cheese. *Foodborne Pathogens and Disease*, *7*. Available from https://doi.org/10.1089/fpd.2009.0412.

Yildirim, S., Röcker, B., Pettersen, M. K., Nilsen-Nygaard, J., Ayhan, Z., Rutkaite, R., ... Coma, V. (2018). *Active packaging applications for food. Comprehensive reviews in food science and food safety*. Available from https://doi.org/10.1111/1541-4337.12322.

Yousef, A. E., & Balasubramaniam, V. M. (2013). Physical Methods of Food Preservation. In M. P. Doyle, R. L. Beuchat, & T. J. Montville (Eds.), *Food Microbiology: Fundamentals and Frontiers* (4th (ed.)). Washington, D.C: ASM Press.

Chapter 7

Food safety knowledge, attitudes, and practices among food handlers in foodservice establishments in the Arab countries of the Middle East

Dima Faour-Klingbeil[1,2]
[1]*Centre for Rural Development, Humboldt University of Berlin, Germany,* [2]*DFK for Safe Food Environment, Food Safety and Regulatory Systems Compliance, Hannover, Germany*

7.1 Introduction

The eating habits and food choices of consumers in the developed and the developing world have changed over the years due to lifestyle changes and the vast selection of food choices made available by advancement in food technology, intensified food production, and globalization. The foodservice industry, such as takeaways, ready-to-eat foods (RTEs), and fast-food chains, has also grown famous as a convenience food source. Such a new trend has emerged due to the increase in consumers' purchasing power (Kearney, 2010) and the Western lifestyle that has become so widespread in developing countries (Hawkes, 2005). The strong influence of the Western culture on consumers' dietary habits has resulted in the accelerated growth in restaurants and food industry, as Arab population is increasingly opting for RTEs and eating out from international food chains (Al-Shabib, Mosilhey, & Husain, 2016). The nutritional transition in food choices from the typical Mediterranean home-prepared diet to the fast-food trend (Yahia, Achkar, Abdallah, & Rizk, 2008) motivated international food chains to continuously expand their stores in many Arab countries (Market Research, 2020).

The restaurant industry is one of the fastest-growing sectors in several Arab countries in the Middle East (e.g., Dubai in the United Arab Emirates, Kingdom of Saudi Arabia (KSA), Bahrain, Lebanon, and others). It has grown exponentially over the last few years, with currently valued at US$13.2 billion

Food Safety in the Middle East. DOI: https://doi.org/10.1016/B978-0-12-822417-5.00002-7

in the UAE alone and expected to grow at a compound annual growth rate of around 8% to reach US$29.3 billion by 2018 (The Restaurant Show, 2018). A case in point, Kuwait has witnessed the growth of various types of restaurants in the last decade with an average consumers' spending of 2 million Kuwait Dinars per day in restaurants (Al-Kandari, Al-abdeen, & Sidhu, 2019).

Along the same line, demand for home delivery is growing popular aided by the increasing internet connectivity and consumer spending, which is projected to become more prominent in the Arab world (McKinsey & Company, 2020). Furthermore, the online food delivery segment is expected to show a revenue growth of 14.6% in 2021. It is estimated that food delivery applications are used by over 6 million people across the KSA alone, making it the largest food delivery market in the Middle East and North Africa (MENA) region. The Kuwaiti food delivery startup "Carriage" has quickly spread across the Gulf region and plans to expand to the broader MENA region (Noureldin, 2020). In parallel to the expansion of the food industry and reliance on prepared meals, opportunities for foodborne diseases may also increase considering that restaurants are a typical setting for reported foodborne disease outbreaks (Angelo, Nisler, Hall, Brown, & Gould, 2017; Gormley, Rawal, & Little, 2012; Rebouças et al., 2017; Todd, Greig, Bartleson, & Michaels, 2007).

Foodborne illnesses threaten public health and cause significant health and economic burdens (Belaya, Hansen, & Pinior, 2012; Scharff, 2012). It is estimated that 33 healthy life years Disability-Adjusted Life Year are lost due to eating unsafe food globally each year, and this number is likely an underestimation (WHO, 2015c). The MENA region has the third-highest estimated burden of foodborne diseases per population, after the African and Southeast Asia regions. The foodborne illnesses are attributed to the use of unsafe water in food preparation and cleaning of premises, poor hygiene and food handling practices, and lack of adequate food storage facilities. Besides, many of these countries have limited foodborne disease surveillance data and poorly enforced food safety laws and control policies (Faour-Klingbeil & Todd, 2019; WHO, 2015c).

The continuous reporting of foodborne disease outbreaks and food scandal substantiates the importance of taking stringent protection measures to ensure safe food and reduce health risks. They were often driving forces for tightening food safety regulations (Marette, Bureau, & ozlan, 2003). For instance, the first Bovine Spongiform Encephalopathy (foodborne-related) case reported in Japan in 2001 triggered far-reaching changes in the regulatory framework of food safety and significant institutional developments, namely the establishment of the Food Safety Commission (Walravens, 2017).

In the Arab world, frequent food poisoning outbreaks also triggered major initiatives. In response to a wave of food poisoning in 2006 and 2007 in Jordan, the strict collaboration between the Ministry of Health in Jordan and the Jordanian Food and Drug Association has enabled efficient and improved control measures in food safety (Qasim, 2011). In Lebanon, frequent incidences of food poisoning and scandals led to the initiation of public–private collaboration for launching training programs in food safety, establishing the Lebanese Food Safety Agency, and ratifying new food law. The latter was stalled in the parliament for years (FAO, 2019; WHO, 2015b) and has not taken effect to date.

The foodborne illnesses can be prevented and minimized; however, dialogs among the different stakeholders to improve policymaking and decisions that foster food safety governance are essential. Government and health agencies should regularly evaluate the regulatory policies to ensure that they are still useful and in line with the current scientific understanding of food safety risks. Simultaneously, compliance inspections should be maintained while providing the necessary and adequate education and resources to the foodservice industry. The food safety governance in Arab countries is relatively new. Compared to the developed countries, food safety governance in Arab countries progresses at a slow pace primarily due to the required budgets, willingness, and expertise to institute a national food safety strategy (Faour-Klingbeil and C D Todd, 2019). Yet, in countries that strive under political and economic instability, any potential progress seems remote.

On the other hand, food safety should be instituted by the food corporations and restaurants through strict policies for preventing food contamination by sourcing safe food ingredients and following strict health and hygiene rules for safe food handling practices in the kitchen. For this reason, appropriate ongoing training of food workers and conveying scientific information on food safety risks in a simple manner are essential to ensure food handlers' awareness, positive attitudes, and compliance with the food safety requirements and operating procedures. This chapter will present an overview of the significant relevance of food safety in the food (catering) service establishments (FSEs) in the Arab countries, with the main focus on the food handlers' responsibilities and knowledge of food safety as essential requirements for food safety. The present chapter will therefore (1) discuss the current findings on food handlers' knowledge, attitudes, and practices (KAP) in food safety and identify common patterns; (2) address the shortfalls in knowledge and practices that may impact consumers' health; and (3) outline recommendations and suggestions for future research.

7.2 The importance of food safety in the foodservice establishments

The reason food safety is important in the FSEs is simply well presented in the definition of food safety, that is, food safety is a scientific discipline describing handling, preparation, and storage of food in ways that prevent foodborne illness. This includes several routines that should be followed to avoid potentially severe health hazards from sourcing the raw ingredients and materials through handling, preparation, serving, delivery, or packing and food. Hence, contamination with biological, chemical, radiological, and physical hazards can occur at any stage of the supply chain. Thus the preparation steps in the FSEs and adhering to safe handling practices and food safety standards significantly reduce the likelihood of food contamination and the chances of causing harm to consumers.

There is a growing body of data globally on the implications of FSEs, that is, restaurants, retail foodservice operations, clubs, assisted-living facilities, nursing homes, child-care centers, schools, and universities, in foodborne disease outbreaks and sporadic cases of gastrointestinal disease (Angulo, Jones, & Angulo, 2006; Gould, Rosenblum, Nicholas, Phan, & Jones, 2013; Sneed & Strohbehn, 2008). It is estimated that 60% of foodborne disease outbreaks worldwide are linked to eating establishments and commercial caterers (OECD/WHO, 2003).

FSEs have been implicated in 78% of the foodborne outbreaks in the United States (Gould et al., 2013). Earlier data showed that of the 9040 foodborne disease outbreaks reported to the CDC from 1998 to 2004, 4675 (52%) were associated with restaurants or delicatessens (including cafeterias and hotels). Of these, 622 (13%) were caused by bacteria, 535 (11%) by viruses, and 3377 (72%) had an unknown etiology (Angulo et al., 2006). Additionally, of the 457 foodborne disease outbreaks reported in 2006 and 2007 by FoodNet sites, 300 (66%) were restaurant-associated. Nearly half of them were caused by *Salmonella* transmitted through food workers (Gould et al., 2013). In one series of restaurant-associated outbreaks of *Salmonella* infection in Minnesota, an infected food worker was identified in 83% of these outbreaks (Medus, Smith, Bender, Besser, & Hedberg, 2006). Norovirus has also been prominently linked to restaurant-associated outbreaks, mainly through transmission by food workers (Todd et al., 2007). Sixty percent of the reported outbreaks between 1975 and 1998 were caused by viral agents, such as noroviruses and hepatitis A and 89% of those outbreaks occurred at retail foodservice operations (Sneed & Strohbehn, 2008).

Similarly, the European Food Safety Authority (EFSA) reported in 2010 that about 48.7% of foodborne diseases were associated with catering establishments (EFSA, 2010). In the United Kingdom (England and Wales), the foodservice sector continues to be the most common vehicle for reported foodborne disease outbreaks with more than half associated with catering establishments. From 1992 to 2009, of the 677 restaurant-associated foodborne outbreaks in England and Wales, 11,795 people were affected, 491 hospitalized, and 7 died. Investigations showed that Chinese, Indian, British, and Italian cuisines were the most frequently and commonly implicated in these outbreaks (26%, 16%, 13%, and 10%, respectively) (Gormley et al., 2012). Consequently, the UK Food Standards Agency (FSA) mandated the UK Food Hygiene Rating Scheme. Commercial food establishments are being inspected and scored with the results made available to the public

(Jones et al., 2017). To decrease the burden of foodborne diseases, the WHO advocates the Five Keys to Safer Food: (1) Keep clean; (2) Separate raw and cooked; (3) Cook thoroughly; (4) Keep food at safe temperatures, and (5) Use safe water and raw materials (WHO, 2015a).

There is a scarcity of officially reported cases on foodborne illnesses in the Arab countries. Only the aggravated incidences are often registered in the national surveillance system and make their way to local news headlines. Shortfalls in the surveillance data on national foodborne disease outbreaks and source investigations are sometimes attributed to the poor communication and cooperation of some hospitals and the lack of investigation and technical skills (Abd-Elhaleem & Abd-Elkarim, 2011; Al-Kandari et al., 2019; Fadlallah et al., 2017; Malaeb, Bizri, Ghosn, Berry, & Musharrafieh, 2016; Rebgui et al., 2013). Consequently, any efforts to transition toward risk assessment along the food supply chain and to understand the hazards sources and risk factors within the local context are undermined.

The Middle East, particularly the Arab countries region, is typically a warm region in the Spring and Summer, which places great importance on food safety. Further, temperature control becomes vital to prevent microbial growth in foods and thus reduce food-related diseases. This fact becomes a peculiar significance in eateries that are expanding informally such as street vendors. Street food vendors present a significant risk to consumers' health both in the absence of adequate (hygienic) water quality and failure to comply with the basic food safety and hygiene practices (El-Sherbeeny, Saddik, & Bryan, 1985; Loukieh et al., 2018; Omar, 2020).

According to Malaeb et al. (2016), data on *Salmonella* infections in Lebanon and many emerging Middle East countries lack crucial information. The reported data do not necessarily represent the actual dimension, incidence, prevalence, and burden of foodborne-related illnesses. Nonetheless, they show that *Salmonella* species are the most prominent bacteria associated with food poisoning. These incidences generally peak during the summer season (June–August) in most Arab countries (Al Arabiya news, 2020; Al-Goblan & Jahan, 2010; ElMeshad, 2011; Malaeb et al., 2016; Rebgui et al., 2013; Saleh, 2011; The Guardian, 2020). For instance, during 2006, 31 foodborne illness outbreaks, accounting for 251 cases, were reported in Saudi Arabia with the highest proportion (64.5%) during the summer months. *Salmonella* species were the common causative agent, followed by *Staphylococcus aureus*. Eating commercial RTE food and Middle-Eastern meat sandwiches were linked to most cases (Al-Goblan & Jahan, 2010).

Also, in Saudi Arabia, approximately 1647 foodborne illnesses were reported in 2010, and 62% of the cases were attributed to the consumption of food from commercial sources. This was followed by 255 incidences of foodborne diseases resulting in sickness of 2066 people in 2011 (Al-Shabib et al., 2016). Gastroenteritis incidences were also reported in the previous years due to the consumption of contaminated RTE foods (Al-Ahmadi, Bushra, & Al-Zahrani, 1998).

In Kuwait, eating Falafel, a traditional Middle-Eastern food, caused 130 cases of food poisoning. Besides, five Salmonellosis cases were reported in a camp of the US army soldiers in 2018 (Kuwait News Agency, 2018; Myers, 2018). In Egypt, more than 2200 cases of food poisoning were reported in 2017 among students who were provided government-subsidized meals, followed by another wave in the same year affecting 98 students (Arab News, 2017). On a list compiled by a British travel illness claim website of holiday destinations worldwide, the renowned Egyptian Red Sea resort of Hurghada recorded the highest rates of food poisoning claims accounting for 95% cases. Many of these cases were traced to foods left out under improper temperature conditions before reheating (Arabian Business, 2019).

The earlier data show that most of the reported cases of foodborne diseases were registered in the last decade, which is likely due to improved surveillance systems and changes in eating habits. Chapter 2, Overview on Food Safety in the Middle East, provides a broader view of the foodborne disease in the Arab countries of the Middle East, such as in Jordan, where series of food poisoning incidences occurred in 1 year (2020), with the highest number reported in the summer (Al Arabiya News, 2020; Qasim, 2011; The Guardian, 2020).

Food scares and scandals receive extensive media coverage, and the common action often entails closure of facilities and legal liabilities. However, the source of the etiological agents and risk factors remain unclear. To prevent the recurrence of massive food safety problems, the foodservice sector should have access to information resources, training, and guidance documents, which are not well established in many countries of the Arab region. The 2014 food safety campaign launched by the Lebanese Ministry of Public Health revealed major and critical violations to the law that could pose health risks to consumers (The Daily Star, 2014; The National, 2018; WHO, 2015b; YaLibnan, 2014). The ministerial campaign focused on a fierce inspection of the FSEs, slaughterhouses, and butcher shops followed by actions such as the closure of facilities or corrective action requirements. But what was not on the campaign plan is adopting an education approach to rectify the root problem, that is, decades of governmental neglect in food safety and lax in law enforcement. The representatives and owners of food businesses were not aware of the local food safety requirements in Lebanon (Middle East Eye, 2015) when clear guidelines and regulatory requirements are not published or available until the date of writing this chapter.

7.3 The common contributing factors of foodborne illnesses and the role of food handlers

Foodborne diseases are caused by bacteria, viruses, parasites, and toxins resulting from unsafe raw materials or ingredients, improper food preparation, inadequate temperature control, and storage conditions, poor sanitation, and personal hygiene. According to the FSA, good food hygiene is all about controlling harmful bacteria, which can cause serious illness through the four pillars of food safety essential for good hygiene and safe food: cross-contamination, cleaning, chilling, and cooking. Hence, lapses in sanitation, hygiene, and temperature controls can render the food unsafe for consumers. It is well recognized that the top five risk factors of foodborne outbreaks in FSEs include improper holding temperatures, inadequate cooking, contaminated equipment, purchase and receipt of food from unsafe sources, and poor personal hygiene. These are all directly related to food handler errors responsible for 97% of all foodborne illnesses associated with the foodservice sector (Egan et al., 2007) and can be prevented if food handlers follow proper food safety practices (Roberts et al., 2008).

There is a large body of evidence on the contribution of those risk factors to foodborne diseases in different parts of the world. Forty-five percent of foodborne disease outbreaks resulted from inadequate temperature control during food processing. More specifically, poor refrigeration and inappropriate storage temperatures of leftover or recently cooked meals accounted for 23.5% and 12.6% of the cases, respectively (Tirado & Schmidt, 2001). In England, multiple risk factors were implicated in food outbreaks including inadequate heat treatment (50%), improper storage (45%), cross-contamination (39%), and infected food handlers (12%) (Evans et al., 1998). Similarly, the FDA (2009) identified improper holding/time and temperature, poor personal hygiene, and contaminated equipment as risk practices and behaviors that contributed to foodborne illnesses.

However, it is strongly evidenced that food handlers through improper personal hygiene or as asymptomatic carriers who may shed pathogens play a critical role in the transmission of infectious diseases thus can be responsible for foodborne outbreaks (Greig, Todd, Bartleson, & Michaels, 2007). A lack of hand hygiene is a significant risk factor in the occurrence of food contamination (Codex Alimentarius, 2003), as it can contribute to transmitting harmful pathogens to foods, such as coagulase-positive staphylococci (Soares, Almeida, Cerqueira, Carvalho, & Nunes, 2012), *Salmonella* (Lee, Abdul Halim, Thong, & Chai, 2017), and viruses (Franck et al., 2015; Stals, Uyttendaele, Baert, & Van Coillie, 2013).

A food handler is anyone who works in a food business and who handles either food or surfaces that are likely to be in contact with food such as cutlery, plates, and bowls, and performs functions such as cooking, preparing, serving, packing, displaying, and storing food. Food handlers can also be involved in manufacturing, producing, collecting, extracting, processing, transporting, delivering, thawing, or preserving food (FSANZ, n.d.). Food handling comprises all stages of food treatment and storage, from the reception of raw items to the distribution of end products, that is, from farm to fork (FAO, 2017). Improper and unsafe food handling practices at any step of the food chain may contribute to food poisoning (McIntyre, Vallaster, Wilcott, Henderson, & Kosatsky, 2013). Hence, It warrants a high level of responsibility and awareness to ensure food safety and prevent food contamination throughout the chain of production, processing, storage, and preparation (Lee et al., 2017). Food handlers can render safe and uncontaminated foods hazardous to eat through cross-contamination. Whereas, proper practices ensure that contaminated foods become safe to eat (e.g., through treatment such as thorough cooking) (Lasky, 2002; Røssvoll et al., 2013). The latter is essential when handling food products with high contamination rates at the point of sale or retail (Jones et al., 2017).

Food workers have a crucial role in ensuring food safety by learning and practicing how and when to wash hands thoroughly, maintain proper personal hygiene, and apply strict preventive and control measures to protect food from contamination and microbial growth. Such a role is mainly achieved through appropriate food safety education and training to improve food safety practices and attitudes. The lack of food safety knowledge could prove to be a major barrier to the effective implementation of food safety principles and practices in catering food-related businesses (Walker, Pritchard, & Forsythe, 2003). It is one of the main reasons responsible for food contamination (Evans et al., 1998).

Although food safety knowledge is necessary for those involved in food handling processes, complex factors could interfere in transmitting this knowledge into safe practices. Knowledge alone does not translate into appropriate behavior modification, hence to explore appropriate strategies that enhance safe practices, researchers have used behavioral theories such as the KAP model. KAP is used to explore human behavior toward a matter in question by assessing what the respondents know about it, how they agree with it or feel about it, and what they do about it. KAP model is based on the assumption that knowledge affects attitudes which in turn can reflect on behaviors.

Researchers have taken an interest in applying KAP studies on food handlers in retail foodservice operations to understand attitudes and practices toward food safety. The findings showed varying levels of deficiencies in knowledge of food handlers in cross-contamination, disease transmission, and temperature control (Martins, Hogg, & Otero, 2012; Ovca, Jevšnik, & Raspor, 2018; Rebouças et al., 2017; Zanin, da Cunha, de Rosso, Capriles, & Stedefeldt, 2017).

In the Arab countries, KAP studies are very few, conducted mainly in the last decade, and slowly building up with the rising interest among researchers given the recurrent reporting of food poisoning or foodborne illnesses. Table 7.1 lists the different studies on food safety knowledge and the few that addressed the KAP.

TABLE 7.1 Extract of the available studies on the food safety knowledge or KAP of food handlers in the FSEs in the Arab countries of the Middle East.

Country	Food production setting	Sample characteristics	Type of survey	Overall food safety knowledge[a]	References
Egypt	Hospitals ($N=4$)	$N=132$ food handlers	Effect of educational program on KAP	9.2 ± 5.3 (before) 18.5 ± 3.9 (after)[b]	Elsherbiny, Sobhy, Fiala, and Abbas (2019)
Lebanon	Restaurants ($N=50$)	$N=80$ food handlers	Observational assessment of food safety practices	N/A	Faour-Klingbeil, Kuri, and Todd (2020)
Egypt	FSEs and street vendors	$N=994$ food handlers	KAP	39.2%	Hamed and Mohammed (2020)
United Arab Emirates	FSEs ($N=88$) restaurants, cafeterias, coffee shops	$N=646$ food handlers	Food safety knowledge	70%	Taha et al. (2020)
Qatar	FSEs ($N=53$)	$N=53$ food safety managers	Food safety practices[c]	No data	Asim et al. (2019)
Qatar	Fast-food restaurants in Qatar University	$N=102$ food handlers	KAP	No data	Elobeid, Savvaidis, and Ganji (2019)
Saudi Arabia	Hospitals ($N=10$)	$N=163$ food handlers	Food safety knowledge and practices	77.9%	Alqurashi, Priyadarshini, and Jaiswal (2019)

(Continued)

TABLE 7.1 (Continued)

Country	Food production setting	Sample characteristics	Type of survey	Overall food safety knowledge[a]	References
Lebanon	Hospitals ($N = 13$)	$N = 254$ food handlers	KAP	59.2%	Bou-Mitri et al.(2018)
Jordan	FSEs ($N = 79$) on 34 university campuses	$N = 520$ food handlers	Food safety knowledge	67.1%	Osaili, Al-Nabulsi, and Allah Krasneh (2018)
Jordan	Hospitals ($N = 37$)	$N = 532$ food handlers and dietitians	Food safety knowledge	62.5%	Osaili, Obeidat, Hajeer, and Al-Nabulsi (2017)
Saudi Arabia	Restaurants ($N = 2$), university canteens ($N = 5$)	$N = 87$ food handlers	KAP	No data	Al-Shabib et al. (2016)
United Arab Emirates	FSEs ($N = 48$)	$N = 48$ PIC (supervisors)	The effect of PIC intervention on knowledge and practice	71.3% (before) to 76.1% (after)	Abushelaibi et al. (2015)
Lebanon	Restaurants ($N = 50$)	$N = 80$ food handlers	KAP	56.6 ± 21.0 on a 100-point scale	Faour-Klingbeil, Kuri, and Todd (2015)
Jordan	Fast-food restaurants ($N = 297$)	$N = 1084$ food handlers	Food safety knowledge	69.4%	Osaili et al. (2013)
Jordan	Hospitals ($N = 7$)	$N = 200$ staff	KAP	84.82%	Sharif, Obaidat, and Al-Dalalah (2013)

Kuwait	Restaurants	$N = 402$ food handlers	KAP	70%	Al-Kandari et al. (2019)
Qatar	Hospital ($N = 1$)	$N = 43$ food handlers	KAP[d]	No data	Kaabi, Lbrahim, and Salama (2010)
Palestine	Restaurants ($N = 202$)	$N = 308$ food handlers	Food sanitation practices	No data	Al-Khatib and Al-Mitwalli (2009)

Notes: The total score of KAP is not reported in all studies. *N/A*, Not applicable; *FSE*, foodservice establishment; *KAP*, knowledge, attitudes, and practices; *PIC*, person in charge.
[a]*Mean percentage score: Overall score of food safety knowledge calculated by summation of correct answers and later converted into a percentage.*
[b]*There is no information on the basis used for calculating the overall knowledge score in this study.*
[c]*The authors referred to the education and training levels of surveyed subjects using the term "food safety knowledge."*
[d]*No details published on the attitudes statements used in this study. Attitude part was omitted in the discussion.*

7.4 Food safety knowledge, attitude, and practice of food handlers

7.4.1 Food safety knowledge

Few of the selected studies followed nearly the same approach by thematically structuring the survey tool into sections: personal hygiene, cross-contamination prevention, sanitation, temperature control, knowledge of foodborne illnesses, and foodborne pathogens (Al-Kandari et al., 2019; Elobeid et al., 2019; Faour-Klingbeil et al., 2015; Osaili et al., 2017, 2018; Taha et al., 2020). Others either did not include all the above themes (Alqurashi et al., 2019) or did not follow a similar approach (Al-Shabib et al., 2016; Bou-Mitri et al., 2018; Hamed & Mohammed, 2020; Kaabi et al., 2010; Sharif et al., 2013).

The overall food safety knowledge, sometimes referred to as the overall score of correct answers on questions, was calculated in most studies by summing up all the correct answers (Table 7.1). Overall scores on each theme were also sometimes calculated separately (e.g., scores on cross-contamination, personal hygiene). The responses for each theme were presented using frequency distribution. The results from the studies that adopted almost the same set of questions and scoring methods are shown in Tables 7.2, 7.3, and 7.4; others will be discussed in context.

In general, the overall food safety knowledge of food handlers in the different Arab countries was reported fair to good (Al-Kandari et al., 2019; Alqurashi et al., 2019; Al-Shabib et al., 2016; Kaabi et al., 2010; Osaili et al., 2013, 2017; Taha et al., 2020) and in some cases low and insufficient (Bou-Mitri et al., 2018; Faour-Klingbeil et al., 2015; Osaili et al., 2018). It is important to note that the assessment level or terms used (e.g., fair, good, poor) in rating the food safety knowledge level varied among the studies because of differences in determining the cut-off point. Comparing countries based on this classification will be inaccurate.

Figures of the overall scores of food safety knowledge in Kuwait, Jordan, and the UAE (Al-Kandari et al., 2019; Osaili et al., 2013; Taha et al., 2020) were higher than those reported in the Lebanese hospitals and the Lebanese and Egyptian food businesses (Table 7.1) (Bou-Mitri et al., 2018; Faour-Klingbeil et al., 2015; Hamed & Mohammed, 2020). The mean score of the food safety knowledge of food handlers in Jordanian restaurants was 69.4%, that is, the correct answers for the food safety tested aspects were 46.47 out of 67 points, compared to the score of food handlers in Jordanian hospitals (62.5%), that is, 56.3 correct answers, indicating an insufficient knowledge in various areas of food safety (Osaili et al., 2013, 2017). On the other hand, the average score of correct answers of food handlers in the Lebanese restaurants and hospitals was 56.6 ± 21.0 on 100 score points and 59.2%, respectively (Bou-Mitri et al., 2018; Faour-Klingbeil et al., 2015).

TABLE 7.2 Food handlers' knowledge on personal hygiene aspect.

Questions on the importance of performing each of the following:	*N* (%)[a]	*N* (%)[b]	*N* (%)[c]	*N* (%)[d]	*N* (%)[e]
Washing hands after touching money	337 (63.3)	378 (72.7)	351 (54.3)	No data	90.5
Washing hands after eating meals	518 (97.4)	500 (96.2)	490 (75.9)	No data	98.1
Washing hands before preparing meals/food preparation	441 (82.9)	502 (96.5)	560 (86.7)	400 (99.5)	95.8
Washing hands after using toilets	528 (99.2)	504 (96.9)	591 (91.5)	400 (99.5)	98.6
Washing hands after handling raw meats or poultry	521 (97.9)	485 (93.3)	459 (71.1)	390 (97.0)	97.6
Washing hands after touching the body	410 (77.1)	472 (90.8)	455 (70.4)	386 (96.0)	92.7
Washing hands during continuous food handling/making salad[b,c]	471 (88.5)	442 (85.0)	318 (49.2)	No data	94.1
Washing hands after touching sanitized countertop	311 (58.5)	384 (73.8)	256 (39.6)	No data	82.2
Washing hands after sneezing and coughing	485 (91.2)	485 (93.3)	521 (80.7)	No data	96.9
Washing hands after cleaning tables	474 (89.1)	472 (90.8)	504 (78.0)	392 (97.5)	97.0
Washing hands after handling the garbage	522 (98.1)	496 (95.4)	559 (86.5)	395 (98.3)	98.0
Washing hands after touching work clothes	405 (76.1)	389 (74.8)	349 (54.0)	No data	89.7
Washing hands after using mobile phone	224 (42.1)	No data	No data	No data	
Washing hands before wearing gloves	392 (73.7)	291 (56.0)	390 (60.4)	No data	
Washing hands after removing gloves	453 (85.2)	375 (72.1)	411 (63.6)	No data	
Duration of handwashing is 20 s or more	157 (29.5)	166 (31.9)	395 (61.1)	264 (65.7)	31.9

Note: The percentage figures represent the % answers as "yes" to questions.
[a] *Osaili et al. (2017).*
[b] *Osaili et al. (2018).*
[c] *Taha et al. (2020).*
[d] *Al-Kandari et al. (2019).*
[e] *Osaili et al. (2013).*

TABLE 7.3 Food handlers' knowledge of cross-contamination prevention and sanitation aspect.

Questions on the appropriateness of each of the following:					
	N (%)[a]	*N* (%)[b]	*N* (%)[c]	*N* (%)[d]	*N* (%)[e]
Wearing gloves before touching RTE food products	503 (94.5)	479 (92.1)	493 (76.3)	373 (92.8)	91.9
Wearing gloves when touching or distributing unwrapped food to patients†/unpackaged food‡/uncovered food*	489 (91.9)	388 (74.6)	473 (73.2)		
Wearing uniform during touching or distributing unwrapped food to patients†/unpackaged food‡	488 (91.7)	413 (79.4)	435 (67.3)		
Wearing mask during touching or distributing unwrapped food to patients/uncovered food*	310 (58.3)	112 (21.5)	330 (51.1)		
Wearing hair net during touching or distributing unwrapped food to patients	468 (88.0)	339 (65.2)	493 (76.3)		
Using the same knife to cut raw meat or poultry and to chop vegetables	17 (3.2)	8 (1.5)	18 (2.8)		
Washing knife used to cut raw meat or poultry with cold water before using it to chop vegetables	24 (4.5)	35 (6.7)	32 (5)		21.0
Washing knife used to cut raw meat or poultry with hot water before using it to chop vegetables	44 (8.3)	77 (14.8)	139 (21.5)	274 (68.2)	55.4
Washing knife used to cut raw meat or poultry with water and soap before using it to chop vegetables	125 (23.5)	138 (26.5)	155 (24.0)	298 (74.1)	48.4
Washing knife used to cut raw meat or poultry with water and soap then applying sanitizer before using it to chop vegetables	227 (42.7)	176 (33.8)	394 (62.0)	276 (68.7)	50.6
Wiping knife used to cut raw meat or poultry with a piece of cloth before using it to chop vegetables	25 (4.7)	30 (5.8)	47 (7.3)		10.9
Changing knife to cut raw meat or poultry and to chop vegetables	232 (43.6)	272 (52.3)	336 (52)		73.6

Using the same cutting board to cut raw meat or poultry and to chop vegetables	13 (2.4)	10 (1.9)	8 (1.2)		3.3
Washing cutting board used to cut raw meat or poultry with cold water before using it to chop vegetables	20 (3.8)	17 (3.3)	26 (4)		16.9
Washing cutting board used to cut raw meat or poultry with hot water before using it to chop vegetables	44 (8.3)	63 (12.1)	141 (21.8)	282 (70.1)	54.0
Washing cutting board used to cut raw meat or poultry with water and soap before using it to chop vegetables	99 (18.6)	120 (23.1)	161 (24.9)		45.0
Washing cutting board used to cut raw meat or poultry with water and soap then applying sanitizer before using it to chop vegetables	215 (40.4)	154 (29.6)	401 (62.1)		51.6
Wiping cutting board used to cut raw meat or poultry with a piece of cloth before using it to chop vegetables	24 (4.5)	27 (5.2)	37 (5.7)		8.0
Changing cutting board to cut raw meat or poultry and to chop vegetables	252 (47.4)	299 (57.5)	391 (60.5)		75.5
Storing vegetable salad on the upper shelf in the refrigerator if raw meat or chicken in the middle shelf	214 (40.2)	165 (31.7)	390 (60.4)		69.0
Storing vegetable salad in the middle shelf in the refrigerator if raw meat or chicken in the middle shelf	13 (2.4)	15 (2.9)	24 (3.7)		9.8
Storing vegetables salad in the lower shelf in the refrigerator if raw meat or chicken in the middle shelf	50 (9.4)	39 (7.5)	53 (8.2)		12.2
Storing vegetables salad in vegetable refrigerator	299 (56.2)	313 (60.2)	359 (55.6)		
Washing surface with water and soap then apply a sanitizer is the most effective method in cleaning and sanitizing food contact surfaces	393 (73.9)	278 (53.5)	339 (52.5)	265 (65.9)	77.1

Notes: Percentage figures represent the % answers as "yes" to questions. *RTE*, Ready to eat.
[a]*Osaili et al. (2017).*
[b]*Osaili et al. (2018).*
[c]*Taha et al. (2020).*
[d]*Al-Kandari et al. (2019).*
[e]*Osaili et al. (2013).*

TABLE 7.4 Food handlers' knowledge of the temperature control aspect.

Questions on the appropriateness and importance of the following:	*N* (%)[a]	*N* (%)[b]	*N* (%)[c]	*N* (%)[d]	(%)[e,f]
Thawing frozen raw meat or poultry on the kitchen counter in an open container	18 (3.4)	16 (31)	21 (3.3)	197 (49.0)	(15.9)
Thawing frozen raw meat or poultry on the kitchen counter in a covered container	65 (12.2)	102 (19.7)	129 (20.0)		(32.5)
Thawing frozen raw meat or poultry in the refrigerator	270 (50.8)	256 (49.2)	351 (54.3)	264 (65.7)	(66.7)
Thawing frozen raw meat or poultry under running tap water		41 (7.9)	323 (50.0)	135 (33.6)	(23.8)
Thawing frozen raw meat or poultry in the microwave	6 (1.1)	42 (8.1)	342 (52.9)		(4.1)
Thawing frozen raw meat or poultry in still water	178 (33.5)	147 (28.3)			
Refrigerator operating temperature is 1°C–4°C		169 (32.5)	339 (52.5)	323 (80.3)	(47.5)
Freezer operating temperature is −18°C	240 (45.1)	175 (33.7)	405 (62.7)	331 (82.3)	(46.4)
Hot ready-to-eat holding temperature is >60°C	165 (31.0)	78 (15.0)	348 (53.9)		
Temperature of internal chicken tissues should reach 74°C during cooking	189 (35.5)	153 (29.4)	373 (57.7)		
Food should reach 73°C during reheating	106 19.9	43 (8.3)	365 (56.5)		(19.6)
Checking poultry is sufficiently cooked when it expels its water	27 (5.1)	47 (9.0)	87 (13.5)		
Checking poultry is sufficiently cooked by appearance	130 (24.4)	140 (26.9)	215 (33.3)		
Checking poultry is sufficiently cooked by thermometer/from its temperature	104 (19.5)	66 (12.7)	370 (57.3)		(31.2)
Checking poultry is sufficiently cooked by experience	201 (37.8)	318 (61.2)	272 (42.1)		
Checking poultry is sufficiently cooked by touching	160 (30.1)	189 (36.3)	176 (27.2)		

Store leftover on steam table	75 (14.1)	79 (15.2)	358 (55.4)		(40.0)
Store leftover in the refrigerator	303 (57.0)	162 (31.2)		196 (48.8)	(53.1)
Store leftover on the countertop or table in the kitchen	12 (2.3)	14 (2.7)	70 (10.8)		(3.8)
Store leftover on the shelf in the kitchen	11 (2.1)	8 (1.5)	34 (5.3)	83 (20.6)	(2.2)
Store leftover in the oven to keep warm	31 (5.8)	63 (12.1)	118 (18.3)		(20.6)
Discard leftover	125 (23.5)	266 (51.2)	348 (53.9)		

Note: Percentage figures represent the % answers as "yes" to questions.
[a] *Osaili et al. (2017).*
[b] *Osaili et al. (2018).*
[c] *Taha et al. (2020).*
[d] *Al-Kandari et al. (2019).*
[e] *Osaili et al. (2013).*
[f] *Number of responses not recorded.*

Several authors identified the limited awareness of food handlers typically on foodborne pathogens, time and temperature control (e.g., thawing, cooking, and reheating of foods) (Al-Kandari et al., 2019; Elobeid et al., 2019; Faour-Klingbeil et al., 2015; Hamed & Mohammed, 2020; Osaili et al., 2013; Sharif et al., 2013), and cross-contamination prevention (Al-Kandari et al., 2019; Elobeid et al., 2019; Faour-Klingbeil et al., 2015; Hamed & Mohammed, 2020). These are discussed in more detail in the forthcoming sections.

7.4.1.1 Personal hygiene

In general, food handlers in all the selected studies possessed a good and satisfactory knowledge of personal hygiene (Al-Kandari et al., 2019; Al-Shabib et al., 2016; Elobeid et al., 2019; Osaili et al., 2013) with a mean score in Kuwait, Qatar, Jordan, Saudi Arabia, UAE, and another study from Jordan of 93%, 90%–95%, 74%, 80%, 70%, and 93%, respectively (Al-Kandari et al., 2019; Al-Shabib et al., 2016; Elobeid et al., 2019; Osaili et al., 2018; Sharif et al., 2013). It is important to note that those percentages do not reflect the scores awarded for answers on the same set and the exact number of questions on personal hygiene across the different studies, hence, comparing countries on that basis is inaccurate. For instance, Bou-Mitri et al., 2018 and Elobeid et al. (2019) did not report the personal hygiene knowledge's total score. Further, Sharif et al. (2013) and Al-Shabib et al. (2016) reported the total scores on personal hygiene, 93.8% and 80.2%, respectively, but with no explicit reference to the type of questions.

The food handlers' knowledge of handwashing occasions was similar across the studies with high scores reported in Kuwait, followed by the UAE (Table 7.2). A great majority of the food handlers in the Kuwaiti hospitals (96.0%–99.5%) knew when to wash their hands, which was similar in other studies (Table 7.2). Also, the highest percentage of correct answers of food handlers in the Lebanese restaurants and Qatar University was obtained on handwashing frequency. The vast majority (90%) was aware of the importance of handwashing after touching raw meat and raw eggs, before handling unwrapped RTE foods (Faour-Klingbeil et al., 2015). Similarly, 95%–96% of food handlers in the Qatar University were aware that frequent handwashing reduces food contamination risk (Elobeid et al., 2019).

On the other hand, only 65.7% were able to tell the correct time for appropriate handwashing, that is, 20 s (Al-Kandari et al., 2019) compared to almost one-third of the Jordanian food handlers in the hospitals (29.5%) (Osaili et al., 2017) and universities canteens (31.9%) (Osaili et al., 2018). In the UAE, the majority ($>90\%$) of the respondents successfully identified that handwashing is necessary after using the toilet, and 86.7%, 86.5%, and 80.7% knew that handwashing is essential before food preparation, after disposing of waste, and after coughing and sneezing, respectively (Taha et al., 2020).

In Qatar, Kaabi et al. (2010) reported that all food handlers followed good hand hygiene before putting on gloves and after taking them off. Besides, 97.7%–100% reported washing hands before and after touching unwrapped raw and cooked meals for the patients.

Despite food handlers' understanding of when to wash hands, the rationale behind the importance of handwashing to prevent foodborne illnesses and that hands act as a vehicle for the disease transmission apparently were unclear to them. For instance, food handlers did not know that handling money can introduce cross-contamination risks to food (Table 7.2). The survival of pathogens on money could represent a potential risk of disease transmission and cause foodborne illnesses (Michaels, 2002). Additionally, only 42.1% of food handlers in the Jordanian hospitals knew that handwashing is necessary after using a mobile phone (Osaili et al., 2017). More than two-thirds (61.8%) of the food handlers in the Lebanese hospitals thought that washing hands with water only before handling food would still reduce contamination risk (Bou-Mitri et al., 2018).

Furthermore, less than half of the food handlers (48.5%) in Saudi Arabia hospitals were able to show why it is vital to wash hands after handling raw meat (Alqurashi et al., 2019). In Egypt, food handlers' knowledge of hand hygiene was not explored. But the authors reported a poor understanding of food handlers (37%) of the contribution of improper hygiene practices to food poisoning (Hamed & Mohammed, 2020).

The relevance of hand hygiene practice to prevent disease transmission is seemingly not well understood. Food handlers' awareness of hand hygiene should be such that hands could shed pathogens and act as a vehicle of disease transmission (Djekic et al., 2016) posing higher health risks to vulnerable people (immune-compromised patients, pregnant women, elderly, children) than healthy people. Additional research on food handlers' misconceptions and the efficacy of training or quality of information they receive would facilitate filling their gaps of knowledge through well-designed educational programs.

7.4.1.2 Cross-contamination prevention and sanitation

The score of the food handlers' knowledge on cross-contamination prevention and sanitation aspects was higher than on other surveyed elements in the Jordanian hospitals (76.3%) (Osaili et al., 2017), Jordanian universities (71.9%) (Osaili et al., 2018) and in Al Madinah hospitals in Saudi Arabia (77.9%) (Alqurashi et al., 2019). Similarly, in the UAE, the cross-contamination prevention score was 76%. Still, only half of the respondents knew the correct procedures for cleaning and sanitizing food contact surfaces (Taha et al., 2020). Whereas food handlers in Kuwait (Al-Kandari et al., 2019) and Saudi Arabia (Al-Shabib et al., 2016) scored lower on cross-contamination and sanitation, 68% and 63%, respectively. But the study by

Al-Shabib et al. (2016) did not elaborate on the kind of questions and respective scores.

In another study in Saudi Arabia, 76.1% of the food handlers in the hospitals correctly indicated that raw and cooked food must be separated during food preparation and refrigeration to prevent cross-contamination. Surprisingly, only half (50.3%) could tell the correct answers when asked to define cross-contamination. Furthermore, 58.3% correctly believed that using gloves during food preparation will prevent the contamination of food (Alqurashi et al., 2019). A lower proportion of food handlers in Egypt (36.0%) correctly identified that food handlers might carry foodborne pathogens and contribute to food contamination (Hamad & Mohammed, 2020).

The overall knowledge scores on cross-contamination may imply high awareness among the majority of food handlers in preventing transfer of disease-causing agents. However, this may not be the actual case as food handlers in general possessed insufficient knowledge in particular areas of cross-contamination. To elaborate further, there was a considerable proportion of food handlers who did not know how to store vegetables safely in the same cold storage units for raw meat or the importance of sanitizing shared utensils and contact surfaces for raw meat or poultry and vegetables (Table 7.3). For instance, less than one-third (25%) of food handlers in the Qatar University correctly knew that adequate cleaning of equipment would reduce cross-contamination risk. Only 51% were aware of the possibility of pathogens transmission from insanitary objects or raw foods to prepared or cooked food (Elobeid et al., 2019).

Furthermore, less than half of food handlers did not know that RTE foods and vegetables should be stored on a shelve above the raw meat or chicken (Osaili et al., 2017, 2018) compared to a higher proportion (69%) in Jordanian restaurants (Osaili et al., 2013) and 60% in the UAE (Taha et al., 2020) (Table 7.3). The food handlers in the hospitals in Saudi Arabia also demonstrated limited knowledge on the safe storage of raw meat (30.7%) and fruit and vegetables (26.4%) in the same refrigerator unit (Alqurashi et al., 2019). When asked why frozen meat should be thawed on the lowest rack of a refrigerator that contains salad, 34% of food handlers in Lebanon believed that the lowest shelf has the least cold atmosphere, so it is more useful for the thawing process. Surprisingly, nearly half of them (47%) received training in food safety (Faour-Klingbeil et al., 2015).

Moreover, separate cutting boards and utensils for fresh produce and raw meat were considered an essential control measure for food safety by 69.3% of the food handlers in Saudi Arabia hospitals. Yet, less than half (46.6%) did not know the appropriate way to clean food and nonfood contact surfaces in the kitchen (Alqurashi et al., 2019). Similarly, Osaili et al. (2017, 2018) observed a lack of knowledge on cleaning and disinfection of kitchen utensils among 33.8% and 53.5% of food handlers in universities. Besides, 42.7% of those in the hospitals knew the correct procedure for cleaning and sanitizing food contact surfaces (knife or cutting board). Whereas in Lebanon, two-third of food handlers considered that the use of disinfection is the appropriate way to clean knives after use with raw meat (Faour-Klingbeil et al., 2015).

In Kuwait, 89.6% of the food handlers knew the importance of using a separate cutting board for raw meat/poultry and vegetables, but fewer (65.9%) were aware of the correct cleaning and sanitizing procedure food contact surfaces (Table 7.3).

The vast majority (95%) in the Lebanese restaurants knew that raw and cooked food should be separated, but one-third of them believed that this is mainly to avoid retaining the flavor/smell of cooked foods from the raw meat or vice versa. Theses misconceptions indicate a critical lack of information and knowledge of cross-contamination routes and source of microbial hazards. Indeed, the authors reported that less than half of respondents (49%) identified the correct answer on the origin of bacterial food contamination (Faour-Klingbeil et al., 2015).

In the Lebanese hospitals, the majority of food handlers (91.7%) knew that incorrect application of cleaning and sanitization procedures on equipment could increase the foodborne illnesses risk. It was known that wearing gloves while handling food would reduce the risk of transmitting infection (66.1%) (Bou-Mitri et al., 2018). Also in the UAE, a small proportion of food handlers, 5%, 21.5%, and 24% considered washing a contaminated knife with cold water, boiled water, and water with soap, respectively, before using for cooked food as appropriate practice (Table 7.3).

In some of the selected studies, questions on the importance of wearing gloves and masks to protect food were addressed under cross-contamination aspect (Bou-Mitri et al., 2018; Kaabi et al., 2010; Osaili et al., 2017, 2018; Taha et al., 2020). There, a high proportion of food handlers recognized that gloves reduce the risk of foodborne illnesses (73%–94.5%) with a lesser proportion of correct answers on wearing masks, 21.5%–58.3% (Table 7.3). Nevertheless, these results do not represent food handlers' proper use of gloves, that is, changing gloves when they turn dirty or damaged. Inappropriate use of gloves could contribute to pathogens transmission to food (Rönnqvist et al., 2014) and might be counterproductive because workers might wash their hands less frequently when gloved (Lynch, Phillips, Elledge, Hanumanthaiah, & Boatright, 2005).

In general, the proportion of correct answers on issues routinely followed or required in the foodservice sector, that is, wearing a hair net, putting on gloves before touching food, wearing a clean uniform, was high (Osaili et al., 2017, 2018; Taha et al., 2020). Thus it has apparently contributed to leveraging the overall score on the cross-contamination aspect in the studies where questions on the importance of wearing gloves and protective clothing fell under the cross-contamination theme. While the same questions were in some studies addressed under personal hygiene aspects (Al-Kandari et al.,

2019; Osaili et al., 2013), in others, cross-contamination aspect was limited to only one question (Alqurashi et al., 2019; Al-Shabib et al., 2016; Bou-Mitri et al., 2018; Sharif et al., 2013).

There is a concerning number of surveyed food handlers who were unaware of specific cross-contamination prevention and sanitation measures despite being trained on food safety. These could unintentionally contribute to food-poisoning incidences. Cross-contamination prevention and sanitation are fundamental preventive controls to protect food from the unintentional transfer of pathogens from contaminated objects, food, and personnel. It is well documented that inadequate cleaning and cross-contamination prevention practices are significantly associated with high levels of hygiene indicators (Faour-Klingbeil, Kuri, & Todd, 2016). Furthermore, inadequate cleaning of cutting boards after use with raw meat and poultry can result in harborage of pathogenic microorganisms on the surface (Doménech-Sánchez, Laso, Pérez, & Berrocal, 2011; Faour-Klingbeil et al., 2016). Such event is likely to contribute to transmitting disease causative agents such as *Campylobacter jejuni* and *Salmonella* (De Boer & Hahné, 1990) even when one single bacteria adhered to the surface (Ravishankar et al., 2010; Soares et al., 2012). Therefore sanitation of food contact surfaces is essential to reduce the chances of pathogens survival and transfer into the food served to consumers.

7.4.1.3 Temperature control and storage of food

Controlling food temperature was generally not well understood by food handlers in all the studied countries. The overall scores were lower than those obtained on personal hygiene questions or foodborne disease pathogens. Almost half (57.5%) of the Lebanese food handlers in restaurants did neither know the danger zone nor the temperature range that is considered optimum for bacterial multiplication. More than two-thirds of trained food handlers (71%) reported they knew about the danger zone. However, when asked to indicate the range, 69% were unable to give correct answers compared to one-third (31%) who answered correctly (Faour-Klingbeil et al., 2015). In Qatar University, only 28% knew the temperature danger zone for food. It is noteworthy that 98% reported having already received food safety training (Elobeid et al., 2019). Similarly, although a great majority was trained on food safety (94%), Al-Shabib et al. (2016) found that food handlers in Saudi Arabia (65.2%) had the lowest score on temperature and time control (44.8%).

By the same token, temperature control was the least known element in food safety by food handlers in the Jordanian restaurants and universities with a percentage of total correct answers of 52.4% and 53.5%, respectively, indicating limited knowledge on the crucial role of temperature in controlling foodborne pathogens in food (Osaili et al., 2013, 2018). Alqurashi et al.

(2019) found that most staff (72.4%) knew the recommended temperature for freezers but obtained a low score (49.7%) for the food handlers' knowledge on the adequate temperature conditions to prevent microbial growth in food.

Overall, the recommended operating temperature for refrigerators and freezers seemed to be better understood by food handlers than temperature control of food and the risks of not achieving or maintaining safe food temperature during preparation, cooking, holding, or storing. Less than half (48%) of food handlers in the Lebanese restaurants were aware of the safe temperature for reheating food. Besides, only 11% identified the correct answer to the hot holding temperature question, although 44% of them were trained (Faour-Klingbeil et al., 2015). This raises doubts about the viability of the training and its frequency and concerns over the lack of temperature control of high-risk foods during preparation, storage, and distribution (Faour-Klingbeil et al., 2015). Al-Kandari et al. (2019) showed that 62.7% of food handlers did not know the importance of the time and temperature control required for preventing the microbial growth in foods and 66% was aware of the correct approach to thaw frozen meat (i.e., in the refrigerator) compared to 54% in the UAE (Taha et al., 2020). In the UAE, the food handlers had insufficient knowledge of the proper cooking, hot holding, and reheating food temperatures, 57.7%, 53.9%, and 56.5%, respectively (Taha et al., 2020). Moreover, less than half (40%) in Egypt knew keeping food leftovers for more than 6 h at room temperature would increase the risk of food poisoning (Hamad & Mohammed, 2020). A lower proportion in Jordan, 19.6% and 31.2%, were aware of the minimum safe temperature for reheating food and cooking poultry, respectively (Table 7.4). Less than half were able to tell the right operating temperatures recommended for refrigerators and freezers (Osaili et al., 2013).

Most concerning, only 33.5% and 45.0% of food handlers in the hospitals in Jordan knew the operation temperatures of refrigerators and freezers, respectively (Table 7.4) compared to 77.5% and 55.0% of food handlers in the Lebanese restaurants, respectively (Faour-Klingbeil et al., 2015). The authors reported that almost one-third (35.5%) knew the safe internal temperature for cooked chicken and one-third (31%) identified the safe hot holding temperature correctly (Table 7.4) (Osaili et al., 2017). In contrast, food handlers in the military hospitals in Jordan were much more knowledgeable in this area (90%). They knew they should not thaw frozen meat and broiler for overnight at room temperature. Additionally, 91.5%–98.5% demonstrated the knowledge of the adequate temperature storage conditions of food. In the Lebanese hospitals, 72.0% knew the recommended refrigerator temperatures in addition to 66.5% and 78.3% who knew the correct temperature for hot holding and reheating food, respectively. In comparison, 58.7% were aware that food preparation in advance could contribute to food poisoning (Bou-Mitri et al., 2018).

The lack of knowledge of foodservice staff on temperature control measures is a critical issue in food safety. Temperature control and monitoring are vital to ensure food sanitation, and inadequate practices in this area are the top reasons for foodborne illnesses resulting from temperature abuse that allows survival and exponential growth of foodborne pathogens and toxin production in foods (Todd, Greig, Bartleson, & Michaels, 2008).

7.4.1.4 Knowledge of foodborne pathogens and related symptoms and illnesses

Poor knowledge of foodborne pathogens was common among food handlers in different countries. Osaili et al. (2013) reported that, except for *Salmonella*, head chefs and catering managers showed poor knowledge about foodborne pathogens and their association with specific foods. In the Jordanian hospitals, a high proportion of food handlers were trained on food safety compared to those working in the restaurants. The results were also unsatisfactory; the food handlers had the lowest score on foodborne pathogens and related symptoms and illnesses (45.3%) compared to their scores on other food safety areas. About 37% and 13% reported that they heard about *Salmonella* and Hepatitis A virus. Less than 10% of the respondents heard about *Listeria monocytogenes*, *S. aureus*, *Bacillus cereus*, *Escherichia coli* O157:H7, and *Shigella*, and were not able to identify common foods associated with these pathogens (Osaili et al., 2017).

In Saudi Arabia, 52.9% knew about *S. aureus* as a food pathogen, and 65.75% were aware of the definition of foodborne illness (Al-Shabib et al., 2016). Like food handlers in the Jordanian hospitals, less than 10% of the Jordanian universities' respondents knew about *S. aureus*, *L. monocytogenes*, *Shigella*, and *B. cereus* but could not mention their food sources. Less than half of them (42%) stated that they heard about *Salmonella*. In comparison, very low percentages (19% and 12.5%) heard about Hepatitis A virus and *E. coli* O157:H7, and they were able to identify one common food source of these pathogens.

Although the majority of the food handlers in the Lebanese hospitals attended a course on food safety, a high proportion did not identify the foodborne pathogens and their sources, that is, Hepatitis A (92.9%), Botulism (92.1%), or brucellosis (89.1%). Only 28% of food handlers in the Lebanese hospitals named correctly the food associated with salmonellosis and 22.0% with cholera (Bou-Mitri et al., 2018). Likewise, when asked about the most common bacteria that cause foodborne diseases, less than half of the food handlers in Saudis hospitals (44.2%) knew about *Salmonella*, *B. cereus*, and *E. coli*, and less than half in Kuwait recognized food pathogens (51%) (Alqurashi et al., 2019). Similarly, in Kuwait, respondents' least knowledge was about foodborne pathogens (51.3%). Only 53.7% knew about *Salmonella*, 40.8% about *S. aureus*, 41.5% about *Shigella*, and 69.4% about Hepatitis A virus and that these pathogens are diseases causing (Al-Kandari et al., 2019).

In Qatar University, 34% recognized *Salmonella* as a foodborne pathogen (Elobeid et al., 2019). On the contrary, Kaabi et al. (2010) reported a higher proportion of respondents in a Qatari hospital familiar with *Salmonella* (95.3%). Yet, very few were able to identify Hepatitis A (20.9%) and *Vibrio cholera* (30.2%) as food pathogens. Food handlers' familiarity with *Salmonella* over other pathogens is likely since *Salmonella* is a well-known causative agent of frequently reported cases of food poisoning in the region.

On the other hand, questions on food-poisoning symptoms recorded a high percentage of correct answers in most studies. More than 90% of food handlers in Jordan's hospitals knew that abdominal pain, diarrhea, vomiting, and nausea are symptoms of foodborne illnesses (Osaili et al., 2017). Along the same line, food handlers in the restaurants (81.7%) and the universities (74.3%) in Jordan identified the most common symptoms of foodborne illnesses (Osaili et al., 2013, 2018). The percentage of correct answers was lower in the UAE and Saudi Arabia with approximately half of the respondents and 52.8% not knowing the food poisoning symptoms, respectively (Alqurashi et al., 2019; Taha et al., 2020); however, 77.9% of food handlers in the Saudi study identified the definition of food poisoning (Alqurashi et al., 2019) correctly.

When asked if contaminated food can be distinguished from safe food, a low proportion (11.5%) of the respondents in the Jordanian hospitals knew that food contamination couldn't be identified by appearance, smell, or taste (Osaili et al., 2017) compared to 52.5% in the UAE (Taha et al., 2020). In comparison, 77.5% of food handlers in the Lebanese restaurants failed to distinguish between food spoilage and food contaminated with pathogens that lead to illnesses (Faour-Klingbeil et al., 2015).

These findings show that inadequate knowledge of foodborne pathogens is common across the studied countries. There is an evident deficiency in learning on the microbial hazards, their sources, factors that contribute to their presence in food, and ways to control and prevent them. The high scores on personal hygiene are not reassuring as indicators of proper food handling. Personal hygiene and health seemed to have been taught or conveyed as instructions to food handlers in isolation from the scientific aspects of the risk involved with unhygienic practices and food mishandling. *S. aureus* is the leading cause of foodborne intoxications worldwide (Kadariya, Smith, & Thapaliya, 2014); understanding this hazard's source would help promote compliance with proper practices. To the same degree, learning about foodborne pathogens, in general, is of significant relevance to manage food safety risks. For instance, *Clostridium perfringens*, *C. jejuni*, and *Shigella* are considered the leading cause of bacterial foodborne diseases (Scallan et al., 2011). The familiarity of food handlers with their characteristics is essential to learn the relevance of the necessary food safety measures during their functions, for example, preparation, cooking, cooling, holding, and storing. There is no effective way to reinforce proper practices on food premises without conveying the science behind the taught messages in an easy-to-understand manner.

7.4.2 Factors affecting food safety knowledge

7.4.2.1 Demographic factors

As few studies investigated the effects of demographic factors on food safety knowledge and KAP, our discussion will address the demographic impacts on food handlers' knowledge and practices.

In Jordan, the KAP scores of food handlers were affected by education level. In the military hospitals, those with college degrees (90.7%) and higher university education (92.1%) scored higher than food handlers who attained an elementary level (79.7%) and secondary education (86.2%) (Sharif et al., 2013). Similarly, food handlers with high education level in the Jordanians universities and the FSEs in the UAE recorded higher food safety knowledge scores than others (Osaili et al., 2017; Taha et al., 2020). Furthermore, in evaluating the effect of person in charge (PIC) intervention on knowledge and practice of food handlers in Dubai, the educational level and former training on food safety were factors that positively enhanced the ability of the PIC to demonstrate knowledge and safer practices (Abushelaibi et al., 2015).

Besides education, age, and income level, Osaili et al. (2018) and Abushelaibi et al. (2015) observed an impact of experience on food handlers' knowledge in food safety. Similarly, Bou-Mitri et al. (2018) reported that the overall KAP scores were significantly higher among those who had been working for more than 21 years in government hospitals (79%) than those who served between 11 and 20 years (70.1%). Also in Lebanon, the overall score on food safety knowledge was higher for food handlers with 10 years of experience or more in the foodservice industry (64.4 ± 18.7, on a 100-point scale) than for those with fewer years of experience (51.1 ± 20.9, on a 100-point scale), also for respondents in higher positions than cook or section chef (Faour-Klingbeil et al., 2015).

While there were no differences in food safety knowledge among the different age groups in the UAE, Taha et al. (2020) reported that food handlers >40 years demonstrated better food safety knowledge (71%) than those <40 years (69%). Furthermore, work experience ≥ 12 years significantly enhanced their knowledge (71%) compared to those with 6–11 years of experience (69%) and <6 years of experience (69%). In contrast, the food handlers' knowledge in the Jordanian hospitals and restaurants was not significantly associated with their levels of experience, age, and income (Osaili et al., 2013, 2017).

In general, a correlation between two variables does not imply causation; this is evident from the contradictory findings on the effect of demographics factors, for example, age, experience, gender, and education, on food handlers' knowledge (Abdul-Mutalib et al., 2012; Acikel et al., 2008; Bou-Mitri et al., 2018; Faour-Klingbeil et al., 2015; Hossen et al., 2020; Ncube, Kanda, Chijokwe, Mabaya, & Nyamugure, 2020; Osaili et al., 2013, 2017). Eventually, when the explanatory factors are not studied, assumptions are made to understand why the age, experience, or position of food handlers brought about a difference in their food safety knowledge. For instance, Osaili et al. (2018) assumed that the longer the food handlers' work experience is the better their food safety knowledge due to better chances for training opportunities. They suggested that those with higher income have had probably better access to higher education and work experience, which explains their improved food safety knowledge compared to those with lower income.

In the Jordanian study, the association of food handlers' experience with their knowledge was insignificant, at the same time, and a great majority of them had not previously been trained on food safety. In Saudi Arabia, 46.6% of food handlers were Saudis and showed a better food safety knowledge than non-Saudis (24.5%) explained by the fact that Saudis had a higher education level than non-Saudi staff (Alqurashi et al., 2019). Unlike other Arab countries of the Middle East, countries of the Gulf Cooperation Council (GCC) region are highly dependent on migrant labor. The GCC area is known to host the highest number of expatriate workforce in the world for contributing to various sectors. The majority of food handlers in GCC countries have a low socioeconomic status from countries with a high illiteracy rate and poor sanitation conditions. Hence, they often have little information about food safety risks (Al-Kandari et al., 2019).

Attribution of changes in food safety knowledge to demographic effects is flawed when confounding factors remain unexplored. Osaili et al. (2017) found that food handlers in private hospitals had significantly higher food knowledge than those working in government hospitals, primarily because private hospitals invest more in food safety training than public hospitals in Jordan. In public hospitals, most foodservice facilities are outsourced to companies that take food safety training a vital issue. Whereas in Lebanon, the food safety management system (FSMS) in the public hospitals were reportedly stringent (Bou-Mitri et al., 2018). In public hospitals, food handlers were more trained and had more extended work experience than those in private hospitals. Hence, the overall KAP was significantly higher among respondents, who served for more than 21 years in government hospitals (Bou-Mitri et al., 2018). The long experience of food workers together with the institutional setup and education resources were the factors that significantly contributed to enhancing their knowledge in food safety.

Furthermore, Faour-Klingbeil et al. (2015) reported significantly higher food safety knowledge scores among food handlers employed by corporate-managed restaurants than those working in sole-proprietor food businesses.

Through the observational assessment of food safety practices, Faour-Klingbeil et al. (2020) found higher adherence levels of food handlers to personal hygiene and safe practices in the corporate-managed restaurants than in the sole-proprietor food businesses. The corporate restaurant businesses provided supportive environment, that is, adequate spaces for food preparation, equipment provisions, staff training on food safety), and a food safety management that oversees the hygiene standards (Faour-Klingbeil et al., 2015).

Along the same lines, the type of FSEs in Qatar was an underlying factor to adherence to food safety practices; compared to fast-food restaurants, food safety managers in fine dining restaurants and hotels chains showed a higher compliance level with safe food handling, implemented and documented food safety management procedures, and enrolled in food safety training (Asim et al., 2019).

Thus the educational background combined with work opportunities and the environment determines the association level of demographics with food safety knowledge. With extended years of work in the food sector, the chances are that food-handling staff may learn more about food safety, provided they have access to adequate resources and opportunities for working under a strong food safety culture. The lack of resources and management commitment to food safety may limit food handlers' accessibility to food safety knowledge and put what they learn into practice. There is already a growing body of evidence on the significant role FSE's management can play in food safety by embracing a food safety culture in their work environment. Management commitment to food safety is a priority to create an enabling environment through frequent communications, support, resources, and continuous updates and refresher courses for all staff to keep the food safety procedures in mind even in the peak hours of food operations. These will be addressed in the coming sections.

7.4.3 Effectiveness of food safety training on food handlers' knowledge

Training is an effective tool for ensuring adequate practices (Hanashiro, Morita, Matté, Matté, & Torres, 2005) through improved knowledge (Choudhury, Mahanta, Goswami, & Mazumder, 2011; McIntyre et al., 2013), while lack of training has been associated with increased frequency in human error (Clayton & Griffith, 2004).

According to existing data, the trained food handlers demonstrated better food safety knowledge than the untrained. In Jordanian restaurants, those who were enrolled in a food safety training course showed higher food safety knowledge level (48.3 out of 67 points) compared with the score of untrained food workers (46.8) (Osaili et al., 2013). Also, the knowledge scores of trained food handlers in the Lebanese hospitals and restaurants, 60.8% and

62.5%, were significantly higher than untrained food handlers, 46.2% and 52.2%, respectively (Bou-Mitri et al., 2018; Faour-Klingbeil et al., 2015).

Similarly, in the UAE, the trained respondents had a significantly higher overall knowledge score (72%) than the untrained (67%) (Taha et al., 2020). However, Osaili et al. (2017) did not find a remarkable difference in scores between untrained (66%) and trained food handlers (69%). In the Medina (KSA) hospital study, 68.1% of all trained staff achieved a food safety knowledge score of 52.8% compared to 18.4% of the untrained counterparts. About two-thirds (63.8%) of the trained respondents were familiar with the Hazard Analysis Critical Control Points system (HACCP) as a preventive food safety system, which indicate an emphasis on food safety training in the hospitals in Al Madinah (Alqurashi et al., 2019). Besides knowledge, food handlers' attitudes toward food safety and their compliance with personal hygiene, safe food handling and storage have improved following participation in an educational program on food safety (Elsherbiny, Sobhy, Fiala, and Md, 2019)

There is no doubt that training enhances knowledge. But there is plenty of evidence that training alone does not necessarily fill gaps in knowledge or improve practices. As shown in the earlier sections 7.4.1.2, 7.4.1.3, 7.4.1.4, food handlers, including the trained, had insufficient knowledge in critical areas of food safety (i.e., temperature control, cross-contamination, food pathogens of public health concerns). The proportion of trained food handlers was notably low in the Jordanian restaurants (15%) and universities (38%), in Kuwaiti restaurants (58%), Palestinian restaurants (37%), and Lebanese restaurants (43%) compared to Qatari FSEs (68%) and 90%, 68%, and 61% in the hospitals in Lebanon, Saudi Arabia, and Jordan, respectively. The data show an interesting trend where an emphasis on staff training in food safety seems much more prevalent in the healthcare sector than the food sector.

The existing data substantiate the effect of training on employees' overall knowledge improvement but had little impact on their understanding of specific and fundamental food safety areas, that is, cross-contamination, sanitation, microbial hazards, and optimum growing conditions. Faour-Klingbeil et al. (2015) observed a higher level of knowledge on temperature control and cross-contamination prevention among trained than untrained food handlers. Nonetheless, respondents could not remember what they had acquired in previous training when asked to indicate the safe temperature for food storage and the danger zone. The reason is very likely a lack of continuous education and refresher training. Food handlers' knowledge gradually decreases over time, indicating a need for regular retraining sessions (McIntyre et al., 2013). Continuous communication and proper ongoing training on the concept of temperature control and monitoring functions are essential for the safety of food and to improve knowledge and foster a culture of food safety.

The common feature of food safety training is that they are based on a standard and framed modular program, narrow in focus, and developed to increase trainees' knowledge of various food safety areas. Such programs that solely focus on theories using facts and knowledge may not be enough to influence behaviors (Hye-Ja, Jaung-Sook, & Tong-Kyung, 2003). Training should address misconceptions and provide the reasoning and rationale and scientific foundation for the food safety requirements to translate the facts into work practices. Otherwise, desirable behavioral changes would be hardly realized without continuous on-premises supervision and routine inspections.

Recent research has shown that knowledge-based training programs were not directly translated into safe food handling, hence investigating other influential factors beyond knowledge is essential to understand food handlers' intentions and behaviors. The best practice for ensuring effective training and follow-through was through continuous food safety training programs that incorporate both knowledge and behavior-based training (Yu, Neal, Dawson, & Madera, 2017).

Behavior-based training is based on identifying and accounting for factors that influence food handlers' behavior, such as workers' allergies, dry skin, dedication to the job, pride in work, or fear of negative consequences, and work environment, that is, time pressure, understaffing, peak service times, and management–coworker relationship (Clayton, Clegg Smith, Neff, Pollack, & Ensminger, 2015; Yu et al., 2017). Hence, it is increasingly considered a more effective strategy than knowledge-based training to retain knowledge and improve employee food safety behavior.

7.4.4 Attitudes toward food safety

Much of the KAP studies are established on understanding the attitude–behavior relationship within the framework of the "Theory of Reasoned Action." According to the theory, the immediate antecedent of any behavior is the intention to perform the behavior in question. The stronger a person's intention, the more the person is likely to try, and hence the greater the likelihood that the behavior will be performed (Ajzen & Madden, 1986). It specifies that attitude is one of the personal factors that determine behavior and refers to the degree to which a person has a favorable or unfavorable evaluation of the behavior in question (Ajzen and Madden, 1986). With the accumulated evidence in support of this theory, food handlers' positive attitudes can mediate their knowledge into appropriate practices in the context of food safety. In other words, food handlers with adequate knowledge of food safety are expected to translate them into practices if they have a strong and favorable attitude.

Studies on food handlers' attitudes and practices are limited in the Arab countries and differ in their approaches. While attitudes scores are measured on a Likert scale (Al-Kandari et al., 2019; Elobeid et al., 2019;

Faour-Klingbeil et al., 2015; Sharif et al., 2013), they were represented as total points on "correct answers" to a set of statements in other studies (Al-Shabib et al., 2016; Bou-Mitri et al., 2018).

The overall attitudes of food handlers tended to be positive toward food safety but to lesser degrees toward specific critical food safety issues. In Kuwait, the food handlers recorded a mean score of 69.1 ± 10.0 (94%) on their food safety attitudes. But only 65% strongly agreed that food safety knowledge is important compared to 98.9% reported by Al-Shabib et al. (2016). Also, 60% of the food handlers in Kuwait showed a strong favor of regular training on personal hygiene and learning on food safety compared to 95.5% in Jordan hospitals (Osaili et al., 2017) and 98.9% in Saudi Arabia (Al-Shabib et al., 2016). The score of food handlers' attitude was higher in Lebanon, 86.3 ± 13.2 over 100 possible points. All food handlers showed strong agreement that they serve safe food to consumers, and that food safety and hygiene training are essential to their work (Faour-Klingbeil et al., 2015).

Compared to a great majority of food handlers in the Lebanese hospitals (94.1%) (Bou-Mitri et al., 2018) and in Saudi Arabia (95.4%) (Al-Shabib et al., 2016), 70% of food handlers in Kuwait and 82.8% in Saudi Arabia agreed with the measures to exclude food handlers with skin injuries, wounds, or cut from handling food (Al-Kandari et al., 2019; Al-Shabib et al., 2016). However, only half of the Lebanese restaurants (57%) agreed that they should not touch and work with food when they have cuts and abrasions on fingers, compared to 37% who disagreed due to staff shortages and work pressures. Unless covered adequately with waterproof bandages, wounds could be infected, and hands become vectors of foodborne pathogens *such as S. aureus* (Faour-Klingbeil et al., 2015).

Also, 72.9% of food handlers in Kuwait showed a strong positive attitude toward wearing personal protective clothing to reduce the risk of food contamination recording on a scale of 1 (strongly disagree) to 5 (strongly agree) a mean score of 4.64 ± 0.678 (Al-Kandari et al., 2019). Nonetheless, they scored substantially lower than the food handlers in the Lebanese restaurants (96.2%) and Qatar University (94.4%) who strongly agreed on the use of appropriate clothing to protect food from potential contamination (Elobeid et al., 2019; Faour-Klingbeil et al., 2015).

Almost all food handlers agreed with separating cooked food from raw food ingredients to prevent cross-contamination risks (Al-Kandari et al., 2019; Al-Shabib et al., 2016; Bou-Mitri et al., 2018; Faour-Klingbeil et al., 2015; Sharif et al., 2013) compared to 44% of food handlers in Egypt (Hamed & Mohammed, 2020). As to how far food handlers agree with controlling food storage temperatures, 64.4% and 60.9% of food handlers in Saudi Arabia agreed with thawing food in the refrigerator and storing leftovers of cooked meals within 2 h at cold temperature are to keep food safe (Al-Shabib et al., 2016) compared to 22.8% and 16.7% in Lebanon, respectively (Faour-Klingbeil et al., 2015). Comparatively, 71.6% in Kuwait demonstrated a favorable agreement on the importance of knowing the "danger zone," to prevent microbial multiplication in perishable foods. Still, only 59.2% believed in the importance of regularly monitoring the cooling and freezing appliances' temperature, compared to a 97.6% in Lebanese hospitals (Al-Kandari et al., 2019; Bou-Mitri et al., 2018). While in Qatar University, the food handlers scored low (69.5%) on their positive attitudes toward safe food handling (Elobeid et al., 2019).

Data from hospitals showed that attitudes' scores were statistically higher among food handlers with long working experience (Bou-Mitri et al., 2018; Sharif et al., 2013), which implies that long-term engagement and work experience in the food sector improve attitudes toward food safety. Work environments have been shown to affect the way food handlers perceive necessary practices in food safety. For instance, food handlers in the corporate-managed restaurants strongly agreed with the management support in promoting safe food handling behaviors than those working in the sole-proprietor businesses. Accordingly, 89.7% of food handlers in corporate-managed food businesses agreed on the importance of monitoring food temperatures compared to 50% in sole-proprietor-managed food outlets. In the latter, food handlers relied on feeling the food temperature (empirically acquired practice) (Faour-Klingbeil et al., 2015).

Despite the effective role of food safety knowledge in enhancing attitudes toward food safety, food handlers may not intend to put these attitudes into practice when a supportive environment, the commitment of management or business owner to food safety, and adequate training programs are lacking (Faour-Klingbeil et al., 2015; Yiannas, 2009). This topic will be discussed within the context of the barriers to food safety practices in the forthcoming section.

7.4.5 Self-reported and observed food safety practices

The high compliance level with personal hygiene was reported in all the studies (Al-Kandari et al., 2019; Al-Khatib & Al-Mitwalli, 2009; Alqurashi et al., 2019; Al-Shabib et al., 2016; Bou-Mitri et al., 2018; Elobeid et al., 2019; Faour-Klingbeil et al., 2015; Kaabi et al., 2010). A high rate of compliance was reported in Saudi Arabia (96%); most of the handlers (95.4%) practiced handwashing after smoking, coughing, and sneezing (Al-Shabib et al., 2016). Likewise, in Palestine, almost all food handlers reported practicing handwashing before food handling, and in the Qatari hospitals, 97%–100% reported proper hygienic practices (Kaabi et al., 2010). In contrast, in Qatar University, the compliance rate ranged from 89.7% to 98.2% (Elobeid et al., 2019). In the latter, besides other studies, self-reported practices focused solely on personal hygiene practices (Alqurashi et al., 2019; Al-Shabib et al., 2016; Elobeid et al., 2019).

In contrast, self-reported practices in Egypt were inadequate as 18.6% wore gloves when touching cooked food, 17.8% washed their hands before food preparation, 20.1% wash their hands after visiting the toilets, and only 21.8% separated raw meat from cooked food (Hamed & Mohammed, 2020).

Concerning temperature control of food and sanitation practices, the overall scores of self-reported practices on food safety in Lebanon were significantly higher in corporate-managed restaurants and among trained food handlers than the overall scores of food handlers in sole-proprietor restaurants and untrained group (Faour-Klingbeil et al., 2015). More than two-thirds of surveyed food handlers (67.6%) did not measure the temperature of incoming cold or frozen high-risk food items. Furthermore, 75.3% and 70.8% never measured foods' temperature during cooling and reheating, and cooking, respectively (Faour-Klingbeil et al., 2015).

In Kuwait, food handlers reported good personal hygiene practices (82.3%) such as washing hands before and after handling foods, wearing protective clothing, and keeping work clothes and surfaces clean. Nonetheless, their self-reported practices concerning cross-contamination prevention and temperature control were poor and consistent with their attitudes; more than half (51.7%) reported touching and handling RTE meals without the use of gloves. Despite the positive attitude of 71.6% toward the importance of maintaining safe temperature conditions for food, 26%–38% did not perform or monitor food temperatures (Al-Kandari et al., 2019). Even though the overall KAP score was satisfactory, it was inadequate in cross-contamination and temperature control (Al-Kandari et al., 2019).

RTE-prepared foods held at improper temperatures during preparation and holding have caused serious outbreaks (Bintsis, 2017; CDC, 2019; CFS, 2020; Todd et al., 2007). From the 17,157 investigated outbreaks in 1993–98, temperature misuse was among the main contributing factors and the primary cause for 32.5% of the cases. Factors such as inadequate refrigeration and insufficient cooking, reheating, or hot holding accounted for a similar percentage (Tirado & Schmidt, 2001).

In the Lebanese hospitals, the majority of the food handlers followed proper handwashing on all necessary occasions. While 94.1% showed positive attitudes toward separating raw food ingredients from cooked food meals, only 77.6% used separate kitchen utensils to prepare raw and cooked food (Bou-Mitri et al., 2018). Moreover, 90% of food handlers in the Jordanian military hospitals separated raw from cooked food during preparation. A great majority (91%) conducted regular checks of the refrigerator temperature (Sharif et al., 2013).

The thorough review of the selected studies uncovered prevalent mishandling practices and shortcomings in keeping food at a proper temperature and safe from cross-contamination. Nevertheless, similar shortfalls could be captured in other areas of practice in food safety. Self-reported practices are subject to employees' beliefs and opinions who may overestimate their actual behavior bias.

Studies that assessed the actual food safety practices offered more reliable data than self-reported surveys (Faour-Klingbeil et al., 2020; McFarland, Checinska Sielaff, Rasco, & Smith, 2019; Park, Kwak, & Chang, 2010). The observational assessment of food safety practices in Lebanon generated substantial evidence on the actual food handling behaviors (Faour-Klingbeil et al., 2020). In their comparison between real-time observed food safety practices and the self-reported data collected from the same surveyed restaurants on the same day of the interviews and the observational survey (Faour-Klingbeil et al., 2015), the authors recorded inconsistency and disparity in practices across the different indicators (i.e., personal hygiene and temperature control). The authors also found discrepancies between the actual practices and self-reported practices concerning the use of protective clothing and gloves, separation of cutting boards for raw meat and vegetables, the application of disinfection, and storing of fresh vegetables in protected areas. Similar inconsistencies in food safety managers' practices were reported by Asim et al. (2019) and Al-Khatib & Al-Mitwalli (2009). In the latter, 76.5% reported proper personal hygiene and handwashing with water and soap despite lacking handwashing liquid dispensers and supplies, protective clothing, gloves, and hairnets.

7.5 The barriers to a food safety culture

Studies have shown that promoting food safety knowledge through training is necessary but not enough to foster safer practices due to various constraints (Clayton & Griffith, 2004; Faour-Klingbeil et al., 2015; Roberts et al., 2008; Soares et al., 2012; Ungku Fatimah, Strohbehn, & Arendt, 2014). According to the Theory of Planned Behavior (TPB), the performance of a behavior is determined by different motivational factors that work together to influence individuals' behavioral intention (Ajzen, 1991). Besides attitude, they include the subjective norm, a social factor, that refers to the perceived social pressure to perform or not to perform a particular behavior, and perceived behavioral control (perceived availability of opportunities and resources required to perform the behavior contributing to the perceived ease or difficulty in its performance) (Ajzen & Madden, 1986; Ajzen, 1991).

The TPB holds that the more favorable the intentions and subjective norms, the greater the perceived control, the more likely individuals' intention is put into action. Hence, the motivating working environment and employee satisfaction, availability of management's support, and resources were essential elements for enacting what has been learned to ensure safe practices on food premises.

Perceived barriers for safe food handling practices were not studied in the Arab countries, except in two studies by Faour-Klingbeil et al. (2015) and Osaili et al. (2018). In Jordan, the principal barriers for not implementing a preventive food safety systems (HACCP) were lack of financial resources, limited knowledge, and unfamiliarity with the good manufacturing practices and standard sanitation operating procedures. The latter are essential prerequisites for a HACCP system. These constraints explain the small percentage (21%) of the surveyed hospitals in Jordan that had a HACCP system and the low proportion (40%) of food handlers who heard about it (Osaili et al., 2018).

Faour-Klingbeil et al. (2015; 2020) found that food-handling behavior is not within the person's sole control. Even when food handlers carried positive food safety attitudes, they did not intend to put it into practice due to other factors than training. Various interfering factors were limiting their behaviors, such as misperceptions of safe and correct practices, misunderstanding of concepts, the workplace environment, and management support.

In other words, food safety is dependent on human behavior that is affected by complex external factors, that is, cultural and social background, resources and space, skills, and national regulatory requirements and law enforcement. These findings paralleled what behaviorists considered additional factors that can influence one or more of the KAP variables, for example, self-esteem, self-efficacy, and misconception (Ajzen, 2002). In Palestine, limited supplies and workspaces in restaurants were common and encouraged unhygienic practices, that is, smoking in food preparation areas and improper handwashing (Al-Khatib & Al-Mitwalli, 2009). Faour-Klingbeil et al. (2020) also found working space on food premises in sole-proprietor restaurants was generally small, increasing the risks of cross-contamination. Furthermore, the limited financial resources were significant barriers for training, improving the working environment and hygiene standards, maintaining the facility and equipment in proper conditions to minimize the risk of contamination, and providing the necessary tools to implement a food safety system. Lack of thermometers for monitoring food and storage temperature and work pressures were found to reduce motivation to comply with the food safety requirements despite positive attitudes and intentions to adhere to safe practices.

There are other factors besides time and resources that influence food safety practices (Phillip & Anita, 2010). The management of food businesses is increasingly viewed as having a crucial role in instilling a food safety culture that fosters safe food handling. The food safety culture has gained researchers' heightened attention in the past years to understand the role of organizational factors in changing food safety behaviors (Mitchell et al., 2007; Pragle, Harding, & Mack, 2007). Griffith et al. (2010) defined food safety culture as the aggregation of the prevailing, relatively constant, learned, shared attitudes, values, and beliefs. Together they contribute to the hygiene behaviors used within a particular food handling environment that it is assessed as employees' perceptions toward the management system and style, leadership, communication, sharing of knowledge and information, accountability, risk perception, and work environment.

Internationally, there is a clear transition toward behavioral-based approaches in training and devising solutions to improve food safety practices and compliance level. The adoption of a food safety culture is increasingly on the agenda of international organization and regulatory agencies with the primary purpose to increase awareness and improve the behavior of employees in establishments.

As such, the adoption of food safety culture within the behavior-based FSMS is gaining ground and has been rapidly expanding in the food industry since the Global Food Safety Initiative (GFSI) has released in 2018 a position paper for embedding and maintaining a positive culture of food safety in any business, regardless of its size or focus. This paper defines a food safety culture as the shared values, beliefs, and norms that affect mind-set and behavior toward food safety across and throughout an organization (GFSI, 2018). The GFSI-recognized certification program, such as the BRC Global Standard for Food Safety, has included food safety culture in the new Global Standard for Food Safety. So the international organizations such as Campden BRI (the United Kingdom's largest independent membership-based organization for research and development in the food and drinks industry) introduced their own Culture Excellence Program for the assessment and improvement of organizational culture (Crew, 2019).

Following the GFSI's updates of its benchmarking criteria, the requirements for food safety culture are now being considered and introduced at the EU level as the EU commission revised the Regulation (EC) No 852/2004 to have the concept of food safety culture instituted in legislation. Furthermore, the Codex Alimentarius Commission revised its standard on General Principles of Food Hygiene, which considered the food safety culture concept as a general principle. The requirements pertain to management commitment, food safety communication and training, and employee feedback on food-safety-related issues and performance measurement.

To help food businesses assess their organizational food safety culture, the FSA developed a voluntary Food Safety Culture Diagnostic Toolkit, which will also help inspectors identify aspects of food safety cultures prevailing in food businesses. Furthermore, the Food Standards Australia and New Zealand have developed self-assessment tools to guide the food industry on understanding the elements and principles of the food safety culture concept.

7.6 Conclusions

The following conclusions are drawn from the selected studies:

Studies on food safety KAP of food handlers in the FSEs in the Arab countries are growing slowly since the last decade. Nevertheless, they are considerably scanty and limited to a few countries (i.e., Lebanon, Jordan, UAE, Qatar, Saudi Arabia, Palestine, Egypt).

The food safety knowledge was inadequate at a broad level with limited awareness of the microbial hazards in food, transmission routes of contaminants, conditions that promote microbial growth, and the necessary control measures.

In general, food handlers with more experience possessed a better knowledge of food safety than those with lesser years of experience. However, this may not be a common finding in all the studies.

The proportion of trained food handlers was relatively low in the studied countries, except for those working in hospitals. Furthermore, food handlers' knowledge and self-reported practices suggested limited access to adequate training and food safety information. The existing data underscore the need for continuous training programs and refresher courses that promote safe food handling practices and integrate learning on foodborne diseases and causative agents and identify food hazards and appropriate control measures.

Food handlers showed a positive attitude toward food safety; however, there was no strong favor for monitoring and controlling food temperature, and this was consistent with the self-reported practices.

7.7 Recommendations

Despite its usefulness as a research tool to identify gaps in knowledge, the KAP is limited in capturing actual food safety behaviors because self-reported practices are subject to biases. Noncompliances with recommended safe food practices could result from several factors other than knowledge alone. There is little research on the barriers to safe food practices in the FSEs in the Arab countries. Future studies could address the motivators and disabling factors to compliance with safe practices. Employing observational survey tools to assess actual practices, organizational food safety culture, and constraints perceived by food handlers is instrumental to craft solutions and food safety interventions that will help overcome the hurdles and improve food safety.

The Codex Alimentarius advises that food handlers must have the necessary knowledge and skills to handle food safely and understand their role and responsibility in protecting food from contamination or deterioration. Specifically, supervisors of food operations must be competent and possess the knowledge to assess the potential risks of foodborne diseases and take necessary actions to remedy any deficiencies in food hygiene principles and practice.

However, to promote safe food handling behaviors, the formal and standard food safety training should be evaluated and customized to the local context and work conditions where certain risks are specific to the food facility and perceived under social and cultural influences. Moreover, instead of only increasing knowledge, the training programs should convey current scientific knowledge by highlighting the rationale of the appropriate food handling practices and the risks of noncompliance, while targeting the barriers, misconceptions, and attitudes of food handlers.

Although surveillance data on food outbreaks are limited in the Arab countries, foodborne illnesses are recurrent on the news, and the Arab citizen has the right to access safe food. For this, food handlers should understand their role and responsibilities in ensuring the safety of the food they prepare and serve. Irrespective, food safety solutions at FSEs level should be within a comprehensive strategy at the national level that functions through regulatory enforcement and guidance. The Emirate of Dubai is a leading example from the region. There is a mandatory requirement for any food establishment to have a PIC, that is, the person who has the overall responsibility for running the establishment is accountable and responsible for the proper food operations and for ensuring that food workers adhere to the established policies and procedures for food safety. Dubai Municipality Food Control Department (DIFC) has mandated the PIC training to enable managers to identify deficiencies and practices that could lead to problems and carry out internal inspections of their premises to take adequate corrective actions. At the same time, to support the foodservice sector in complying with the requirements, free education and training resources were made available on DIFC website. Among other international examples, the FSA provides the industry with guide documents, HACCP generic models, information packs to assist small FSEs in improving compliance with food hygiene regulations, and developing their food safety management procedures. Across the supply chain, the US Food and Drug Administration passes from Food Safety Modernization Act rulemaking to implementation with the concept of "we regulate while we educate" providing the industry across the supply chain access to continuous support and educational information to facilitate and improve compliance to food safety regulations. There are plentiful examples to work by on national regulatory agencies that promote food safety education and provide know-how materials to the food industry.

It may not be reasonable to suggest regulatory solutions that equally fit all the Arab countries in the Middle East given the different social, economic and political structures, institutional setups, and challenges. Yet, it is evident that collaborative efforts through partnerships among public, academic, and private sectors are the cornerstone of a successful integrated national food safety systems and for fostering technical and educational support to stakeholders while addressing challenges and understanding local circumstances. Collaborative efforts are the pathways for successful food safety policies and improving food safety and protecting consumers' health.

References

Abd-Elhaleem, Z. A., & Abd-Elkarim, M. A. (2011). Pattern of food poisoning in Egypt: A retrospective study. *Journal of Pharmacology and Toxicology*, *6*(5), 505–515. Available from https://doi.org/10.3923/jpt.2011.505.515.

Abdul-Mutalib, N.-A., Abdul-Rashid, M.-F., Mustafa, S., Amin-Nordin, S., Hamat, R. A., & Osman, M. (2012). Knowledge, attitude and practices regarding food hygiene and sanitation of food handlers in Kuala Pilah, Malaysia. *Food Control*, *27*(2), 289–293. Available from https://doi.org/10.1016/j.foodcont.2012.04.001.

Abushelaibi, A. M., Jobe, B., Afifi, H. S., Mostafa, B.-E., Murad, A. A., & Mohammed, A. K. (2015). Evaluation of the effect of person-in-charge (PIC) program on knowledge and practice change of food handlers in Dubai. *Food Control*, *50*, 382–392. Available from https://doi.org/10.1016/j.foodcont.2014.09.013.

Acikel, C. H., Ogur, R., Yaren, H., Gocgeldi, E., Ucar, M., & Kir, T. (2008). The hygiene training of food handlers at a teaching hospital. *Food Control*, *19*(2), 186–190. Available from https://doi.org/10.1016/j.foodcont.2007.03.008.

Ajzen, I. (1991). The theory of planned behavior. *Theories of Cognitive Self-Regulation*, *50*(2), 179–211. Available from https://doi.org/10.1016/0749--5978(91)90020-T.

Ajzen, I. (2002). Perceived behavioral control, self-efficacy, locus of control, and the theory of planned behavior. *Journal of Applied Social Psychology*, *32*(4), 665–683. Available from https://doi.org/10.1111/j.1559-1816.2002.tb00236.x.

Ajzen, I., & Madden, T. J. (1986). Prediction of goal-directed behavior: Attitudes, intentions, and perceived behavioral control. *Journal of Experimental Social Psychology*, *22*(5), 453–474. Available from https://doi.org/10.1016/0022-1031(86)90045-4.

Al-Ahmadi, K. S., Bushra, H. E. E., & Al-Zahrani, A. S. (1998). An outbreak of food poisoning associated with restaurant-made mayonnaise in Abha, Saudi Arabia. *Journal of Diarrhoeal Diseases Research*, *16*(3), 201–204. Available at:. Available from https://www.jstor.org/stable/23498604.

Al Arabiya News. (2020). Jordan shuts down 11 restaurants following new wave of food poisoning | *Al Arabiya English. Alarabya.Net*. https://english.alarabiya.net/en/News/middle-east/2020/08/02/Jordan-shuts-down-11-restaurants-following-new-wave-of-food-poisoning. Accessed October 30, 2020.

Al-Goblan, A. S., & Jahan, S. (2010). Surveillance for foodborne illness outbreaks in Qassim, Saudi Arabia, 2006. *Foodborne Pathogens and Disease*, *7*(12), 1559–1562. Available from https://doi.org/10.1089/fpd.2010.0638.

Al-Kandari, D., Al-abdeen, J., & Sidhu, J. (2019). Food safety knowledge, attitudes and practices of food handlers in restaurants in Kuwait. *Food Control*, *103*, 103–110. Available from https://doi.org/10.1016/j.foodcont.2019.03.040.

Al-Khatib, I. A., & Al-Mitwalli, S. M. (2009). Food sanitation practices in restaurants of Ramallah and Al-Bireh district of Palestine. *Eastern Mediterranean Health Journal*, *15*(4), 951–958.

Alqurashi, N. A., Priyadarshini, A., & Jaiswal, A. K. (2019). Evaluating food safety knowledge and practices among foodservice staff in Al Madinah Hospitals, Saudi Arabia. *Safety*, *5*(1), 9. Available from https://doi.org/10.3390/safety5010009.

Al-Shabib, N. A., Mosilhey, S. H., & Husain, F. M. (2016). Cross-sectional study on food safety knowledge, attitude and practices of male food handlers employed in restaurants of King Saud University, Saudi Arabia. *Food Control*, *59*, 212–217. Available from https://doi.org/10.1016/j.foodcont.2015.05.002.

Angelo, K. M., Nisler, A. L., Hall, A. J., Brown, L. G., & Gould, L. H. (2017). Epidemiology of restaurant-associated foodborne disease outbreaks, United States, 1998–2013. *Epidemiology & Infection*, *145*(3), 523–534. Available from https://doi.org/10.1017/S0950268816002314.

Angulo, F. J., Jones, T. F., & Angulo, F. J. (2006). Eating in restaurants: A risk factor for foodborne disease? *Clinical Infectious Diseases*, *43*(10), 1324–1328. Available from https://doi.org/10.1086/508540.

Arab News. (2017). Ninety eight students in Egypt treated for food poisoning. *Arab News.* Available at: https://www.arabnews.com/node/1072526/middle-east. Accessed October 29, 2020.

Arabian Business. (2019). Egyptian resort tops global list for worst holiday locations for food poisoning. *ArabianBusiness.Com.* Available at: https://www.arabianbusiness.com/travel-hospitality/426234-egyptian-resort-tops-global-list-for-worst-holiday-locations-for-food-poisoning. Accessed October 29, 2020.

Asim, H. S., Elnemr, I., Goktepe, I., et al. (2019). Assessing safe food handling knowledge and practices of food service managers in Doha, Qatar. *Food Science and Technology International, 25*(5), 440–448. Available from https://doi.org/10.1177/1082013219830843.

Belaya, V., Hansen, H., & Pinior, B. (2012). Measuring the costs of foodborne diseases: A review and classification of the literature. *52nd Annual conference, Stuttgart, Germany, September 26–28, 2012.* Available at: https://ideas.repec.org/p/ags/gewi12/138195.html.

Bintsis, T. (2017). Foodborne pathogens. *AIMS Microbiology, 3*(3), 529–563. Available from https://doi.org/10.3934/microbiol.2017.3.529.

Bou-Mitri, C., Mahmoud, D., Gerges, N., & Jaoude, M. A. (2018). Food safety knowledge, attitudes and practices of food handlers in Lebanese hospitals: A cross-sectional study. *Food Control, 94*, 78–84. Available from https://doi.org/10.1016/j.foodcont.2018.06.032.

Codex Alimentarius Commission (CAC) (2003). Food Hygiene Basic Texts. 3rd Edition, Roma, 68 p.

CDC. (2019). *Salmonella saintpaul* infections linked to raw produce. Available at: https://www.cdc.gov/salmonella/2008/raw-produce-8-28-2008.html.

CFS. (2020). Review of food poisoning outbreaks related to food premises and food business in 2019. Available at: https://www.cfs.gov.hk/english/multimedia/multimedia_pub/multimedia_pub_fsf_164_01.html.

Choudhury, M., Mahanta, L. B., Goswami, J. S., & Mazumder, M. D. (2011). Will capacity building training interventions given to street food vendors give us safer food?: A cross-sectional study from India. *Food Control, 22*(8), 1233–1239. Available from https://doi.org/10.1016/j.foodcont.2011.01.023.

Clayton, D. A., & Griffith, C. J. (2004). Observation of food safety practices in catering using notational analysis. *British Food Journal, 106*(3), 211–227. Available from https://doi.org/10.1108/00070700410528790.

Clayton, M., Clegg Smith, K., Neff, R. A., Pollack, K., & Ensminger, M. (2015). Listening to food workers: Factors that impact proper health and hygiene practice in food service. *International Journal of Occupational and Environmental Health, 21*(4), 314–327. Available from https://doi.org/10.1179/2049396715Y.0000000011.

Crew, S. (2019). Certifying food safety culture. *Food Science and Technology, 33*(1), 26–29. Available from https://doi.org/10.1002/fsat.3301_8.x.

De Boer, E., & Hahné, M. (1990). Cross-contamination with *Campylobacter jejuni* and *Salmonella* spp. from raw chicken products during food preparation. *Journal of Food Protection, 53*(12), 1067–1068. Available from https://doi.org/10.4315/0362-028X-53.12.1067.

Djekic, I., Kuzmanović, J., Anđelković, A., Saračević, M., Stojanović, M. M., & Tomašević, I. (2016). Relationships among hygiene indicators in take-away foodservice establishments and the impact of climatic conditions. *Journal of Applied Microbiology, 121*(3), 863–872. Available from https://doi.org/10.1111/jam.13211.

Doménech-Sánchez, A., Laso, E., Pérez, M. J., & Berrocal, C. I. (2011). Microbiological levels of randomly selected food contact surfaces in hotels located in Spain during 2007–2009.

Foodborne Pathogens and Disease, *8*(9), 1025–1029. Available from https://doi.org/10.1089/fpd.2011.0856.

EFSA. (2010). The community summary report on trends and sources of zoonoses, zoonotic agents and food-borne outbreaks in the European Union in 2008. *EFSA Journal*, *8*(1), 1496. Available from https://doi.org/10.2903/j.efsa.2010.1496.

Egan, M. B., Raats, M. M., Grubb, S. M., Eves, A., Lumbers, M. L., Dean, M. S., & Adams, M. R. (2007). A review of food safety and food hygiene training studies in the commercial sector. *Food Control*, *18*(10), 1180–1190. Available from https://doi.org/10.1016/j.foodcont.2006.08.001.

ElMeshad, S. (2011). Summer food poisoning: Concerns and prevention. *Egypt Independent*. Available at: https://egyptindependent.com/summer-food-poisoning-concerns-and-prevention/. Accessed October 29, 2020.

Elobeid, T., Savvaidis, I., & Ganji, V. (2019). Impact of food safety training on the knowledge, practice, and attitudes of food handlers working in fast-food restaurants. *British Food Journal*, *121*(4), 937–949. Available from https://doi.org/10.1108/BFJ-01-2019-0066.

El-Sherbeeny, M. R., Saddik, M. F., & Bryan, F. L. (1985). Microbiological profiles of foods served by street vendors in Egypt. *International Journal of Food Microbiology*, *2*(6), 355–364. Available from https://doi.org/10.1016/0168-1605(85)90026-1.

Elsherbiny, N. M., Sobhy, S. A., Fiala, L., & Abbas, M. A. (2019). Knowledge, attitude and practices of food safety among food handlers in Ismailia city hospitals, Egypt. *Int J Adv Community Med*, *2*(2), 96–102. Available from https://doi.org/10.33545/comed.2019.v2.i2b.13.

Evans, H. S., Madden, P., Douglas, C., Adak, G. K., O'Brien, S. J., Djuretic, T., Wall, P. G., & Stanwell-Smith, R. (1998). General outbreaks of infectious intestinal disease in England and Wales: 1995 and 1996. *Communicable Disease and Public Health*, *1*(3), 165–171.

Fadlallah, S., Shehab, M., Cheaito, K., Saleh, M., Ghosn, N., Ammar, W., El Hajj, R., & Matar, M. (2017). Molecular epidemiology and antimicrobial resistance of Salmonella species from clinical specimens and food Items in Lebanon. *The Journal of Infection in Developing Countries*, *11*(01), 19–27. Available from https://doi.org/10.3855/jidc.7786.

FAO. (2017). Food handler's manual: Instructor. FAO. Available at: http://www.fao.org/documents/card/en/c/82035acd-32e6-4d95-987b-86dafc9f7297/. Accessed October 19, 2020.

FAO. (2019). Food safety and quality: Country page. Available at: http://www.fao.org/food/food-safety-quality/gm-foods-platform/browse-information-by/country/country-page/en/?cty = TUN. Accessed October 23, 2020.

Faour-Klingbeil, D., & Todd, E. C. D. (2019). Prevention and control of foodborne diseases in Middle-East North African Countries: Review of national control systems. *International Journal of Environmental Research and Public Health*, *17*(1), 70. Available from https://doi.org/10.3390/ijerph17010070.

Faour-Klingbeil, D., Kuri, V., & Todd, E. (2015). Investigating a link of two different types of food business management to the food safety knowledge, attitudes and practices of food handlers in Beirut, Lebanon. *Food Control*, *55*, 166–175. Available from https://doi.org/10.1016/j.foodcont.2015.02.045.

Faour-Klingbeil, D., Kuri, V., & Todd, E. (2016). The transfer rate of *Salmonella typhimurium* from contaminated parsley to other consecutively chopped batches via cutting boards under different food handling scenarios. *Food Research International*, *89*, 495–503. Available from https://doi.org/10.1016/j.foodres.2016.09.001.

Faour-Klingbeil, D., Kuri, V., & Todd, E. (2020). Comparison of hygiene standards and food safety practices between sole-proprietor and corporate-managed restaurants in Lebanon.

British Food Journal, *122*(4), 1112–1129. Available from https://doi.org/10.1108/bfj-01-2019-0018.

FDA. (2009). Retail risk factor study—FDA report on the occurrence of foodborne illness risk factors in selected institutional foodservice, restaurant, and retail food store facility types [Web Content]. Center for Food Safety and Applied Nutrition. Available at: https://wayback.archive-it.org/7993/20170406023004/; https://www.fda.gov/Food/GuidanceRegulation/RetailFoodProtection/FoodborneIllnessRiskFactorReduction/ucm224321.htm. Accessed October 19, 2020.

Franck, K. T., Lisby, M., Fonager, J., Schultz, A. C., Böttiger, B., Villif, A., Absalonsen, H., & Ethelberg, S. (2015). Sources of Calicivirus contamination in foodborne outbreaks in Denmark, 2005–2011—The role of the asymptomatic food handler. *The Journal of Infectious Diseases*, *211*(4), 563–570. Available from https://doi.org/10.1093/infdis/jiu479.

FSANZ. (n.d.). Health and hygiene responsibilities of food handlers. Available at: https://www.foodstandards.gov.au/consumer/safety/faqsafety/pages/foodsafetyfactsheets/healthandhygieneresp101.aspx. Accessed October 30, 2020.

GFSI. (2018). A culture of food safety. Available at: https://mygfsi.com/wp-content/uploads/2019/09/GFSI-Food-Safety-Culture-Full.pdf. Accessed October 30, 2020.

Gormley, F. J., Rawal, N., & Little, C. L. (2012). Choose your menu wisely: Cuisine-associated food-poisoning risks in restaurants in England and Wales. *Epidemiology and Infection*, *140*(6), 997–1007. Available from https://doi.org/10.1017/S0950268811001567.

Gould, L. H., Rosenblum, I., Nicholas, D., Phan, Q., & Jones, T. F. (2013). Contributing factors in restaurant-associated foodborne disease outbreaks, FoodNet Sites, 2006 and 2007. *Journal of Food Protection*, *76*(11), 1824–1828. Available from https://doi.org/10.4315/0362-028X.JFP-13-037.

Greig, J. D., Todd, E. C., Bartleson, C. A., & Michaels, B. S. (2007). Outbreaks where food workers have been implicated in spread of foodborne disease, part 1. Description of the problem, methods, and agents involved. *Journal of Food Protection*, *70*, 1752–1761.

Griffith, C. J., Livesey, K. M., & Clayton, D. A. (2010). Food safety culture: the evolution of an emerging risk factor? *British Food Journal*, *112*(4), 426–438. Available from https://doi.org/10.1108/00070701011034439.

Hamed, A., & Mohammed, N. (2020). Food safety knowledge, attitudes and self-reported practices among food handlers in Sohag Governorate, Egypt. *East Mediterr Health Journal*, *26*(4), 374–381. Available from https://doi.org/10.26719/emhj.19.047, PMID: 32338355. Accessed April 16, 2020.

Hanashiro, A., Morita, M., Matté, G. R., Matté, M. H., & Torres, E. A. F. S. (2005). Microbiological quality of selected street foods from a restricted area of São Paulo city, Brazil. *Food Control*, *16*(5), 439–444. Available from https://doi.org/10.1016/j.foodcont.2004.05.004.

Hawkes, C. (2005). The role of foreign direct investment in the nutrition transition. *Public Health Nutrition*, *8*(4), 357–365. Available from https://doi.org/10.1079/phn2004706.

Hossen, M. T., Ferdaus, M. J., Hasan, M. M., Lina, N. N., Das, A. K., Barman, S. K., Paul, D. K., & Roy, R. K. (2020). Food safety knowledge, attitudes and practices of street food vendors in Jashore region, Bangladesh. *Food Science and Technology*, *41*(suppl. 1). Available from https://doi.org/10.1590/fst.13320.

Hye-Ja, C., Jaung-Sook, L., & Tong-Kyung, K. (2003). Effectiveness of HACCP-based training on the food safety knowledge and behavior of hospital foodservice employees. *Nutritional Sciences*, *6*(2), 118–126. Available at: https://kmbase.medric.or.kr/KMID/1012320030060020118.

Jones, A. K., Cross, P., Burton, M., Millman, C., O'Brien, S. J., & Rigby, D. (2017). Estimating the prevalence of food risk increasing behaviours in UK kitchens. *PLoS One*, *12*(6), e0175816. Available from https://doi.org/10.1371/journal.pone.0175816.

Kaabi, S. K. A., Lbrahim, A. a E., & Salama, R. E. (2010). Assessment of knowledge, attitude and practice of food safety among food service staff at Hamad General Hospital in 2006. *Qatar Medical Journal*, *2010*(2), 8. Available from https://doi.org/10.5339/qmj.2010.2.8.

Kadariya, J., Smith, T. C., & Thapaliya, D. (2014). *Staphylococcus aureus* and Staphylococcal food-borne disease: An ongoing challenge in public health. *BioMed Research International*, *2014*, 827965. Available from https://doi.org/10.1155/2014/827965.

Kearney, J. (2010). Food consumption trends and drivers. *Philosophical Transactions of the Royal Society B: Biological Sciences*, *365*(1554), 2793–2807. Available from https://doi.org/10.1098/rstb.2010.0149.

Kuwait News Agency. (2018). 130 Foreign workers affected by food poisoning. Available at: https://www.kuna.net.kw/ArticleDetails.aspx?id = 2757655&language = en.

Lasky, T. (2002). Foodborne illness—Old problem, new relevance. *Epidemiology (Cambridge, Mass.)*, *13*(5), 593–598. Available from https://doi.org/10.1097/01.EDE.0000025309.37329.C1.

Lee, H. K., Abdul Halim, H., Thong, K. L., & Chai, L. C. (2017). Assessment of food safety knowledge, attitude, self-reported practices, and microbiological hand hygiene of food handlers. *International Journal of Environmental Research and Public Health*, *14*(1), 55. Available from https://doi.org/10.3390/ijerph14010055.

Loukieh, M., Mouannes, E., Abou Jaoudeh, C., Hanna Wakim, L., Fancello, F., & Bou Zeidan, M. (2018). Street foods in Beirut city: An assessment of the food safety practices and of the microbiological quality. *Journal of Food Safety*, *38*(3), e12455. Available from https://doi.org/10.1111/jfs.12455.

Lynch, R. A., Phillips, M. L., Elledge, B. L., Hanumanthaiah, S., & Boatright, D. T. (2005). A preliminary evaluation of the effect of glove use by food handlers in fast food restaurants. *Journal of Food Protection*, *68*(1), 187–190. Available from https://doi.org/10.4315/0362-028X-68.1.187.

Malaeb, M., Bizri, A. R., Ghosn, N., Berry, A., & Musharrafieh, U. (2016). Salmonella burden in Lebanon. *Epidemiology & Infection*, *144*(8), 1761–1769. Available from https://doi.org/10.1017/S0950268815003076.

Marette, S., Bureau, J., & ozlan, E. (2003). Regulating food safety in the European Union. In A. G. J. Velthuis, L. J. Unnevehr, H. Hogeveen, & R. B. M. Huirne (Eds.), *New approaches to food-safety economics*. Kluwer Academic Publishers.

Market Research. (2020). Saudi Arabia pizza restaurants market—Growth, trends and forecast (2020–2025). No. MOI16350439; p. 68. Mordor Intelligence LLP. Available at: https://www.marketresearch.com/Mordor-Intelligence-LLP-v4018/Saudi-Arabia-Pizza-Restaurants-Growth-13600934/. Accessed October 20, 2020.

Martins, R. B., Hogg, T., & Otero, J. G. (2012). Food handlers' knowledge on food hygiene: The case of a catering company in Portugal. *Food Control*, *23*(1), 184–190. Available from https://doi.org/10.1016/j.foodcont.2011.07.008.

McFarland, P., Checinska Sielaff, A., Rasco, B., & Smith, S. (2019). Efficacy of food safety training in commercial food service. *Journal of Food Science*, *84*(6), 1239–1246. Available from https://doi.org/10.1111/1750-3841.14628.

McIntyre, L., Vallaster, L., Wilcott, L., Henderson, S. B., & Kosatsky, T. (2013). Evaluation of food safety knowledge, attitudes and self-reported hand washing practices in FOODSAFE trained and untrained food handlers in British Columbia, Canada. *Food Control, 30*(1), 150–156. Available from https://doi.org/10.1016/j.foodcont.2012.06.034.

McKinsey & Company. (2020). Consumer sentiment and behavior continue to reflect the uncertainty of the COVID-19 crisis. Available at: https://www.mckinsey.com/business-functions/marketing-and-sales/our-insights/a-global-view-of-how-consumer-behavior-is-changing-amid-covid-19#.

Medus, C., Smith, K. E., Bender, J. B., Besser, J. M., & Hedberg, C. W. (2006). Salmonella outbreaks in restaurants in Minnesota, 1995 through 2003: Evaluation of the role of infected foodworkers. *Journal of Food Protection, 69*(8), 1870–1878. Available from https://doi.org/10.4315/0362-028x-69.8.1870.

Michaels, B. (2002). Handling money and serving ready-to-eat food. *Food Service Technology, 2*(1), 1–3. Available from https://doi.org/10.1046/j.1471-5740.2002.00030.x.

Mitchell, R. E., Fraser, A. M., & Bearon, L. B. (2007). Preventing food-borne illness in foodservice establishment: Broadening the framework for intervention and research on safe food handling behaviors. *International Journal of Environmental Health Research, 17*, 9–24. Available from https://doi.org/10.1080/09603120601124371.

Middle East Eye. (2015). Lebanon's food safety scandal refuses to go away. *Middle East Eye*. Available at: http://www.middleeasteye.net/news/lebanons-food-safety-scandal-refuses-go-away.

Myers, A. (2018). Army looking into food poisoning outbreak at Kuwait base. Available at: https://www.armytimes.com/news/your-army/2018/07/25/army-looking-into-food-poisoning-outbreak-at-kuwait-base/.

Ncube, F., Kanda, A., Chijokwe, M., Mabaya, G., & Nyamugure, T. (2020). Food safety knowledge, attitudes and practices of restaurant food handlers in a lower-middle-income country. *Food Science & Nutrition, 8*(3), 1677–1687. Available from https://doi.org/10.1002/fsn3.1454.

Noureldin, M. (2020). The rise of food delivery platforms in the Arab world. *Arab America*. Available at: https://www.arabamerica.com/the-rise-of-food-delivery-platforms-in-the-arab-world/.

OECD/WHO. (2003). *Foodborne disease in OECD countries*. OECD/WHO. Available from https://doi.org/10.1787/9789264105386-en.

Omar, S. S. (2020). Food safety knowledge of street food vendors in downtown Amman-Jordan. *Eurasian Journal of Biosciences, 14*(2), 3601–3606. Available at: http://www.ejobios.org/article/food-safety-knowledge-of-street-food-vendors-in-downtown-amman-jordan-7979.

Osaili, T. M., Abu Jamous, D. O., Obeidat, B. A., Bawadi, H. A., Tayyem, R. F., & Subih, H. S. (2013). Food safety knowledge among food workers in restaurants in Jordan. *Food Control, 31*(1), 145–150. Available from https://doi.org/10.1016/j.foodcont.2012.09.037.

Osaili, T. M., Al-Nabulsi, A. A., & Allah Krasneh, H. D. (2018). Food safety knowledge among foodservice staff at the universities in Jordan. *Food Control, 89*, 167–176. Available from https://doi.org/10.1016/j.foodcont.2018.02.011.

Osaili, T. M., Obeidat, B. A., Hajeer, W. A., & Al-Nabulsi, A. A. (2017). Food safety knowledge among food service staff in hospitals in Jordan. *Food Control, 78*, 279–285. Available from https://doi.org/10.1016/j.foodcont.2017.02.057.

Ovca, A., Jevšnik, M., & Raspor, P. (2018). Food safety practices of future food handlers and their teachers, observed during practical lessons. *British Food Journal, 120*(3), 531–548. Available from https://doi.org/10.1108/BFJ-05-2017-0292.

Park, S.-H., Kwak, T.-K., & Chang, H.-J. (2010). Evaluation of the food safety training for food handlers in restaurant operations. *Nutrition Research and Practice, 4*(1), 58–68. Available from https://doi.org/10.4162/nrp.2010.4.1.58.

Phillip, S., & Anita, E. (2010). Efficacy of the theory of planned behaviour model in predicting safe food handling practices. *Food Control*, *21*(7), 983–987. Available from https://doi.org/10.1016/j.foodcont.2009.12.012.

Pragle, A. S., Harding, A. K., & Mack, J. C. (2007). Food workers' perspectives on hand washing behaviors and barriers in the restaurant environment. *Journal of Environmental Health*, *69*(10), 27–31.

Qasim, N. (2011). An epidemiological study of food poisoning outbreaks, Jordan 2009–2010. *TEPHINET*. Available at: https://www.tephinet.org/an-epidemiological-study-of-food-poisoning-outbreaks-jordan-2009-2010.

Ravishankar, Sadhana, Zhu, Libin, & Jaroni, Divya (2010). Assessing the cross contamination and transfer rates of Salmonella enterica from chicken to lettuce under different food-handling scenarios. *Food Microbiology*, *27*(6), 791–794, ISSN 0740-0020. Available from https://doi.org/10.1016/j.fm.2010.04.011.

Rebgui, H., Nekkal, N., Benlarabi, S., El Hattimy, F., Hadrya, F., Soulaymani, A., Soulaymani-Bencheikh, R., & Mokhtari, A. (2013). Food poisoning in Morocco: Evolution and Risk factors. *International Journal of Scientific & Engineering Research*, *4*(11), 1015–1021. Available at: https://www.ijser.org/paper/Food-poisoning-in-Morocco-Evolution-and-Risk-factors.html.

Rebouças, L. T., Santiago, L. B., Martins, L. S., Rios Menezes, A. C., Araújo, M. da P. N., & Almeida, R. C. de C. (2017). Food safety knowledge and practices of food handlers, head chefs and managers in hotels' restaurants of Salvador, Brazil. *Food Control*, *73*, 372–381. Available from https://doi.org/10.1016/j.foodcont.2016.08.026.

Roberts, K. R., Barrett, B. B., Howells, A. D., Shanklin, C. W., Pilling, V. K., & Brannon, L. A. (2008). Food safety training and foodservice employees' knowledge and behavior. *Food Protection Trends*, *28*(4), 252–260. Available at: https://krex.k-state.edu/dspace/handle/2097/806.

Rönnqvist, M., Aho, E., Mikkelä, A., Ranta, J., Tuominen, P., Rättö, M., & Maunula, L. (2014). Norovirus transmission between hands, gloves, utensils, and fresh produce during simulated food handling. *Applied and Environmental Microbiology*, *80*(17), 5403–5410. Available from https://doi.org/10.1128/AEM.01162-14.

Røssvoll, E. H., Lavik, R., Ueland, Ø., Jacobsen, E., Hagtvedt, T., & Langsrud, S. (2013). Food safety practices among Norwegian consumers. *Journal of Food Protection*, *76*(11), 1939–1947. Available from https://doi.org/10.4315/0362-028X.JFP-12-269.

Saleh, M. (2011). Salmonellosis in Lebanon, 2010. *TEPHINET*. Available at: https://www.tephinet.org/salmonellosis-in-lebanon-2010.

Scallan, E., Hoekstra, R. M., Angulo, F. J., Tauxe, R. V., Widdowson, M.-A., Roy, S. L., & Griffin, P. M. (2011). Foodborne illness acquired in the United States—Major pathogens. *Emerging Infectious Diseases*, *17*(1), 7–15. Available from https://doi.org/10.3201/eid1701.P11101.

Scharff, R. L. (2012). Economic burden from health losses due to foodborne illness in the United States. *Journal of Food Protection*, *75*(1), 123–131. Available from https://doi.org/10.4315/0362-028X.JFP-11-058.

Sharif, L., Obaidat, M. M., & Al-Dalalah, M.-R. (2013). Food hygiene knowledge, attitudes and practices of the food handlers in the military hospitals. *Food and Nutrition Sciences*, *4*(3), 245–251. Available from https://doi.org/10.4236/fns.2013.43033.

Sneed, J., & Strohbehn, C. H. (2008). Trends impacting food safety in retail foodservice: Implications for dietetics practice. *Journal of the American Dietetic Association*, *108*(7), 1170–1177. Available from https://doi.org/10.1016/j.jada.2008.04.009.

Soares, L. S., Almeida, R. C. C., Cerqueira, E. S., Carvalho, J. S., & Nunes, I. L. (2012). Knowledge, attitudes and practices in food safety and the presence of coagulase-positive Staphylococci on hands of food handlers in the schools of Camaçari, Brazil. *Food Control*, *27*(1), 206–213. Available from https://doi.org/10.1016/j.foodcont.2012.03.016.

Stals, A., Uyttendaele, M., Baert, L., & Van Coillie, E. (2013). Norovirus transfer between foods and food contact materials. *Journal of Food Protection*, *76*(7), 1202–1209. Available from https://doi.org/10.4315/0362-028X.JFP-12-392.

Taha, S., Osaili, T. M., Saddal, N. K., Al-Nabulsi, A. A., Ayyash, M. M., & Obaid, R. S. (2020). Food safety knowledge among food handlers in food service establishments in United Arab Emirates. *Food Control*, *110*, 106968. Available from https://doi.org/10.1016/j.foodcont.2019.106968.

The Daily Star. (2014). Abu Faour adds, removes from supermarkets, eateries blacklist. Available at: https://www.dailystar.com.lb/News/Lebanon-News/2014/Nov-26/278976-abu-faour-adds-removes-from-supermarkets-eateries-blacklist.ashx.

The Guardian. (2020). More than 800 hospitalised in Jordan food poisoning outbreak. Available at: https://www.theguardian.com/world/2020/jul/30/more-than-800-hospitalised-in-jordan-food-poisoning-outbreak.

The National. (2018). Dubai health authorities report 800 cases of food poisoning this year. *The National*. Available at: https://www.thenational.ae/uae/health/dubai-health-authorities-report-800-cases-of-food-poisoning-this-year-1.766542. Accessed October 19, 2020.

The Restaurant Show. (2018). Middle East restaurant project report 2019–2020. The Restaurant Show. Available at: https://www.restaurantshowmiddleeast.com/news6. Accessed October 20, 2020.

Tirado, C., & Schmidt, K. (2001). WHO surveillance programme for control of foodborne infections and intoxications: Preliminary results and trends across greater Europe. *The Journal of Infection*, *43*(1), 80–84. Available from https://doi.org/10.1053/jinf.2001.0861.

Todd, E. C. D., Greig, J. D., Bartleson, C. A., & Michaels, B. S. (2007). Outbreaks where food workers have been implicated in the spread of foodborne disease. Part 3. Factors contributing to outbreaks and description of outbreak categories. *Journal of Food Protection*, *70*(9), 2199–2217. Available from https://doi.org/10.4315/0362-028x-70.9.2199.

Todd, E. C. D., Greig, J. D., Bartleson, C. A., & Michaels, B. S. (2008). Outbreaks where food workers have been implicated in the spread of foodborne disease. Part 4. Infective doses and pathogen carriage. *Journal of Food Protection*, *71*(11), 2339–2373. Available from https://doi.org/10.4315/0362-028x-71.11.2339.

Ungku Fatimah, U. Z. A., Strohbehn, C. H., & Arendt, S. W. (2014). An empirical investigation of food safety culture in onsite foodservice operations. *Food Control*, *46*, 255–263. Available from https://doi.org/10.1016/j.foodcont.2014.05.029.

Walker, E., Pritchard, C., & Forsythe, S. (2003). Food handlers' hygiene knowledge in small food businesses. *Food Control*, *14*(5), 339–343. Available from https://doi.org/10.1016/S0956-7135(02)00101-9.

Walravens, T. (2017). Food safety and regulatory change since the 'mad cow' in Japan: Science, self-responsibility, and trust. *Contemporary Japan*, *29*(1), 67–88. Available from https://doi.org/10.1080/18692729.2017.1256987.

WHO. (2015a). The five keys to safer food programme. Available at: https://www.who.int/foodsafety/consumer/5keys/en/ Accessed October 20, 2020.

WHO. (2015b). WHO | From kebabs to fattoush – Keeping Lebanon's food safe. World Health Organization. Available at: https://www.who.int/features/2015/lebanon-food-safety/en/. Accessed October 20, 2020.

WHO. (2015c). WHO estimates of the global burden of foodborne diseases: Foodborne disease burden epidemiology reference group 2007–2015 (ISBN 978 92 4 156516 5). Available at: https://www.who.int/foodsafety/foodborne_disease/ferg/en/. Accessed October 30, 2020.

Yahia, N., Achkar, A., Abdallah, A., & Rizk, S. (2008). Eating habits and obesity among Lebanese university students. *Nutrition Journal*, *7*(1), 32. Available from https://doi.org/10.1186/1475-2891-7-32.

YaLibnan. (2014). Lebanon food scandal: The health minister took action against violators. Available at: https://yalibnan.com/2014/11/15/lebanon-food-scandal-the-health-minister-took-action-against-violators/. Accessed October 30, 2020.

Yiannas, F. (2009). *Food safety culture: Creating a behavior-based food safety management system* (pp. 1–8). Springer. Available from https://doi.org/10.1007/978-0-387-72867-4_3.

Yu, H., Neal, J., Dawson, M., & Madera, J. M. (2017). Implementation of behavior-based training can improve food service employees' handwashing frequencies, duration, and effectiveness. *Cornell Hospitality Quarterly*, *59*(1), 70–77. Available from https://doi.org/10.1177/1938965517704370.

Zanin, L. M., da Cunha, D. T., de Rosso, V. V., Capriles, V. D., & Stedefeldt, E. (2017). Knowledge, attitudes and practices of food handlers in food safety: An integrative review. *Food Research International*, *100*, 53–62. Available from https://doi.org/10.1016/j.foodres.2017.07.042.

Chapter 8

Legislation for food control in the Arab countries of the Middle East

Dima Faour-Klingbeil[1,2], Moza Abdullah Al-Busaidi[3] and Ewen C.D. Todd[4]

[1]DFK for Safe Food Environment, Food Safety and Regulatory Systems Compliance, Hannover, Germany, [2]Centre for Rural Development, Humboldt University of Berlin, Germany, [3]Research and Innovation Sector, Ministry of Higher Education, Research and Innovation, Sultanate of Oman, [4]Ewen Todd Consulting, LLC, Okemos, MI, United States

8.1 Introduction

Access to adequate food is a human right regardless of race, color, sex, language, religion, political or other opinions, national or social origin, property, birth, or other status. This right is recognized since the 1948 Universal Declaration of Human Rights and enshrined in the international human rights law, the 1966 International Covenant on Economic, Social and Cultural Rights (OHCHR, 2010). The latter lay downs the state's obligation to respect, protect, and fulfill the right to food by creating an enabling environment within which people are able to meet their food needs. Heads of State and Government reaffirmed these rights during the World Food Summit organized by the Food and Agriculture Organization (FAO) in 1996.

The right to food is also recognized implicitly in other international conventions protecting specific groups, in other rights, and nonlegally binding international human rights instruments, including recommendations, guidelines, resolutions, or declarations relevant to the right to food. Following the World Food Summit, the FAO adopted in 2004 a set of Voluntary Guidelines, one of the nonlegal instruments, as a useful guide to United Nations Member States on how they can implement their existing obligations.

The human right to adequate food implies that the food must satisfy the different population groups' dietary needs, be culturally acceptable and safe for human consumption. Safe food means free from adverse substances, such

Food Safety in the Middle East. DOI: https://doi.org/10.1016/B978-0-12-822417-5.00007-6

as contaminants from industrial or agricultural processes, including residues from pesticides, hormones, or veterinary drugs (OHCHR, 2010). According to §9 p19–20 ¶9.1–9.9 of the Voluntary Guidelines, States should establish comprehensive risk-based food control systems, promote safe practices in the food chain, and adopt science-based standards to ensure the safety of locally and imported food and feed, and to reduce the risk of foodborne diseases from farm to fork (FAO, 2005).

On this basis, the FAO and the World Health Organization (WHO) established an intergovernmental body, the Codex Alimentarius Commission, in 1962. The commission was created to develop a collection of internationally recognized standards, codes of practice, guidelines, and other food quality and safety recommendations under the Joint FAO/WHO Food Standards Programme, known as the Codex Alimentarius or the Food Code. This program aims to protect consumers' health, ensure fair practices in the international food trade, and promote coordination of food standards adopted by international governmental and nongovernmental organizations.

Driven by food safety concerns, the World Trade Organization (WTO) mandated the Sanitary and Phytosanitary (SPS) Agreement in 1995, which sets out the global agricultural trade's basic rules. The SPS recognizes three standard-setting bodies: the International Plant Protection Convention for plant health, the International Office of Epizootics for animal health, and Codex Alimentarius Commission for Food Safety formed to ensure conformity of imported goods with health standards based on internationally agreed rules, foundations, and scientific evidence. Hence, exporting countries are required to certify exported consignments in compliance with SPS requirements and are encouraged to adopt Codex standards as a benchmark for harmonization to ensure alignment with the SPS measures and Technical Barriers to Trade (TBT) agreements (UNIDO, 2017).

The global trade in food products has increased in the last decades, rising to US$1.5 trillion by 2017 (WHO, 2019). The dynamic rise in international food trade has made available a wide variety of food products yet eroded the borders to spread the risks. Local hazards are capable of traversing boundaries through a globalized food network (Ercsey-Ravasz, Toroczkai, Lakner, & Baranyi, 2012) and causing international havoc and enormous economic and public health burdens (Karch et al., 2012). Fraudulent activities such as using melamine in food, banned additives, falsified claims, and mislabeling, as well as ongoing incidents in food contamination, e.g. mad cow disease agents (prions), dioxins and polychlorinated biphenyls in poultry, egg, and meats, excessive pesticides residues, unsafe levels of mycotoxins, emerging hazards such as *Escherichia coli* O121 in flour, acid-resistant strains of *E. coli* O157: H7 along local and global supply chains unequivocally show that unsafe imported foods are challenging issues in food safety.

In April 2019, the FAO, WHO, and WTO joint statement at the International Forum on Food Safety and Trade highlighted the need for continued investments in institutions and infrastructure and effective food safety systems to meet the magnitudes of food safety challenges. The statement addressed the importance of technology and massive data that allows for better detection, investigation, monitoring and surveillance tool, and food safety risk assessment. Additionally, it emphasized the crucial role of digital technologies in improving transparency and traceability in food supply chains, thus, can contribute to enhancing food safety and facilitating safe trade (WHO, 2019). The international food safety regulatory landscape has matured and progressed over the years to respond much more efficiently to food safety problems. The significant progress in food research, and advanced molecular technology for testing food and tracing hazards such as the next-generation genome sequencing forms an essential basis to well-informed risk assessment and risk management and to adapting legislation and policies to continuously evolving food production technology and changing consumers' food preferences.

All countries should establish national standards and be responsible for ensuring that all necessary local or international standards are met to curb the costly health problems and strengthen multilateral trade. Food safety regulations aim primarily to safeguard public health and reduce the risk of illnesses and associated health costs (Ragona & Mazzocchi, 2008). Globally, these concerns were translated into significant reforms and legislation development by importing countries such as the European Union (EU), the United States, Japan, and others. Along the same line, the WHO Member States of the Eastern Mediterranean Region passed a resolution in 1999 to (1) assess their current infrastructure at a national level and prepare a comprehensive country profile for food safety; (2) establish or strengthen the national food safety committee or similar body, and make it operational to implement the national food safety program; (3) develop legislation and keep it up-to-date following the latest scientific developments; (4) promote preventive food safety management systems based on hazard analysis critical control point (HACCP); (5) ensure effective education of food handlers and training of workers in food safety issues; and (6) carry out research and data collection, including foodborne disease surveillance and exchange information on food which does not comply with health standard (WHO, 2001).

Many Arab countries in the Middle East have been reviewing their national food safety systems and initiating reforms in recent decades. National food control systems are crucial to protect consumers' health and ensure the safety and quality of foods being traded nationally and internationally; their organizational structures differ among countries and may fall under one of the three structures: (1) a system based on multiple agencies responsible for food control—multiple-agency system; (2) a system based on a single, unified agency for food control—single agency system; (iii) a system based on a national integrated approach—integrated system.

The national food control systems generally consist of the national food laws and regulations, food control management, inspection services, laboratory services (food monitoring and epidemiological data), information, education, communication, and training (FAO/WHO, 2003; Faour-Klingbeil & Todd, 2019). In this chapter, we mainly focus on the national food laws and regulations. We examine the extent to which the food safety regulatory framework and operational structures in the Arab countries of the Middle East have progressed to adapt to global regulatory requirements and ensure consumers' right to adequate food. Our review is limited by the data available, with some countries having extensive documentation and others with scarce material to make many comments.

8.2 Global direction toward a comprehensive food safety system

Intentional and unintentional food contamination can occur at any stage of the food chain, necessitating a comprehensive farm-to-fork approach in food control. These opportunities of food adulteration become more complex in a global market where controlling the source of raw materials and goods is vital to protect consumers' health and ensure food safety following SPS measures and national and international requirements.

The global food trade has substantially increased food products' rapid movements through a dense network of suppliers and stakeholders. Consequently, more countries are imposing strict regulatory requirements and controls over food imports to reduce the public health and economic burden of foodborne diseases and food recalls, and ensure product conformity with national standards. There is a worldwide trend for governments to adopt stricter and more rigorous food safety control systems such as in the EU, China, Japan, United States, United Arab Emirates (UAE), Saudi Arabia (Al-Kandari & Jukes, 2011, 2012; Jia & Jukes, 2013; Matsuo, 2013).

The US Food Safety Modernization Act (US FSMA) is one of the most recent regulatory reforms to the US food laws in 70 years. In the aftermath of high-profile food outbreaks, US Congress signed FSMA into a food law in 2011. Under this law, the Food and Drug Administration (FDA) released seven rules that spanned across the supply chain. It mandated implementing a science and risk-based system to prevent food safety hazards from farm to table. Additionally, the US FSMA has given the FDA an expanded authority to shift focus toward preventive strategies, including inspection of foreign facilities that export food for human and animal consumption in the United States. The effect of this transition from reactive to preventive approach outreached international processors, as it addresses controlling domestic and imported goods by imposing equivalent regulatory requirements.

The European Commission (EC) food regulation has also undergone significant changes in response to increasing health risks following a series of food incidents, such as the bovine spongiform encephalopathy (BSE) in cattle, mainly in the United Kingdom. To achieve a higher level of protection for the consumers, EC adopted the integrated approach to food safety "from farm to fork" covering all food chain sectors, including feed production, primary production, food processing, storage, transport, and retail sale. Furthermore, the European Parliament and the Council adopted Regulation (EC) No 178/2002 in 2002, which outlines the general principles and requirements of food laws (General Food Law Regulation). The General Food Law Regulation is the foundation of food and feed law. It sets out an overarching and coherent framework for developing food and feed legislation both at the EU and national levels (European Commission, 2016). It also lays down general principles, requirements, and procedures that underpin decision-making in matters of food and feed safety, covering all stages of food and feed production and distribution. The General Food Law Regulation sets up an independent agency responsible for scientific advice and support, the European Food Safety Authority responsible for risk assessment and risk communication. Through this system, reform and the Rapid Alert System for Food and Feed (RASFF) was created in 1979 to enable taking swift reaction when risks to public health are detected in the food chain. The EU has therefore enhanced its capability in controlling food safety risks and managing local and global emerging hazards (European Commission, 2016).

The international competition in the feed and food industry paved the way for fraudulent activities, which is likely to increase when more stakeholders are involved in the global supply chain. Thus, understanding the source and origin of food and raw materials, identifying vulnerabilities, and determining preventive measures are essential requirements entrenched in international regulatory requirements (e.g., United States, EU) and private standards to counteract food fraud. Extensive efforts have been directed toward enhancing analytical tests for the detection of microbial and chemical contaminants. The US Pharmacopeial Convention (USP) sets standards for the identity, strength, quality and purity of medicinal drugs, food ingredients, and food supplements produced, distributed and consumed worldwide (USP, 2016). The USP also established the Intentional Adulteration Expert Panel to develop a Food Fraud Mitigation Guidance. This guidance provides manufacturers and retailers with a comprehensive, practical four-step approach to conduct vulnerability analysis and develop a mitigation plan. To this end, this panel has created a food fraud database on current analytical technologies to detect counterfeits in specific products and substances (Moore, Spink, & Lipp, 2012; USP, 2016).

Many Arab countries are strongly dependent on food imports to meet the growing demands that exceeded domestic production (Arab Development Portal, 2020). The climate change effects and limited access to water resources, including the complex social and political factors, economic challenges and poverty, shrinkage in agricultural lands, and the rising in food prices, continue to pose significant food security challenges that will likely last for the coming decades (FAO/ESCWA, 2017). Achieving food self-sufficiency and sovereignty in the Arab region is particularly challenging in the Gulf Cooperation Council (GCC) region, where arable lands are limited. Hence, ensuring the safety and quality of imported foods and local goods is vital not only for public health concerns and trade participation but also for waste reduction, representing a significant threat to food security (Baig, Al-Zahrani, Schneider, Straquadine, & Mourad, 2019; Irani et al., 2018). For instance, the UAE rejected 6%–7% of imported shipments in 2001–03 due to their inconsistency with local food safety standards. In Bahrain, over 6 months in 2003, 379 tons of imported food products, unfit for human consumption, were confiscated due to their contamination with lead, mercury and cadmium, or foodborne pathogens (FAO, 2004a).

For the non-oil-producing Arab countries such as, Jordan, Egypt, Morocco, and Lebanon, the EU, and the United States represent crucial and lucrative markets for their food products; however, compliance to SPS measures and the high food safety standards of importing countries and its associated costs, market competition by other Mediterranean countries, and weak infrastructure undermine food trade opportunities (Brunel, 2009; Faour-Klingbeil & Todd, 2018; Hufbauer & Brunel, 2009; Torayeh, 2013). Improving food safety performance along the supply chain to meet the mandated international requirements is vital for boosting international and regional food trade, access higher-end niche markets, and maintaining competitiveness, promoting job opportunities and social stability.

Food safety represents a global public health issue. According to a report of WHO (2015), around 600 million people become ill, and 420,000 die each year from foodborne-related diseases. Such an enormous health burden requires food safety regulations and food control systems to effectively address the risks at all points along supply chains both locally and internationally. In 2001, 27% of food exports from Egypt, Jordan, Lebanon, and Syria to the United States were rejected by the FDA due to noncompliance with US national food laws (CSPI, 2005). In 1998, Egyptian potato exports to the EU were banned due to contamination from brown rot. To resume exports, Egypt had to submit files to prove that the Egyptian potato cultivation areas are completely free of the disease, caused in most cases by fungi (*Monilinia fructicola*). However, the EU authorities recognized only 23 of the 133 files submitted, claiming that the documentation was insufficient (the maps could not be thoroughly inspected and also the translation from the Arabic language to English was lacking), and only five regions were considered disease-free areas and were granted this status (FAO, 2004a).

Based on the review of the RASFF, a number of notifications have identified high aflatoxin content of some ground nuts and other exports from Egypt to the EU (Torayeh, 2013). The EU banned fish and fish products from Gulf countries for not meeting environmental and quality control requirements in the same year. This rejection led to a loss in exporters' market share. The public and private sectors subsequently incurred enormous costs to meet the health requirements, established laboratories and trained capacities, obtained technical assistance and implemented risk-based food safety systems to demonstrate compliance. The EU lifted the ban on Oman in 1999, on Yemen in 2002, and on UAE in 2003, when certificates were issued confirming that fish exports were fully compliant with the rules and standards (FAO, 2004a).

Food commodities are often subjected to a complex set of legislation to fulfill national and international food safety and quality requirements. In the context of international trade, importing countries determine the food safety objectives (FSO) as a regulatory requirement. The Codex standards, guidelines, and codes of practice have raised awareness on food safety in Arab countries and serve as a reference for setting their food legislation and national regulations, trade and dispute settlement, and strengthening agencies responsible for monitoring compliance with laws. Egypt, Jordan, Morocco, Sudan, Syria, and Tunisia have established national Codex committees (FAO, 2004a); also, of the twenty two Arab countries, nine are WTO members (Bahrain, Djibouti, Egypt, Kuwait, Mauritania, Morocco, Qatar, Tunisia, UAE) and eight are in the process of accession: Algeria, Comoros, Iraq, Lebanon, Libya, Somalia, Sudan, and Syria, whereas Palestine has participated in all WTO ministerial conferences as *ad hoc* observer since 2005 (WTO, 2020). Nonetheless, given the limited scientific, technical, and financial resources, their participation in the Codex technical committee meetings is not effective. To a certain extent, standards and regulations in several Arab countries are not entirely in line with the Codex Alimentarius and the WTO agreements; the lack of harmonization of national standards of most countries with international food safety standards has been a significant constraint to their access to developed country markets and leads to increased costs for exporters (Faour-Klingbeil & Todd, 2018).

8.3 National regulatory framework

Countries need to establish food safety regulations, apply appropriate food control systems to ensure safe local food production, and meet the FSO of importing countries. National regulatory frameworks are an essential pillar for any countries seeking an effective food control system. In recent years, updating national regulations and standards has received attention in some Arab countries. They brought their national food standards in line with Codex requirements and initiated reform and modernization of their systems and infrastructures for food control to incorporate risk analysis into their approaches. Some countries drafted new food legislation to meet the international requirements, such as Egypt, Jordan, Lebanon, Oman, UAE, and others integrated a risk-based approach,e.g. UAE and established an independent agency responsible for monitoring and controlling food safety, i.e. Saudi Arabia, Jordan, Oman). The pace of regulatory transformations and countries' capabilities to realize institutional reform and technological advancements in their national food control systems is primarily influenced by the existing political and economic conditions, which differ significantly among the Arab countries. The following sections describe the latest developments concerning the national food standards in both the Middle East and the GCC countries.

8.4 Egypt and the Levant States

These can be considered low- and middle-income with little in the way of oil revenues because the oil fields do not exist in these countries or they are not effectively managed. It is a typical case that favorable transformations in the food safety regulatory arena are slow in countries exposed to ongoing political stresses and upheaval, such as Syria, Lebanon, Palestine, and Iraq, and to some extent Egypt. These countries are exposed to constant political chaos or actual conflicts and lack a supportive environment that hinders any chances for progress and development (Faour-Klingbeil & Todd, 2019).

8.4.1 Egypt

Egypt intensified efforts to bring the national food standards in harmonization with Codex, at the same time shifting toward a risk-based approach in managing food safety through legislative reforms. The responsibility for food safety has long been divided between several agencies with overlapping spheres of authority, including the Ministries of Environment, Agriculture, Health, and Industry, with no apparent risk management structure and systems to handle significant food safety crises and traceability.

In 2017 the Egyptian parliament approved law number 1/2017 to establish the new National Food Safety Authority (NFSA), whose management constitutes the Board of Trustees, Board of Directors, and the Executive Manager. This step is a major leap to institute a new regulatory framework that consolidates the national food safety system and eliminate the overlapping functions of multiple agencies overseeing food safety regulation. The NFSA is an independent organization reporting directly to the Prime Minister's office and the only authority responsible for food safety regulation for domestic production, import and export through undertaking inspection, licensing, and certification (Ibrahim & Abdel-Haleem, 2016). It is mandated to establish the regulatory framework for food safety and modernize, strengthen, maintain the food safety system, capacity of analytical laboratories, and risk-based food inspection. The authority also ensures food handlers' compliance with the NFSA regulatory requirements, sets the necessary risk assessment procedures, analysis, management, communication, and awareness, including setting inspection priorities with the relevant international organizations' norms. Moreover, NFSA is responsible for conducting studies and research related to food safety to collect relevant scientific and technical data (FAO, 2019b). the authority management is distributed amongst the Board of Trustees, Board of Directors, and the Executive Manager.

Among many ministerial decrees, amendments and laws governing food and livestock production, import and export, some of the primary national legislations are shown in Table 8.1 (FAOLEX, n.d.).

Guided by the FAO/WHO Codex Alimentarius Commission and international food standards-setting bodies, the NFSA has embarked on modernizing the food import control systems that were initially mandated to the General Organization for Export and Import Control. The new system was established based on a risk-based approach in food import control and inspections so the consignments would be subject to different levels of sampling and verification at the borders according to a set of criteria. The criteria include the inherent risk factors of the food products, the robustness of the regulatory authority of the food consignment's country of origin, compliance of the shipment through a registered third-party or recognized foreign competent authority, and the history of compliance of the food importer (NFSA, 2020).

On the other hand, the Central Administration for Plant Quarantine (CAPQ) is the competent authority responsible for controlling phytosanitary issues and harmful organisms, issuing phytosanitary certificates, controlling exports of agricultural commodities and coordinating the activities relating to imports and exports of commodities of plant origin. CAPQ prohibits the food from export if it does not meet Egyptian food standards and can take legal actions against farms and packaging houses under decree No 670/2017 that do not comply with legislation (EC, 2019).

NFSA is a key factor in SAFE Project, an initiative implemented by the United Nations Industrial Development Organization (UNIDO) in partnership with several international organizations to facilitate trade. SAFE has been providing technical support to improve the ability of the NFSA under the Country Support Program in Egypt and assistance to build its capacity and support its mandate for effective implementation of the national food control system and the food safety agenda in Egypt. Under this initiative, Egypt will advance its national food safety and contribute to regional efforts of enhanced coordination and harmonization of food safety interventions (UNIC, 2018).

Meanwhile, the NFSA has moved toward coordinating the operational food control system by signing several memoranda with government entities to harmonize and streamline regulatory implementation and clearly define the various institutional responsibilities. Until the NFSA assumes its full responsibility, entities charged with overseeing food safety will continue to

TABLE 8.1 An unexhaustive list of the Egyptian national legislations.

Law/Decree	Scope
Resolution No. 2721 of 2004 prohibiting the use of antibiotics as a growing stimulator for animal, poultry, and fish.	It provides for the absolute prohibition of antibiotics as a growing stimulator, anabolic steroids, and thyrostatic treatment in forage and fodder used for animal, poultry, and fish feed.
Agricultural Law No.53 of 1966 amended by Law No.34 of 2018 for some provisions	
Law No. 124 of 1983 regarding fishing, aquaculture and fish farms regulations.	
Law No 10/1966 on food control	It controls the circulation of harmful/unfit food in the market and lays down the hygienic conditions for food production.
Law No.1 of 2017 establishing the National Food Safety Authority.	
Ministerial Decree No 3007/2001 of the MARL	It defines the export procedures for the export of plants and agricultural products.
Decree of the Minister of Health and Housing No. 204 of 2015	It defines the food additives authorized for use in the food industry.
Ministerial Decree No 757/2010	It lays down the requirement of all food and beverage processing establishments to apply Egyptian Standard (ES) No 4884/2008. This standard required HACCP or International Organisation for Standardization 22000, as from January 2011.
The joint Ministerial Decree No 670/2017	It defines the system of inspection and monitoring of Egyptian fresh fruits and vegetables export requirements to be applied on farm.
	It lays down the obligation that the farms obtained Global Good Agriculture. Practices certification before being officially inspected. For pack houses and exporters, Good Hygiene Practice/Good Manufacturing Principles systems inspected and certified by private bodies are required.
Egyptian standard 1546 (2011)	Labeling guidelines

Data from, EC (2019). Final report of an audit carried out in Egypt from 28 January 2019 to 07 February 2019 in order to evaluate the systems in place to control microbiological contamination in food of non-animal origin intended for export to the European Union (DG(SANTE) 2019-6697). *European Commission, Directorate-general for health and food safety.* https://ec.europa.eu/food/audits-analysis/act_getPDF.cfm?PDF_ID = 14389. Accessed 17.02.21;
FAOLEX (n.d.). FAOLEX Database—Egypt. *Food and Agriculture Organization of the United Nations.* Retrieved February 18, 2021, from http://www.fao.org/faolex/country-profiles/general-profile/en/?iso3 = EGY. Accessed 17.02.21;
GOEIC (n.d.). *General Organization for Export and Import Control.* https://www.goeic.gov.eg/en/documents/default/category/id/4/m/6-35. Accessed 18.02.21.

function, i.e. Ministry of Trade and Industry, Ministry of Health (MoH). The CAPQ and The General Organization for Veterinary Services under the Ministry of Agriculture (MoA) and Land Reclamation functions do not conflict with the NFSA responsibilities (GAIN, 2020).

While the recent developments in Egypt contribute to improving local products' food safety, the extent to which the new authority has advanced the planned agenda and realized the objectives are not broadly reported. Nonetheless, the 2019 audit report of the European Commission Directorate-General for Health and Food Safety in Egypt (EC, 2019) shed light on Egypt's efforts through a series of law amendments to bring the food standards up to the EU requirements and to foster and support food exports. The report reflected the clear transition to a gradual adoption of good agricultural practices and strict control over the food exports to ensure compliance with the importing countries requirements. For instance, the joint Ministerial Decree No 670/2017 concerning the production and export system of the vegetable and fruits crops requires all farms to be Global GAP[1] certified and all processing facilities and packaging stations to be ISO 22000[2] or BRC[3] certified (EC, 2019; GOEIC, n.d.), in addition to enforcing standards of hygienic practices (ES No 3586/2006) and food safety management systems (ES No 4884/2008). It also specifies standards for fresh strawberries (ES No 1704/2006) and for herbs and spices (ES No 7155/2010) (EC, 2019; FAO, 2004a). The EC audit reviewed the controls at the different stages of the production chain and export, besides the national legislation, the organization and operation of the competent authorities (CAs). It also reviewed the applied controls over food business operators' compliance with hygiene rules and the effectiveness of the response of the CAs to the RASFF notifications related to goods originating in Egypt.

The report concluded that the control system of microbiological risks of food of non-animal origin (FNAO) intended for exports to the EU is in a phase of transition and reform. At the processing stage of the food chain, official controls of FNAO are in place. The CAs demonstrated awareness of the requirements of EU legislation on FNAO. Hygiene practices at farms and exporters/processing facilities the audit team visited were in line with the relevant EU requirements. Some of the major findings were as follows:

- Legal provisions are in place to authorize the CAs to implement official controls and enforce corrective measures regarding microbiological risks in FNAO to be exported to the EU for all stages of production.

1. GAP is an acronym for Good Agricultural Practices. It is now the world's most widely implemented farm certification scheme. https://en.wikipedia.org/wiki/GLOBALG.A.P
2. ISO 22000 is a standard developed by the International Organization for Standardization dealing with food safety. It is a general derivative of ISO 9000
3. https://www.fda.gov/food/food-safety-modernization-act-fsma/full-text-food-safety-modernization-act-fsma

- The CAs have a structure, organization, powers, staff and resources which can adequately support the official control system covering the production chain of FNAO to be exported to the EU. For instance, the Egyptian Organisation for Standardisation and Quality is responsible for communication with CODEX and other organizations. It has issued many Egyptian Standards (ES), based mainly on international equivalent standards.
- The official control system addressing microbiological risks covers the primary production stage, processors, and exporters of FNAO intended for EU export, including documented follow-up/enforcement and follow-up action.
- The laboratories involved in official controls can carry out microbiological analysis with reliable and consistent results; however, only two official laboratories are involved in the control of microbiological contamination.

The CAs operate under a structured organization and with adequate resources which can support the official control system covering the production chain of FNAO to be exported to the EU.

On the other hand, Egypt has embarked on bringing food safety and hygiene information and knowledge to stakeholders and raising public awareness through the 5-year agreement between the NFSA and the World Food Program (WFP). This program signed in 2018 aimed to support the government's efforts to ensure access to safe, nutritious food by establishing an online training platform for food safety inspectors on critical issues related to food safety (i.e., Good Manufacturing Practices (GMPs) for food, food handling, and supply chains efficiency and launching several public awareness campaigns in hypermarkets, public parks and public transportation. The WFP was also tasked to develop the current NFSA website as a platform for sharing public awareness messages on food safety measures (WFP, 2018)

The NFSA improved the inspection and control systems, built the organization's management capacity, helped to train food safety inspectors, and created food regulations/standards that align with international norms, with the support of the United States Agency for International Development (USAID) and the US Department of Agriculture (USDA). Additionally, the USAID supports the NFSA to implement WTO-compliant food safety policies and scale up its domestic and international food trade through the five-year project "Transforming the Assessment and Inspection of Food Businesses." This project provides NFSA with the necessary technical and financial support responsive to the developing regulatory authority's evolving needs. Assistance will aim to harmonize Egyptian food laws and regulations and international standards, implement robust inspection systems, manage outbreaks, conduct science-based risk assessments, monitor Egyptian Food Safety systems, and reduce foodborne illnesses (GAIN, 2020).

8.4.2 Jordan

Being the country's standard-setting body, the Jordan Standards and Metrology Organization (JSMO): (1) prepares, approves, revises, and amends mandatory and voluntary standards and monitors their application; (2) adopts and approves other countries, regional, and international organizations' (Arabic or English language) standards, and; (3) cooperates and coordinates standardization and metrology issues with regional and international institutions. It is also the Codex inquiry point and a corresponding member of the International Organization for Standardization (ISO) and the International Organization for Legal Metrology. Jordan is a member of the WTO. Its accession to the WTO (April 11, 2000) coincides with economic and legislative structural reforms, bringing it in line with international standards and requirements (GAIN, 2017). Jordan's food control regime is governed by two laws: The Agriculture Law 44 (2002) and the Jordan Food Law 30 (2015), replacing the Jordanian Food Control Law 32 (2003). The new food law was enacted in May 2015 and entered into force within 30 days after being published in the official journal at the end of June 2015. The law gave the Jordan Food and Drug Administration (JFDA) the authority to supervise food imports and control processed foods' safety and quality issues. The statute was designed to ease the processed food importation and eliminate the deleterious effect of multiagency territorial disputes. The impact of the unification of the regulatory authority has been positive. Under the new food law, pertinent regulations are being revised, updated, and drafted by JFDA. The JFDA consists of a technical committee comprising of members that are representing various stakeholders, whose responsibility is to lay down technical instructions for food quality and safety and define control measures and risk assessment procedures. The new food law also establishes a high committee to adopt the instructions and measures issued by a technical panel of experts committee, outlining the food quality and safety control programs, testing methods, and selecting laboratories for food analysis (MAS, 2017). Accordingly, pertinent regulations have been revised, updated, and drafted by JFDA.

Furthermore, the food safety standards are now harmonized with the Codex Alimentarius requirements and revised to integrate into a risk-based food safety risk management. Jordan maintains a three-tier inspection rate system for imported food products based on the product's health risk. A document review is mandatory regardless of the level of inspection with different rates depending on the risk: high-risk products, 80%–100%; medium risk products, 25%–50%; and low-risk products, 5%–10%.

According to Agriculture Law 44, which stipulates the MoA responsibility for the safety of live animals and plants, importing raw food items is also subject to advance approval of import license from the MoA. The reasons for the up-front approval are to ensure compliance with SPS requirements and for keeping records or statistical tracking. Preliminary approval may be denied to protect domestic producer interests. As the JFDA and other Jordanian authorities have a very low tolerance for food standard violations, any consignment not meeting the official standard will be rejected and either destroyed or re-exported at the expense of the importer. It should be noted that Jordanian authorities stipulate that all meat products are halal as defined by the Jordanian government, and packaging requirements are being used as a barrier to trade in poultry parts. The maximum package size for poultry parts is set to 2.5 kg in an attempt to protect local producers from US poultry suppliers. Any food or feed including grains fall within the jurisdiction of MoA, yet the JFDA has the authority for the final decision. In the absence of a local standard, Jordan applies internationally recognized standards to locally processed food. Enabling laboratories capabilities is essential in a modern national food control system for adequate monitoring of food contamination along the food supply chain. Consumption of any such contaminants may lead to foodborne diseases. Through the USDA's extended support, the JFDA and the MoA improve their laboratories and scale up the testing methodology's scope to advance the national food safety agenda (GAIN, 2021).

8.4.3 Lebanon

A new food safety law 35-2015 was ratified by the Lebanese parliament in 2016. The new law proposes establishing an independent agency, the Food Safety Lebanese Commission (FSLC), and enforces food standards for alignment with the SPS measures and TBT. The Commission includes a board of directors comprising seven members assigned by the Council of Ministers. It will be responsible for setting food safety policy, risk assessment, testing process, the norms and technical standards related to food, pesticides, fertilizers, and fodder (MAS, 2017). It will also draft the by-laws and prepare the food safety plan in cooperation with the nine agencies currently responsible for food safety (Cortas, 2018). However, Lebanon's economic development, infrastructure, and political stability have been profoundly impacted by decades of internal and regional conflicts, albeit a post-civil war period that witnessed a resurge in its economy.

Consequently, FSLC has not been formed yet, which hinders the food safety law's implementation. This fact leaves food safety governed by nine government agencies of the different ministries without clear and defined responsibilities and coordination (Cortas, 2017, 2018; El-Jardali, Hammoud, Kamleh, & Jurdi, 2014). Lebanon made some improvements to the food control system's efficiency and capacity through a comprehensive review and qualifying trainers on the HACCP system with the FAO's support. Moreover, several internationally funded projects have been launched to leverage institutional capacities. For instance, the MoA, which has the sole mandate to regulate crops and animal products' safe production, established with the FAO's support a national project to push forward the GAP implementation for strengthening production and marketing of Lebanese agricultural products. This project aimed at improving institutional and producers' capacities and formulating a new framing law and registration decree for pesticide management (FAO, 2013). International donors' projects such as the Lebanon Investment in Quality Program, funded by USAID, also focused on enhancing food safety and quality expertise in the agribusiness and fresh products sectors (Land O'Lakes, 2018). All this has resulted in the revision and modernization of food standards and improved quality control systems. More than 1673 standards adapted from international standards are issued by the Lebanese Standards Institution (LIBNOR) of the Ministry of Industry (MoI) (CCIB, 2012). Nevertheless, to date, there is no food policy and actual law enforcement in Lebanon. Unclear institutional responsibilities and lack of a risk management structure weaken Lebanon's operational framework, which renders the solutions provided through funded programs or projects rather unsustainable in the long run.

Lebanon's seeking accession to WTO since 1999 has been hindered for the limited compliance with international standards and sanitary measures. The lax management in food control is a long-standing problem caused by poor coordination among the different agencies, duplication of functions, shortage in inspection staff, and antiquated system. This fragmentation in the regulatory system and the lack of science-based policies to match global food safety challenges lead to inefficient identification of food safety issues along the supply chain (Faour-Klingbeil & Todd, 2019) (Fig. 8.1) and limit enhancement of the existing testing capacities tasked to FSLC. At this stage, the food authorities rely on the Food Safety Research Institute, the Laboratories of the Industrial Research Institute, and the American University of Beirut Laboratories to control domestic and imported food (Cortas, 2017).

To address recurrent food safety problems and scandals, MoA and the MoI jointly issued in January 2011 regulation number 950/1, which stipulates that food and beverages manufacturing establishments should register with the MoA and be inspected for their compliance with health and technical standards (CCIB, 2012). This regulation addresses the implementation of food safety and hygiene along the various steps of the processed food destined for local consumption or exports in harmony with international practices and guidelines (i.e., GMP, HACCP and local regulations and standards such as the Lebanese standard number 656 "General Food Safety Rules"). Through the decision, the stated aim of the MoA is to motivate processors to voluntarily adopt the HACCP approach as the ministry does not seek to impose HACCP certification. Today, the private sectors rely on LIBNOR to obtain technical and educational support on food safety, HACCP, and other related areas to improve compliance with the local and international market

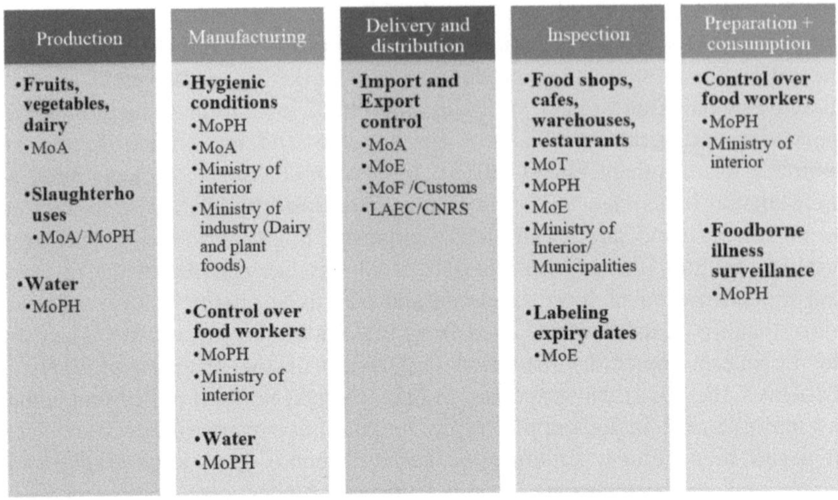

FIGURE 8.1 The functions of various national institutions along the food chain in Lebanon (Faour-Klingbeil, 2017). *MoPH*, Ministry of Public Health; *MoE*, Ministry of Economy and Trade; *MoT*, Ministry of Tourism; *MoF*, Ministry of Finance.

requirements (CCIB, 2012). Nonetheless, Lebanon's Food Safety system structure and operating mechanism are still underdeveloped to meet the challenges of emerging food hazards and international requirements.

8.4.4 Iraq

The food control system in Iraq is based on a multiagency approach. It involves different Ministries and Departments, e.g. MoA, MoH, Ministry of Trade, Ministry of Planning, Central Organization for Standardization and Quality Control (COSQC), MoI, Ministry of Environment, Radiation Protection Center, Ministry of Science and Technology, Ministry of Higher Education and Scientific Research, in addition to laboratories of factories, private sector laboratories, and consumer protection societies (Hasan & Gheni, 2011). Given that the implementation of the current food legislation in Iraq falls under these ministries with a lack of coordination, there are overlaps and duplication of effort and functions (El Haddad et al., 2011; Hasan & Gheni, 2011). For instance, the certification and testing of meat products for import and export controls fall under the jurisdiction of the veterinary services division of the MoA, MoH, COSQC_KSQCA/MoP, Ministry of Trade, and Ministry of Environment. The inspection and certification of foods and feed at ports of entry, warehouses and retailers are under the MoA, MoH, COSQC – KSQCA/MoP, Ministry of Trade, and Ministry of Environment (Hasan & Gheni, 2011).

Furthermore, the lack of trained staff, low fines, and limited financial resources hinder law enforcement and stakeholders' compliance. In 2004 the FAO (2004b) shed light on the importance of improving coordination between the various departments, ministries, and civil societies participating and implementing food control at the national level to achieve a coherent joint achievement. To this end, it emphasized the importance of avoiding duplication in functions and improving the food law. Similarly, the WHO experts's visit to Iraq in 2019 to assess the current state of food safety revealed critical gaps and weaknesses that need to be addressed in the national food control system with respect to (1) inter-sectoral coordination; (2) laws, regulations, and implementation of food safety policy; (3) emergency preparedness and response; (4) foodborne disease surveillance and response; (5) food safety monitoring and inspection; (6) information and communications; and (7) human resources and finances (WHO EMRO, 2019).

The Iraqi government is working on improving the level of preparedness for emergencies related to food safety through an emergency prevention system. In this respect, the FAO and WHO extend support for the government to identify areas for improving food quality control and control efforts. The food safety emergency prevention system shall ensure rapid exchange of information during food safety emergencies through the international network of authorities (WHO, 2021).

Risk assessment and risk management capabilities are essential for countries accession to WTO. The WTO Agreement requires compliance with SPS measures which currently is not fulfilled. There is a lack of a proper system to facilitate traceability of food of animal and plant origin from farm to fork, and the testing and inspection system is inadequate. The current system would not allow rapid testing and evaluation of goods to implement timely corrective actions. Besides, the existing food control system needs to be upgraded, mainly that the Iraqis rely on food import in the absence of adequate laboratories (ElAddad, 2011; Hasan & Gheni, 2011).

There are various laws and instructions to govern food safety in Iraq, but they are scattered among multiple ministries.

The current food safety legislation in Iraq consists of:

1. The Central Organization for Standardization and Quality Control (COSQC) Law No. 54/1979
2. General Health Law No. 89/1981
3. Food Law No. 29 /1982
4. Consumer Protection Law No. 1/2010
5. Plant Development and Protection Law No. 71/1978
6. Agriculture Quarantine Law No. 17/1966
7. Slaughtering Arrangement Law No. 22/1972
8. General Trade Laboratory Law

9. National Quality Control System/1988
10. Food Standards IQS/230/1989 on Labelling Requirements for Prepackaged and Canned foods were drafted in 1973 and were updated in 1978 by the COSQC.

The COSQC is an independent government agency established by Law no.54 in 1979 to manage quality control and standardization issues for government ministries and state-owned enterprises. Food standards in Iraq are established based on Codex Alimentarius and regulations and standards of neighboring countries such as Egypt, Jordan and GCC countries. The guidelines for shelf-life of foodstuffs were first established in 1986 and later updated in 1999 under Iraq General Standardization number 1847/1994, as published in the National Gazette issue number 3868 on March 5, 2001, (GAIN, 2011).

8.4.5 Palestine

Palestine, a country struggling for many decades with shortages of resources, deficient economic capabilities, and restricted trade, has a multiple-agency food control system. Like the countries mentioned above, food safety in Palestine is an issue dealt with by overlapping powers and conflicting functions of multiple institutions working to protect the consumers. Currently, the legal framework for food safety is fundamentally composed of Public Health law No 20 of 2004, Agriculture law No 2 of 2003, the Palestinian Standards and Measurements law No 6 of 2000, the Decree on the law of industry No. 10 of 2011, and the Consumer Protection law No 21 of 2005 (MAS, 2017).

There are considerable gaps in what form a robust regulatory structure, that is, well-trained inspectors, equipped laboratories, regulatory legislation, technical and logistical capabilities. At present, the regulatory framework governing food safety is fragmented, not harmonized, and does not match modern food safety legislation requirements in line with international standards (MAS, 2013, 2017). These shortcomings in the current legal and regulatory systems, together with the lack of routine inspections, legal deterrent sanctions and low fines, the weakness of the Consumer Protection Association's capacities, the absence of a judicial committee as outlined in the regulations of the Consumer Protection Act (MAS, 2013), all encourage non-compliance and fraudulent activities along the food chain.

Notwithstanding these challenges, the government is strengthening the control systems for food safety and national food products' competitiveness. In 2017 the Council of Ministers approved the National Food Safety Strategy (2017–22), which comes within the framework of capacity building and support in the field of SPS measures, including building the capacities of official inspectors in the field of food control (SAMA news, 2019). With the support of international donors, the Cabinet endorsed the National Quality Policy for Palestine in 2014. Accordingly, a national steering committee for implementing the assistance policy, chaired by the Minister of National Economy and composed of representatives of the MoH, MoA, Public Works and the Palestine Standards Institution, was established to fulfill the objectives for a "Quality Infrastructure." The quality infrastructure is defined as the totality of the institutional framework required to develop and implement standardization, metrology (scientific, industrial, and legal), accreditation and conformity assessment services (inspection, testing, and certification) necessary to provide acceptable evidence that products and services meet defined regulatory criteria and food trade requirements (MAS, 2017).

8.4.6 Syria

Food safety governance in Syria resembles in its approach that in Lebanon and Iraq. Syria has embarked on updating its food standards and regulations. Several activities undertaken with FAO's support have contributed to improving food control systems in Syria by strengthening quality control measures and coordinating tasks among the various national agencies involved in food control (FAO, 2004b). Furthermore, in 2008, law no. 19 of 2008 related to food safety was issued to ensure the safety, health, and quality of locally produced, imported, exported, and traded food in Syria, in addition to regulating the control of imports, exports and local food products following the national specifications and international agreements, including the Codex Alimentarius (Syriandays, 2021).

The new law is a fundamental shift in food control and safety aligned with the national and global food requirements to protect the consumer and the national economy. It stipulates the general requirements for controlling food production, export and import control to ensure the safety, health, and quality of locally produced, imported, exported, and traded food following national and international standards adopted by the Competent Authority. More specifically, the provisions address all the conditions and processes during the production, processing, storage, and distribution of food to ensure its safety or suitability for human consumption. It consists of 40 articles that aim to bring the national standards in line with international requirements and define the responsible bodies for law implementation.

According to the new law, a National Food and Drug Authority is set to be created to monitor the food products' safety in its various stages and unify all regulatory bodies' efforts (Aliqtisadi, 2011). For instance, under this law, the Ministry of Economic and Trade is the responsible entity for ensuring implementation of the law, compliance with the standards and recommendations of the Codex Alimentarius Commission, and verifying that food conforms to the technical rules approved by the Food Safety Authority (AlJaml, 2008).

The national food authority has an expanded power to ensure all production stages are monitored by applying science-based solutions. The authority will provide the laboratories with modern equipment, tighten control over imported foods, and take measures to ensure the entry of safe food according to the national specifications and promote adequate awareness among producers, owners of food establishments and consumers. However, the current overlapping and multiplicity of regulatory agencies in Syria are still a problem that undermines the practical operability of the food control system. The customs monitor imported food, the MoE monitors food Markets, and the MoT is responsible for food safety in tourist establishments, restaurants, and hotels. Besides, the MoH, MoA, local administration, the pharmacist's union and authority of Standards and the Atomic Energy Commission have also essential roles in food safety.

Meanwhile, besides establishing a national Codex committee, national laboratories' analytical capabilities for food control were upgraded and improved for their performance with the FAO' support to reach the levels required by international certification bodies. Yet, in its current state, the regulatory oversight appears fragile and weak given the shortage of qualified food inspectors and lack of communicating food safety as an area of public health concern with all stakeholders (Aliqtisadi, 2011). According to available news (2011), food fraud has increased in recent years, with meat retailers and distributors selling expired goods in the markets and smuggled meat, in particular, being a constant concern for the Syrian consumers. Also, inadequate storage and holding conditions of meat are common in the market and generally not adherent with the sanitary requirement.

8.5 Gulf Cooperation Council countries

8.5.1 Introduction

The GCC countries enjoy political stability and economic strength, which help provide a supportive environment for advancement at all levels, including food safety governance. In 1993 the GCC countries adopted the Gulf Standard 150/1993, Part I, for shelf-life durations of food products, which was an initial step toward the regulatory harmonization. Harmonizing food policies, regulations and standards, including labels and shelf-life, have achieved milestone development in member countries of the GCC with the formulated joint procedures for food exports that allow for common inspection policies and standards. Food produced in or imported from any member countries enjoys the freedom of movement in the various GCC countries. The GCC countries have also formed food safety committees to serve as a forum for all relevant Ministries and Agencies to cooperate in food control and legislation in this field.

In 2005, the GCC Standardization Organization (GSO), a standards organization for the member states of the Gulf Cooperation Council and Yemen, was established and headquartered in Riyadh. It comprises seven national standards bodies of the Arabian Gulf countries (UAE, Saudi Arabia, Kuwait, Bahrain, Oman, Qatar, and Yemen), with the Saudi Arabia being the most influential member.

As a group, GSO strives to create a common set of food regulations and standards. The GSO's Food Standards Committee (FSC) is responsible for drafting new food regulations and standards and updating existing ones. Chairmanship of the GSO FSC rotates among member states. All GSO draft standards are submitted for review and approval to the GSO Board of Directors (BOD), which is composed of Ministers responsible for standardization of each Member State and meets twice a year to deliberate on standards and other related issues. Once the GSO's BOD approves a new standard, it is supposed to be implemented in each member state after a grace period of six months from the date of approval (GAIN, 2014).

In practice, GCC countries differ concerning the timing of implementation and the enforcement of new GSO technical regulations. GSO issues two types of official documents that govern food and agricultural products:

1. GSO technical regulations: all technical regulations are approved unanimously by all member countries, they replace existing national standards, and their implementation is mandatory in all member counties.
2. GSO standards: a majority vote adopts GSO standards, and their implementation is voluntary in member countries, unless it is legalized in the national law. Technical regulations that address high priority topics are mandatory in performance (GSO, 2018).

GSO standards[4] are typically based on Codex Alimentarius and some extent, on European and US standards but are modified to reflect local religious, cultural, and climatical conditions. GSO often adopts existing member countries standards after updating them to conform with Codex Alimentarius guidelines and ISO standards. GSO Ministerial Board has authorized GSO to adopt International Standards in their original language as a fast track measure to develop and increase the total number of Gulf standards. As such, the GSO has adopted several ISO and Codex technical regulations and standards in their original language in the past few years.

The fourth meeting of the GCC Ministerial Committee on food safety hosted in the Sultanate of Oman in 2019 has urged the execution of the provision of a proposed GCC Unified Food Law applied across the member states; Sultanate of Oman, Saudi Arabia, UAE, Qatar, Bahrain and Kuwait, as follow-up of the decision made in the previous Ministerial Committee back in 2017 and 2018 (Gulf News, 2003). Furthermore, a GCC Guide for Control on Imported Foods unifying the monitoring procedures for imported

4. http://www.gso.org.sa/standards/public/standardsList.seam.

foodstuffs was approved by WTO and is used as a voluntary guideline to regulate the import requirements for all member states (Cooperation Council for the Arab States of Gulf, 2016). Currently, the GCC's CAs apply an integrated and harmonized import inspection and certification system that is risk-based and conforms with the obligations of the relevant WTO agreement (Cooperation Council for the Arab States of Gulf, 2016).

Moreover, in 2012, the Gulf Rapid Alert System for Food, formed by the GCC Food Safety Committee linking all the GCC member states, was set up to facilitate the rapid exchange of information on food-related emergency cases. Notification on food contaminants, the safety of food contact materials, foodborne diseases, and product withdrawals are communicated among the member states to prevent such products from entering their borders, as a preventive measure to protect their consumer's safety and well-being (SFDA, 2015). At a country level, most of the GCC countries, such as Oman, UAE, Saudi Arabia, and recently Kuwait, have adopted a unified food control system based on the single agency approach or the integrated approach (Alrobaish et al., 2021). This restructuring process of national food safety governance has led such countries to upgrade their food legislation and adhere to international food safety and quality standards (Jia & Jukes, 2013).

The GCC Guide for Control on Imported Food (2015) documents the factors taken into account in applying the risk-based food control system. Foods are classified according to their potential to transmit foodborne disease relative to their intended end-use. Risk profiles for classification of foods will include reference to (1) likelihood of contamination with biological, chemical and/or, physical hazards; (2) likelihood of significant levels of contamination persisting throughout the food chain; (3) potential risks to human health for the general population; (4) potential risks to human health for susceptible subpopulations; (5) effect of consumer food suitability demand on modifying risks. Based on these criteria, food will be classified into three general categories: high, medium, or low potential risk to human health. The number of risk categories may be increased based on risk assessments conducted. The CAs of the GCC countries will interact with CAs in other countries to identify and manage the risk of new or emerging hazards in the food supply. Where the GCC countries do not have the technical ability to monitor imported foods for new or emerging hazards, it is expected that the competent authority in the exporting country will have applied the same tests and safeguards as for food in their domestic market.

8.5.2 Bahrain

In the Kingdom of Bahrain, the majority of consumed foods is imported from all over the world. Therefore, the Bahrain government has established the Food Control Section, which is responsible for controlling and protecting food from contamination and taking care of consumers' health through assurance of a high level of food safety. Thus, to achieve the desired goals, the Food Control Section is divided into two groups: (1) the Imported Food group and (2) the domestic food safety and licensing group. Bahrain has a role in developing policies and guidelines and participating in the standards formulation, implementation, and evaluation, particularly with the GCC Food Safety Committee and other relevant activities. For instance, Bahrain is a member of the GCC Technical Sub-Committee on GCC legislation of organic, functional and Genetically Modified Food since 2008. So far, there are eight legislations on GM food and feed. More specifically, the Public Health Directorate, MoH, in conjunction with the Directorate of Standards and Metrology, Ministry of Commerce (MoC) are responsible for formulating food regulations (GAIN, 2012). The Directorate of Agencies and Industrial Property, MOC, is responsible for formulating and enforcing trademark and agency laws. The Directorate of Customs and Ports, Ministry of Finance and National Economy, is responsible for enforcing local agency laws. The Public Health Directorate, Food & Water Control Section (FWCS), MoH, is responsible for enforcing food safety regulations. For example, the FWCS is responsible for inspecting all imported fresh fruits and vegetables and processed food products, ensuring compliance with label regulations and, if deemed necessary, drawing samples and laboratory testing the products. Live plants and live animals are the responsibility of the Agricultural Affairs, Ministry of Municipalities Affairs and Agriculture. The Food Safety Committee, an interagency committee composed of representatives from the MoH, the Directorate of Standards and Metrology, Director of Consumer Protection, MOC and the Directorate of Agriculture, Ministry of Municipal Affairs & Agriculture, oversee all food safety and control issues, including the imposition of product bans.

The mission of food safety in the MoH in the Kingdom of Bahrain is to protect the health of the consumers from any health hazard and ensure that food, whether imported, prepared, or manufactured locally, is safe and fit for human consumption. The Public Health Law No. 3 of 1975 gives authority to the MoH to carry out inspections and issue notifications and warnings, fines, with closure notices for offenders with litigation before forwarded to the courts (Bahrain Ministry of Health, 2014). Along the same lines, the Green Sticker project was launched in 2013, where the Green Sticker is displayed on the front window of assessed restaurants that have shown 80% or more compliance to health standards. The project includes awarding food outlets that achieve a 100% food safety standard, a blue sticker, while those meeting 80% of the standard are awarded a green sticker. Outlets that fail to achieve basic standards are warned with a red sticker. The total number of outlets assessed between August 2013 and February 2015 was 241, 17 of which were presented with blue stickers, 174 with green stickers and 50 of them received red stickers. This informs the consumer of the relative safety of the establishment and reflects the tendency to provide safer food and protect consumers from food poisoning. The sticker is valid for 6 months after which, it is reassessed to ensure that it maintains compliance with our requirements. The project has encouraged participating restaurants to reach and maintain a very high safety level. In 2013/14, 67%–77% of restaurants received a green sticker status. A total of 54,968 inspection visits were conducted in 2014 by 25 inspectors from the food safety and licenses group, which closed 41 of around 7000 registered outlets (Anonymous, 2015). A total of 71,886 visits revealed around 883,584 tons of imported food was consumable, compared with almost 1873 tons rejected as nonconsumable during the same period. It was also reported in 2015 that many homes sell food without a license, and some people even had barns where they slaughtered livestock and sold the meat illegally. A recommendation was made to have a new Public Health Law that would impinge harsh punishments for outlets that neglected food safety.

In January 2003, the "GCC Unified Customs Law and Single Customs Tariff" (UCL) was released (GAIN, 2012). The UCL established a unified customs tariff of 5% on nearly all processed food products. Under the UCL, some food products, including live animals, fresh fruits and vegetables, seafood, grains, flour, tea, sugar, spices and seeds for planting, are exempt from tariffs. It also established a single-entry point policy. In other words, a product entering any GCC member market would pay the appropriate duty only at the point of entry. It would then be permitted duty-free transit among GCC member countries.

This same report states that the Imported Food Safety Group (IFSG) is responsible for the safety and authenticity of all imported foods that enter through various ports in the Kingdom of Bahrain, being Air Cargo, Khalifa Bin Salman and King Fahad Causeway Ports. Besides National Standards and Regional Standards, IFSG follows the SPS and TBT Agreements as guides to international trade regarding food safety topics. IFSG is responsible for inspecting foods to determine whether they conform to relevant criteria and food standards regarding standards for raw materials, food additives, foods labeling, and hazardous substances such as pesticides, veterinary drugs, etc. As mentioned IFSG is responsible for controlling and monitoring all types of foods and drinks from being contaminated with pathogenic bacteria, viruses etc. or any other chemical and physical contaminants that could make foods unsuitable for human consumption. The main achievements for this group up to November 2014 were as follows:

- The Food Microbiology unit contributing the majority of this group with a total work load of 11503 tests (4002 food samples).
- Water analysis conducted for 2343 water samples.
- Analyses on treated sewage water parasites for 188 samples.
- Food Poisoning Samples analyses conducted for 393 suspected samples.

8.5.3 Kuwait

In four of the GCC countries, namely Kuwait, Qatar, Oman and the UAE, food control is spread across several government ministries and agencies (Al-Kandari & Jukes, 2009). In Kuwait, Oman, and Qatar, issues directly related to public health, such as food hygiene and sanitation and foodborne disease surveillance, are dealt with by the health authorities at central and local municipal levels. Matters related to food production, processing, and distribution, including controlling the quality and safety of foods of animal origin, fall under the municipal authority. In Kuwait, there are several governmental authorities and agencies involved in food safety and control. The enforcement of food control regulations is divided among the Kuwait Municipality (KM), the MoH, the Public Authority for Industry (PAI), the Public Authority for Agriculture Affairs and Fisheries Resources and the MoC. However, primary authority for food control comes under the jurisdiction of the KM, which has responsibility for all domestic and imported foods and food establishments. It seeks to ensure that foods from these sources are safe, nutritious and adequately labeled (Alomirah et al., 2010). Kuwait consists of six governments, each has a KM Food Control/Inspection regional office (Al-Mazeedi, Abbas, Al-Jouhar, Al-Mufty, & Al-Mendicar, 2015). In addition, there are five regional KM slaughterhouses and five regional KM food import offices. All of the sixteen regional KM offices are supported by food inspectors that act as another technical arm for all KM routine food inspection activities enforcing food inspection laws. Other agencies involved in food safety control are the department of imported foods and the department of sanitary municipal services control of KM and the food control laboratory at MoH. University (Health) Colleges provide technical advice, labor, and supports the local food industry. Scientific research is also provided to support KM, the MoH, and Public Authority for Applied Education and Training (PAAT) on strategic issues to help in improving the functional role of agencies and authorities. In Kuwait, major research activities are carried out by a governmental body mainly by the Kuwait Institute for Scientific Research (KISR), Kuwait University (KU) and PAAT which provide research and technical support to the food sector. The Kuwaiti Food Safety and control system aims to safeguard Kuwaiti's food supply with high-quality and safe standards.

The reported decline in foodborne illnesses may be due to a lack of reporting systems or underreporting even with reporting systems in place. Food laws will need to specify the responsibilities of national authorities in integrating food controls at all stages of production and in all sectors in the context of the farm-to-fork supply chain (Al-Kandari & Jukes, 2009). Currently, food safety and control system regulations are set by PAI, KM, MoH, PAAF, and KISR as mandatory for food businesses and food handlers being subjected to inspection according to these food regulations. The primary food laws are KM 21/92, which addresses the general food safety; KM 25/92 is related to mobile (street vendor type) shops of convenient and cooked food; KM 26/92 pertaining to shops and factories that sell or manufacture food; GCC food standard 21/1984 specifies food factories must establish hygiene rules (prerequisite programs) that must be established by food factories; GCC food standards 150/1993 set the expiry date of packaged foods; PAI food standard 42/1973 deals with food labeling; GCC food standard 23/1998 that deals with food colors; MoH food standard 231/1989 that deals with particular foods. Before harvest, of animal or plant origin, foods are controlled by the PAAF (Al-Mazeedi et al. 2015). Imported live animals and plants, feedstuffs or horticultural products are being inspected at the port of entry to determine if quarantine is warranted. Boxes containing imported fresh fruits and vegetables are also regulated, but no special packaging type or size is required for other food products unless incorporated in processed food regulations. Imports of irradiated food products are permitted, as long as labels indicate irradiation. Kuwait enforces GCC shelf-life standards for food products and recognizes manufacturer-established shelf-life standards for all mainly imported food items from either neighboring Gulf countries or from abroad others.

Kuwait is becoming more involved in the international food trade, bringing new challenges for coping with international food control systems trends. In the past five years, Kuwait has increased its efforts to strengthen its food control system. Based on the WTO and Codex Alimentarius, Kuwait's national legislation is in compliance with the SPS and TBT Agreements, and all food standards in Kuwait are based on the Codex Alimentarius. There are 556 standards, of which more than 25% are mandatory. In Kuwait, food inspection is largely the responsibility of the KM with the department of imported foods and the department of sanitary municipal services control, also being responsible for inspection of imported food at all points of entry on land, air or sea, and also for the locally produced food products, respectively. For imported foods, Kuwait is increasingly using a system based on risk assessment to allow more targeted inspections. To eliminate inconsistencies, overlaps, and gaps, a centralized system for food control for inspection and laboratories, which acts as an independent governmental entity for food safety and quality has been established. As in other Gulf countries, a national rapid alert system to interlink all of the agencies, ministries, and organizations involved would enable the authorities to provide a comprehensive estimate of each hazard, an evaluation of emerging issues and new trends and finally, an assessment of the increasing risks in foods and feed from the raw material through to the finished product. Encouragement of training and education of food handlers would help in increasing knowledge and raising awareness of issues affecting the safety of the food they prepare and serve. Explaining their legal responsibilities and developing their skills and knowledge would allow government to promote correct hygiene practice at all steps in the food chain. In Kuwait, in its supplementary session in the second deliberation, the National Assembly approved the draft amendment of law No. (112) of 2013 for establishing the General Authority for Food Safety and Nutrition to ensure and protect consumers' health from foodborne diseases and epidemics. The law stipulates the intensification and detail of penalties and transferred responsibility for food control from the Kuwait Municipality to the General Authority for Food Safety and Nutrition. Moreover, Article No. (12) outlines explicitly the Food and Nutrition Authority's obligation to establish laboratories for inspecting imported foods that constitute a significant share of consumers' daily food consumption. Strengthening laboratory capacities is also necessary to facilitate the review process of imported goods and ensure the protection of goods when on hold. It also allows Kuwait to comply with the GCC Customs Union agreement. The agreement specifies any single-entry point, meaning land, sea, or air customs, and the GCC states should inspect and examine the imported goods. These goods will be exempted from reinspection at any other port in the GCC states (Kuna, 2019).

Al-Mazeedi et al. (2015) recommended more consistency among local health departments and their interpretations of the state food service rules by forming a Food Safety Review (FSR) panel of experts, a partnership between industry, government, academia, and the consumer. The mission of the FSR would be to work together with the department of health in developing advisory technical interpretations of the state food service regulations and other matters, relating to the Kuwait Administrative Code. FSR experts should also provide information on food handling practices and processes, guidance on "equivalency" determinations, providing recommendations for revisions to the Kuwait State Board of Health, and finally facilitating communications to all stakeholders regarding FSR activities and actions. Knowledge of food safety appears to be limited, based on a university survey study in which only 29% of students achieved a score of 5 or more out of 10 (Al-Khamees, 2007). Education status of the mother, but not of the father, was a significant factor in both knowledge and reported behavior concerning the storage, handling, and processing of foods. It is possible today, that the population is more aware of food safety issues, especially as there are several food safety courses available and widely accessible on the internet.

8.5.4 Oman

The Sultanate of Oman is going through a major transition with government reforming and restructuring. Food safety legislation is well constructed in Oman to ensure food and consumers' integrity and safety. Fig. 8.2 illustrates the various laws and regulations spanning over a wide range of the food supply chain.

Food in General

- Food Safety Law RD (84/2008)*and its Executive Regulations MD (2/2010)
- Food Control Regulation (29/2016) amending MD (241/1999)
- Muscat Municipality's Regulation on Health Requirements for Activities Related to Public Health MD (219/2019) amending MD (168/2011)

Agriculture, Animal and Fisheries Wealth

- Plant Quarantine Law RD(47/2004) and its Executive Regulations MD (32/2006) amending RD(91/2000)
- Veterinary Quarantine Law RD (45/2004)* and its Executive Regulations MD (107/2008)
- Pesticide Law RD (64/2006) and its Executive Regulations MD (41/2012) repealing MD (194/2007)
- Fishery Quality Control Regulation MD (12/2009)*repealing MD (136/98 & 4/97)
- Aquaculture & Quality Control Reg. MD (177/2012)* amending MD (36/2004)
- Fish Market Organization Reg. MD (312/204)
- Marine Aquatic Resources Transportation and Marketing Reg. MD (29/2004)

Relevant Laws

- Consumer Protection Law RD(66/2014) and its Executive Regulations MD (77/2017) amending RD (81/2002)
- GCC Unified Customs Law (67/2003)

FIGURE 8.2 Legislation governing the food safety in the Sultanate of Oman. *Under revision.

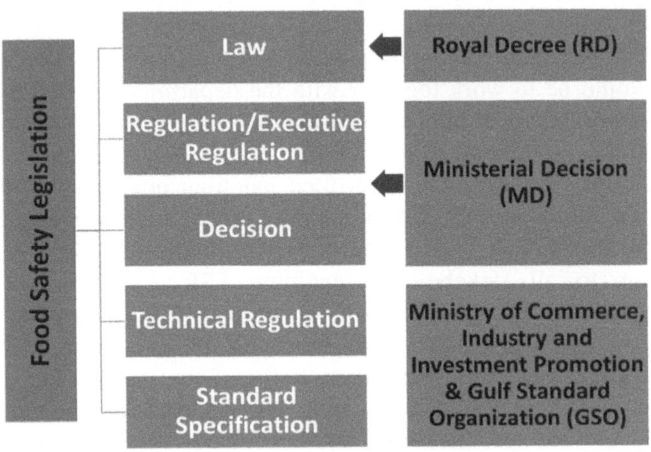

FIGURE 8.3 The Omani Food Safety Legislation Framework.

The primary legislation is the Royal Decree (RD), which is promulgated by the Sultan of the country. Secondary legislation is the Ministerial Decision (MD) and issued following specific powers that royal decrees delegate to the competent executive or ministerial body. Therefore, laws are promulgated by RD and regulation and executive regulations by MD as shown in Fig. 8.3. As for standards and technical regulations, they are issued by the Directorate-General for Standards and Metrology (DGSM), the country representive in the GSO, within the MoC, Industry and Investment Promotion, the national standard organization in Oman.

A Food Safety Committee comprising members from the various governmental entities was established by Article 13 of the Food Safety Law (84/2008) and later amended by the MD (272/2009), to coordinate the various authorities managing food safety in the country and assuring the implementation of an effective and competent system, given the complexity of the existing one (MJLA, 2019). To unify the effort and overcome the overlapping responsibilities of the various governmental authorities enforcing food safety law and regulation in Oman, the Council of Ministers approved establishing a national Centre for Food Safety and Quality under the auspices of the Ministry of Regional Municipalities and Water Resources in 2013 (Al-Busaidi & Jukes, 2015). By 2019, a RD 24/2019 was issued to establish the "Centre for Food Safety and Quality" within the Ministry of Regional Municipalities and Water Resources at a general directorate level. The decree stipulates all domain related to food safety and quality in terms of laws, royal decrees, regulations, employees and related departments shall be transferred to the stated ministry (MJLA, 2019). This effort aims to raise the country's food safety measures throughout the farm to plate continuum and ensure a high level of consumer protection and public health with a principal goal of transitioning gradually from a multi-agency system into an integrated one and subsequently a single food safety authority in the upcoming years. This approach will allow time for the consolidation system to work effectively before unifying the entire system into one entity.

The strategic approach "Oman Vision 2040" was set to promote decentralization in governance. In this context, the new RD 92/2020 was issued to allocate all the provisions, origins, rights, obligations, and assets of the Public Authority for Stores and Food Reserve, the divisions of Water Resources, and the Food Safety and Quality Centre (FSQC) at the Ministry of Regional Municipalities and Water Resources to the newly renamed Ministry, e.g. MoA, Fisheries Wealth, and Water Resources (MAFWR) (MJLA, 2019). Equally, RD No. 101/2020 on regulating governorates and municipal affairs was promulgated, assigning all allocations, assets, rights, obligations, duties, and holdings of the regional municipalities to three governorates, Muscat, Mussandam and Dhofar, whereas other governorates duties are carried out by the Ministry of Internal Affairs (MIA) (MJLA, 2019). The reformed management and enforcement system will coordinate among the different authorities within an integrated approach to facilitate a comprehensive food safety system covering the farm-to-fork continuum, as shown in Fig. 8.4. MoA, MAFWR will govern food safety and quality. This approach adopts a risk-based system meeting the food safety challenges for domestic, import, and potential export markets.

MoA, MAFWR, according to RD (92/2020) is the competent authority for food safety; therefore, the issuance of all legislation will be its primary responsibility. FSQC, a directorate under the MAFWR designated as the national regulatory authority in governing and fulfilling all the national and international

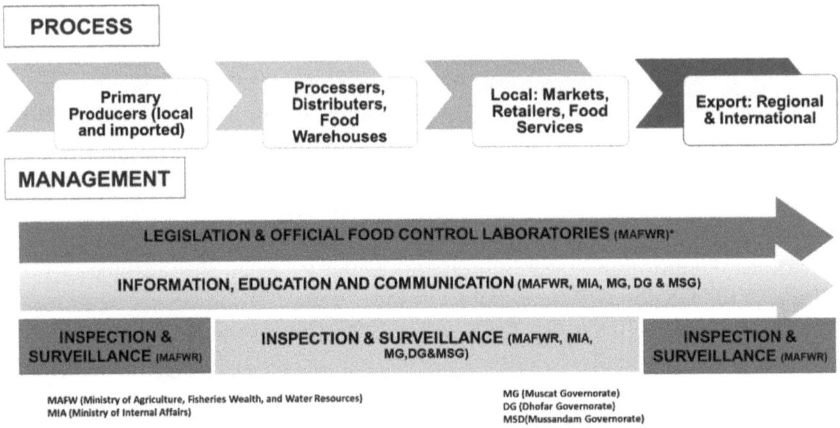

FIGURE 8.4 The process and management of the food supply chain from farm to fork in Oman.

requirements of food and safety and quality. Other authorities will abide by this legislation, a step that will standardize legal codes in the country.

FSQC manages the official food control laboratories at the central level with subdivisions in the different governorates. All official laboratories are accredited with ISO 17025 and recognized internationally. Food safety laws and regulations enforcement will be carried out in an integrated manner with more than one entity involved. MAFWR will lead the shared responsibilities among these entities with effective coordination with its counterpart, the MIA, Muscat, Mussandam and Dhofar Governorates. Seafood safety, on the other hand, will under the jurisdiction of MAFWR. The latter was the primary regulator in the country besides being bound by international agreements with the European Commission (EC), Eurasian Economic Union, the United States, and others designating it as the CA representing the Omani Government in the global fisheries market (Busaidi, 2017).

The Communicable Diseases and Surveillance Control within the MoH is in charge of the surveillance of foodborne diseases outbreaks in the country by liaising with governmental and private hospitals at the different governorates.

Information, Education and Communication (IEC) activities have been crucial for the national food control authorities. Food safety conferences, seminars, and workshops are conducted annually to raise awareness and educate the different stakeholders in the food supply chain. These platforms have provided a mean for informative forum for learning, networking and opportunity to share information, education and communication among government officials, academia, food industry and consumers. A Food Safety Week is held every April of each year throughout the country to raise public awareness of the importance of food safety and quality. This awareness campaign consists of various programs ranging from mobile awareness seminars, exhibitions highlighting various topics related to the safety of food and foodborne diseases and their causes, school lectures, educational, cultural, and recreational events, inspection campaigns and ending the week with an international conference. The conferences address the latest developments in the field, and share scientific and practical experiences of experts worldwide.

8.5.5 Qatar

In its Qatar Public Health Strategy 2017–22, the Ministry of Public Health (2021) states that food safety control plays a critical role in quality assurance and observance of standards for the import, production, processing, preparation, and disposal of food products. Food safety control is essential, given that approximately 90% of foods available in Qatar is imported. Rapid population growth continues to increase pressure on food inspection services and port authorities and the importance of having adequate control to prevent the potential risk of foodborne disease outbreaks. The ministry admits that foodborne diseases occur, mainly caused by various pathogens, including *E. coli, Salmonella* spp. (nontyphoidal and typhoidal) and more recently, norovirus in seafood products. The number of reported cases of food poisoning has increased since the beginning of this century. However, a large proportion of this increase may be due to population growth mainly driven by a continual influx of multicountry expatriates representing more than 80% of the population and globalization of food trade and increased tourism. However, like in other countries, underreporting of foodborne infections remains an issue that requires further attention in Qatar (Farag et al., 2016).

The ministry has specific goals related to food safety, as follows:

- Promote public awareness of nutritional and health risks from consuming unsafe foods by employing various effective mass media communication channels.
- Strengthening the capabilities of the food safety management system to provide services that conform to international best practices in important functional areas, such as inspection services, laboratory services, risk analysis, and setting standards for oversight, supervision, and regulation.
- Creating an integrated food safety device whose work is in line with international best practice standards for food safety management throughout the food supply chain, from farm to consumer.
- Create an integrated risk-based inspection service that is in line with relevant international standards, such as ISO/IEC 17020: 2012 specifications for imported, home-made and exported food products, backed by modern electronic management systems, effective diagnostic services, and control and supervision systems.
- Promote a culture of food safety among all parties involved in the food supply chain by implementing effective public-private partnership programs to enhance awareness of the need to take responsibility for managing food risks.

The Department of Public Health (DPH), is part of the MoPH involved in most functions related to food safety. The DPH, in coordination with the General Organization for Standards and Metrology and the Ministry of Economy & Commerce, is responsible for establishing food safety regulations. Additionally, the National Food Safety Committee (FCC) decides on all food safety and control issues, including import bans. Qatar also has its central food laboratories established in the early 1970s. Qatar's municipality inspectors randomly check food products in wholesale and retail markets typically unannounced. In addition to the visual inspection of labels, samples are collected and analyzed to ensure product ingredients match those listed on the label. If a discrepancy is found, the product is removed and destroyed at the importer's expense.

Over the years, several laws related to food and food establishments were introduced in the State of Qatar (Eltai, El-Obeid, Kassem, & Yassine, 2018). Law No. 8 (1990) organizes and controls human foods and the process of food trade in the State of Qatar and sets associated penalties and fines, including food labeling. Law No. 4 (2014) amended specific provisions of Law No. 8 to give the State the ability for judicial enforcement on offenses that violate Law No. 8, including the power to shut down facilities and stores and post signage on the premises to indicate violations of food safety regulations. These provisions grant the authority to oversee all imported foods, including fruits, vegetables, spices, meat and meat products, milk, and fish . Most food products were imported via trucks from UAE and Saudi Arabia before the 2017 embargo by many Arab states. These border crossings were reopened in 2021. But alternative routes were developed to include seaport and air transportation and mainly engage fresh fruits and vegetables and chilled meat. Other essential regulations include Packaging and Container Regulations: GS 839/1999; Food Additives Regulations; and Pesticides and other contaminants: QS 382/1996 and QS 383/1996. Eltai et al. (2018) conclude that, because of the importance of food safety in the country, published awareness guidelines (that provide stakeholders in food processing facilities and food service establishment with information) must be followed during food handling to reduce transmission of foodborne illnesses. Such food safety awareness programs are developed by the Ministry of Municipality and Urban Planning to target several different sections of society, including workers in food establishments, officials, school students, consumers, and tourists/holidaymakers.

8.5.6 Saudi Arabia

Much of the information on the Food Laws in the Kingdom of Saudi Arabia (KSA) is based on the GAIN system (Gain, 2014). For religious reasons, Saudi Arabia bans imports of alcoholic beverages, biotech-based animal products, live swine, pork and food ingredients or additives that contain pork products, including pork fat, rennet, and gelatin. Meat and poultry shipments must be accompanied by a "Halal" slaughter certificate issued by an Islamic center in the country of origin. Saudi Arabia also bans cattle, meat, and meat products imports from countries implicated in the past (e.g., the United Kingdom) in foodborne diseases such as BSE, Foot and Mouth, and Cattle Plaque. Such imported products are banned until the affected countries have declared free of the diseases by the World Organization for Animal Health (OIE) and proof is provided. Imports of live poultry, poultry meat and hatching eggs are banned from countries that were affected by bird flu. Imports of live poultry are also banned from countries that were affected by the West Nile Virus epidemic. In 2003 the Saudi Ministry of Commerce and Industry issued Ministerial decree number 2436 to all Chambers of Commerce in the country, requiring a new clause in health certificates. According to this decree, all meat and meat products processed in foreign abattoirs should comply with the HACCP system to be exported to the Kingdom of Saudi Arabia. Saudi Arabia is one of the countries that comply with Codex Alimentarius and SPS and TBT Agreements. KSA has adopted a strongly worded resolution that recognizes food safety as an essential component of a Public Health function and priority. The development of an interdisciplinary approach with direct interaction between the monitoring, surveillance and risk analysis systems could be a potential basis for improved foodborne disease prevention in KSA (El Sheikha, 2015).

The Saudi Food and Drug Authority (SFDA) was established under the Council of Ministers resolution no (1) dated January 1, 2003, as an independent body chaired by the Crown Prince and reports directly to the King well as the Prime Minister. The SFDA is responsible for regulating, overseeing, and controlling food, drug, medical devices, and setting mandatory standard specifications thereof, whether imported or locally manufactured. The control and testing activities can be conducted at the SFDA or any other agency's laboratories. Moreover, the SFDA is in charge of consumers' awareness of food, drug, and medical devices and associated other products and supplies. All food, drinks, and edible agricultural products, including food ingredients and processed animal feed, whether locally manufactured or imported to Saudi Arabia, must comply with regulations and standards laid down by SFDA or GSO.

The SFDA's Food Sector has nine Executive Departments: (1) Imported Foods Control, (2) Technical Regulations and Specifications, (3) Laboratories, (4) Control of Local Markets, (5) Risk Assessment, (6) Animal Feed, (7) Monitoring and Crisis Management Centers, (8) Awareness and Communication, and (9) Pesticides. The SFDA's Executive Department for Control of Local Markets is responsible for registering, licensing and license renewal of local food establishments (factories, distribution centers, warehouses of food and food products). It also conducts periodic inspections of facilities to ensure the implementation of licensing requirements. The agency works with the Environmental Protection Department at the Ministry of Municipality and Rural Affairs (MOMRA) to issue nationwide food sanitation laws and guidelines. MOMRA's inspectors at the municipality levels are responsible for monitoring food products already in the market. They inspect retailers, wholesalers, restaurants, bakeries, fast food chains, vegetable and meat markets for expiration dates, sanitary and storage conditions, as well as product handling. Outlets found selling unhygienic or expired products are subject to stiff financial fines or closure of facility (Gain, 2014).

On the other hand, biotech agricultural products exported to Saudi Arabia as well as to the GCC countries must have been approved in the country of origin for human or animal consumption or planting seeds and should meet all relevant Saudi and GSO approved regulations and standards requirements. Each shipment must be accompanied by an official health certificate issued by a competent government agency, stating that the GE ingredient(s) used in the foodstuff, grains or seed exported is/are approved in the country of origin for human or animal consumption or for planting seeds. SFDA accepts health certificates issued by the FDA, federal or state departments of agriculture for high value and processed feed products. All imported foodstuffs are inspected by the SFDA's Executive Department for Imported Food Control at Saudi ports of entry or Border Inspection Posts[5]. The majority of Saudi food imports enter the country via Jeddah port on the Red Sea or Dammam port on the Arabian Gulf. About 70% of all foodstuffs enter via Jeddah port (Al-Kandari & Jukes, 2012). Imports from nearby countries enter the Kingdom by trucks. King Khalid International Airport in Riyadh and King Abdulaziz International Airport in Jeddah also receive significant quantities of food items, particularly fresh fruits, vegetables and chilled meat. Fresh and chilled products are usually cleared within 24 h of arrival. Imported processed feed and feed ingredients are inspected by SFDA's EDAF. Shelf-life can only be shown by clear and unambiguous production and expiration dates. The use of any of the following statements for expressing expiration date is permissible: Expiration Date, Use by (date), Fit for (from the day of production), Use Before (date), Sell by date (for food products having an expiration period exceeding three months).

The Environmental Protection Department at the Ministry of Municipality and Rural Affairs is responsible for establishing national food sanitation laws and guidelines. The authorities inspect retailers, wholesalers, restaurants, bakeries, fast food chains, vegetable and meat markets for expiration dates, sanitary and storage conditions, and product handling. Outlets found selling unhygienic or expired products are exposed to stiff financial fines, temporary closure or bot (GAIN, 2017).

5. https://old.sfda.gov.sa/en/food/Pages/default.aspx

Updates on SFDA regulations and activities are found on their website[6] where there is a current list of food facilities exported to Saudi Arabia from around the world and a reference to the Journal "Food and Medicine in Saudi Arabia" concerned with publishing news and reports on the activities of the Authority, in addition to awareness topics and the latest scientific studies and discoveries worldwide in the field of food, medicine and medical devices. For instance, in June 2020, the authority implemented a national food monitoring program that includes the analysis of more than 10,000 food samples to ensure their safety from pollutants and create databases on the quality and quantity of food consumed by Saudi society. In addition, Food and Medicine carried out 51,756 inspection visits to food facilities, collected 29,645 samples and conducted more than 73,000 laboratory analyses. A further 136 scientific opinions were studied and prepared on various topics related to the safety of food products and an assessment of the safety of more than 277 food products. The SFDA also has periodic podcasts on different topics. For instance, the head of the Epidemiological Investigation Department, Mazen Al-Saghir, talked about food poisoning and its symptoms, contamination, and its relation to food poisoning, on measures and strategies to avoid food poisoning to occur. El Sheikha (2015) recommends improving tracking and traceability systems to be incorporated into information systems where consumers can receive information on any product. Traceability systems enable efficient product recall and allow fewer products to be recalled if they are prevented from reaching the retail level.

8.5.7 United Arab Emirates

The UAE depends largely on imports to secure up to 90% of its food demands. The UAE opted for the integrated approach and centered its food safety system around HACCP and risk analysis by developing a national food safety committee, consisting of representatives from different ministries and agencies (The Official Portal of the UAE Government, n.d.). This reference covers all the following section. In January 2016, Federal Law No. 10 of 2015 on food safety was approved. The law imposes standards and regulations for maintaining the safety and quality of food and ensuring the protection of public health and consumers. The law imposes strict penalties on those found to be endangering food safety across the UAE. Some aspects of the UAE food laws are no food may be imported into the country for the first time without the approval of the Ministry of Climate Change and Environment. Those dealing in food or products that contain pork or alcohol or any of their by-products without permission, face a prison term of not less than a month and a fine of up to AED 500,000 (AED 1 = USD 0.27). Misleading consumers by publishing a false description of food or using

6. General Standards for Food (sfda.gov.sa)

incorrect labels will attract a fine ranging from AED 10,000 to 100,000. The law authorizes MoE to impose fines of up to AED 100,000 for other offenses, provided that the Cabinet regulates these offenses. Through its National Food Safety Committee, the Ministry of Climate Change & Environment works with its partners on implementing the law on safety of food and its executive regulations, which includes strict controls and standards to ensure food safety throughout the food chain.

The National Food Accreditation and Registration System of 2018 states that food, whether imported or locally produced, or modified on its food label or ingredients or composition, must be registered in the electronic system, which is an integrated smart platform for food products data, before being handled in the UAE's markets. The National Rapid Alert System for Food launched in 2017 ensures proper implementation of response measures when serious food risks are detected. The system identifies the mechanisms of managing food risk alerts and banning and lifting bans on adulterated and misbranded food. The system components include assignment of responsibilities and roles, identifying types of food alerts, identifying the criteria to report food incidents, including border rejection of food and adulterated products in the market. The system applies a classification matrix to the food incidents as either high, medium, or low. It also includes the triggers for the classification, namely the severity of the risk to public health, the size and scale of an incident and the number of people affected.

According to Ministerial Decree No. 14 of 2016 on Controlling of Imported Food for Non-trading Purpose, personal food is allowed to be imported through the country's borders with a restriction on specific types and quantities. Food packages should have clear and nonremovable labels that include the names of stakeholders except for the passengers' food. Imported foods should enclose documents issued by the producer/manufacturer in the country of origin. The documents must provide full details of the imported foods.

The UAE is a signatory to the WTO SPS Agreement, which sets provisions on how governments can apply food safety and animal and plant health measures. In 2020, the Ministry of Food Security launched a national Food Security strategy with support from local authorities in each Emirate. The efforts to enhance food security through strengthening local production, improving trade, investing in technology, and reducing food waste have been further accelerated during the coronavirus pandemic. Today, the risk management system to control food safety risks of locally produced and imported food has been substantially modernized. The UAE has invested in upgrading food analysis laboratory techniques, introduced new methods and equipment/instruments for rapid testing of food pathogens, and new software programs to manage the food samples being analyzed and communicate the results. Updates on food safety laws and regulations can be found on the Ministry of Climate Change and Environment's website.

Within the UAE local entities have additional procedures to ensure food safety. Abu Dhabi Agriculture and Food Safety Authority ensures food safety in the emirate of Abu Dhabi and guarantees that the food is fit for human consumption. It also conducts the necessary research and studies on safe food and issue rules, regulations and standards on food items sold or offered for human consumption. The Department of Health, Abu Dhabi publishes a list of adulterated products. In the emirates of Dubai and Sharjah, food safety falls under the scope of the respective municipal authorities. Municipalities oversee food safety requirements and ensure that products have correct labels and expiry dates for consumption. The staff of the municipalities conduct random inspections of all foods and food products available in supermarkets or retail chain stores and within restaurants, food catering premises to ensure the quality of foods and guarantee the safety of foods being suitable for human consumption. The Department of Health, Abu Dhabi also conducts analyses for other emirates, including Ras Al Khaimah (RAK), Ajman, Fujairah, and UAQ municipalities. Recently, Abu Dhabi has been active in initiating risk assessment programs with the FAO's support and providing tips for safe food; RAK released a new set of requirements for food businesses, which serve as a reference guide for practices in food safety. Dubai has a food code and has specifically made major investments in technology. Dubai has gone fully digitalized in managing its food safety programs and services and registering food businesses. All registration of food items passes through an integrated digital portal that can trace all foods back to importers (based on a Food Traceability approach).

Additionally, every food business can manage its food safety system entirely online. To enhance compliance, a revised training program has been launched for food handlers and managers, such as designated person-in-charge with E-learning options made available free for all users. Moreover, Dubai made significant changes in the testing of goods at the port of entry and adjusted the testing requirements based on 12 years of monitoring data, which brought down food sampling to 80%. Testing for verification of processes will continue in place.

8.5.8 Yemen

Yemen, the poorest country in the Arab world, has been embroiled in conflict since early 2015, with nearly 10 million Yemenis are acutely food insecure (WFP, 2020). It is currently suffering the worst humanitarian crisis in the world (World Bank, 2021). Fighting has devastated its economy, leading to food insecurity, verging on famine, and destroying critical infrastructure. Since 2015 following 6 years of conflict, the value of food imports has risen sharply from <20% to 200% because the infrastructure has been incapable of supporting the populations' food needs, with malnutrition present for much of the population. The UN has estimated that 24.3 million people in

2020 were "at-risk" of hunger and disease. In February, the World for Food Program reached over 273,000 beneficiaries with cash transfers to participate in food assistance for assets (WFP, 2021). New activities for over 6000 new participants started in Hajjah and Sana'a governorates. This brings the total of active sites to 410, including rural road rehabilitation, water harvesting schemes, and agricultural projects. Tandon and Vishwanath (2020) demonstrated that violence could affect supply chains and impact food security beyond the location where the violence occurs. Specifically, the geographic location of violence has been used to target food assistance during the active conflict.

Nevertheless, there are structures in place to promote food safety. In 2010, a National Committee was created in Yemen to be responsible for food safety (FAO, 2019a), consumer protection, food production control, organizing and unifying all the activities and the executive decrees related to food safety. This committee is set to create a solid relationship between all the interested bodies, individuals, and Codex's international organization (FAO, 2018). The committee aims to achieve the following: (1) responsible for developing food laws to protect the consumer and oversee food producers, including auditing their performance. (2) Organizing and unifying all the activities and the executive decrees related to food safety. (3) Creation of a strong relationship between all the interested bodies and individuals in Yemen and the international food organization, such as Codex Alimentarius.

Yemen is a member of the GSO and conducts safety assessment by the National Commission to regulate food safety in consultation with all relevant authorities and to include estimates of studies on the potential for adverse effects and food allergies and regulation of genetically modified food. However, little oversight is probably being done today, and this is mainly due to the ongoing conflict over the last years.

Some provisions of the Republican decree of law No. 38 of 1992 regarding food control and regulation of its trade were amended by law No. (13) of 2002 (FAOLEX, 2002). Nonetheless, while Yemen has food laws, they are not sufficiently applied to locally produced and consumed foods, rather directed toward controlling imported and exported foods. The fisheries sector represents a great advantage to Yemen for contributing to global trade. In recent years, Yemen has intensified its efforts to integrate into the international trade system and join the WTO. To benefit from the trade, it has also recognized that it has to focus on exports to access the lucrative global markets. Today, Yemen is a member of the WTO since 2014 and is represented in the Gulf states as a GSO member. The Gulf Standardization and regulation of genetically modified food occur at the Gulf countries level and conduct safety assessment by the National Commission to regulate food safety in consultation with all relevant authorities (FAO, 2018).

However, several non-tariff barriers exist to access the profitable markets in the EU and United States, mainly stemming from ever more stringent product quality standards Standard and Trade Development Facility and Yemeni Seafood Exporters Association (STDF/YSEA, 2010). Three main issues represent main challenges to trade with the EU:

- EU standards for SPS measures;
- EU legislation on residue levels and heavy metals in fishery products; and
- EU legislation on labeling and traceability.

Considerable efforts were made by the development agencies, notably the World Bank, the International Development Association and Integrated Framework, to improve public sector capacity and help Yemen overcome these hurdles. Recognizing the private sector's need for technical support, the Standards and Trade Development Facility has been tasked with improving the capacity of private and public sector organizations involved in trade development through the project "Improving Capacity for Ensuring the Quality of Yemeni Seafood Products." This project focused on improving the private sector processing capacity and delivering safe and high-quality products to regional and international markets (STDF/YSEA, 2010).

Yemeni Seafood Exporters Association (YSEA) is an organization formally established in February 2005 to enable the weaker producers to meet the European markets' exacting standards, improve the quality of their production, and raise the overall expectations of Yemeni fish production. To overcome these barriers, a trust fund was established in 2002 by FAO, OIE, World Bank, WHO, and the WTO to enhance their expertise and capacity to analyze and implement international SPS standards food safety. The project focuses on developing the YSEA's capacity to deliver safer and higher quality products by influencing the activities and practices of its members. In addition to YSEA, the project will also enhance the capacity of the Ministry of Fish Wealth in several areas, including (1) risk assessment, (2) product quality development and inspection, (3) training needs assessment, and (4) regulatory frameworks governing access to key overseas markets (STDF/YSEA, 2010).

8.6 General synopsis and conclusion

Most Arab countries in the Middle East have initiated upgrades to their existing legislation and regulations or have reformed their food laws. Along with the institutional and organization's restructuring, it is expected that the level of compliance with the food safety measures and effectiveness of food control systems would rise. However, there is limited information on the outcomes since governments have initiated reforms to their food laws or transitioned into a single authority. In comparing the different countries' regulatory framework, governments responses to food safety challenges are variables in pace and approaches as influenced by the availability of technical assistance, resources, funds, national plan, and supportive environment.

There is a glaring disparity in the regulatory structure and the coordination mechanism between the GCC countries and other Arab countries of the Middle East, with Jordan being an exception. Like UAE, Jordan made significant and fast progress in modernizing its control system and shifting toward a science-based risk management approach. In contrast, in some countries, such as Lebanon, Syria, Iraq, and Palestine, despite the positive changes and varying degrees of building capacities, their national food control systems are inconsistent with the current global food production developments and international requirements. These countries' progress is seemingly hindered by the fragmentation of the regulatory framework, governments' inability to implement their policies and enforce amended laws, limited resources, and internal conflicts. All this will compromise the effectiveness of law enforcement and control measures.

In general, compared to domestic food products sold for local consumers, strict controls over those destined for exports have accentuated in Arab countries, mainly in low- and middle-income countries (e.g., Yemen, Egypt, Lebanon, Syria), where efforts are intensified with international donors' supports to improve their systems and comply with international food safety requirements for expanding food trade opportunities but also for enhancing food security. Simultaneously, little progress has been made to develop food safety policies and enforce a risk-based approach whereby the safety of products traded locally should also be prioritized.

The implementation of risk-based and preventive food safety systems is generally voluntary and still far from being addressed in regulating the safety of the locally sold foods (e.g., Syria, Lebanon, Egypt, Palestine). In Oman, UAE, and Yemen, their implementation becomes essential and de-facto-mandatory to access international markets. At the same time, Egypt and the GCC countries rolled out their new science-based import control systems and clearance procedures based on potential risks to consumers considering the emerging food safety risks that may be introduced through the global food supply.

Notwithstanding the significant steps toward reforming and updating regulations, the national institutions and surveillance laboratories' capacity still needs to be improved. The testing capacities and identification of hazards and risk profiling are crucial for preventing foodborne diseases and developing national risk-based control strategies. While the whole-genome sequencing is used in epidemiological investigations of foodborne outbreaks to identify and characterize pathogens, it is still not a standard tool or used in many countries, including the Middle East, due to limited skills or resources (Faour-Klingbeil & Todd, 2019).

Continued efforts are needed to leverage food safety and consumer protection in the Arab countries through laws and regulations established based on the current scientific understanding and monitoring hazards and implementation of systems. While upgraded laws and legislations are necessary, they would be of little value when not complemented with governmental support and commitment to enact and implement them. Arab countries can benefit from the successful experience of others in modernizing their systems and leveraging the interregional coordination in their food safety policies. They can make effective use of the Codex standards, guidelines, and code of practice to adapt their national legislation.

Recently, the Arab Food Safety Initiative for Trade Facilitation funded by the Swedish International Development Cooperation Agency was launched to enhance regional trade capacity in food commodities and create an advanced food safety environment in the Arab region. To this end, the project is implemented to strengthen the conformity assessment systems for food safety in joint regional-international cooperation through the General Secretariat of the League of Arab States and technical support from the UNIDO (United Nations Industrial Development Organization). A team of representatives of organizations, ministries, and agencies involved in food safety in the member states of the League of Arab States within the agreement of "Facilitating and developing trade exchange between Arab countries" is formed to provide technical advice to each of the League of Arab States, the Arab Organization for Industrial Development and Mining, and the Arab Organization for Agricultural Development, to reach the coordination and suitability of conformity and food safety assessment systems.

In this context, representatives of Arab regulatory agencies (e.g., Saudi Arabia, Morocco, Lebanon, Sudan, Egypt, and Kuwait) emphasized the importance:

- to enhance collaboration between Arab and international food safety regulators, as well as sustaining capacity building efforts,
- to improve the food regulatory system in the Arab region and maintain and work toward progressing the convergence of food safety regulatory measures adopted by Arab food regulators,
- to establish effective communication with regional and international partners, represented by the FAO and the Codex Working Groups.

Regulating food products' safety requires laws and regulations to be updated based on risk analysis and current scientific understanding of the transmission mechanisms of food hazards, and root cause analysis. Hence, it is of significant relevance for the public sector in the Arab countries to foster communication between the scientific communities and the regulatory authorities, and food industry to foster research and develop a scientific database for initiating and advancing regional risk assessment studies, practical and reasonable food safety policies and risk management strategies.

Globalization means food commodities can be shared throughout the world but to do so requires sufficient safety standards for consumer confidence in these products. One example of preventive control is specified in the FSMA. These mandates apply to food manufacturing plants and the value chain product as an integrated policies within the country and from other countries exporting to the United States. These require (1) a written food safety plan; (2) a hazard analysis; (3) preventive controls; (4) monitoring of the operation for hazards; (5) have corrective actions in place; (6) verification of these actions; and (7) keeping secure associated records. Arab countries in the business of exporting local-produced foods need to comply with all of the aforementioned requirements and also other mandatory international regulations, such as the nutritional labeling requirements, EU or US pesticides Acts, food additives regulations, etc., or they may risk in losing a share in the global food market.

Acknowledgment

We thank Mr. Bobby Krishna (Senior Specialist, Food Permit Control Section, Food Safety Department Dubai Municipality) for his valuable inputs and appreciated the information on the recent developments in the United Arab of Emirates.

References

Al-Busaidi, M. A., & Jukes, D. J. (2015). Assessment of the food control systems in the Sultanate of Oman. *Food Control, 51*, 55–69. Available from https://doi.org/10.1016/j.foodcont.2014.10.039.

Aliqtisadi (2011). *Syria officially begins implementing the Food Safety Law: Multiple regulatory authorities*. https://aliqtisadi.com/79024-%d8%b3%d9%88%d8%b1%d9%8a%d8%a9-%d8%aa%d8%a8%d8%af%d8%a3-%d8%b1%d8%b3%d9%85%d9%8a%d8%a7%d9%8b-%d8%aa%d8%b7%d8%a8%d9%8a%d9%82-%d9%82%d8%a7%d9%86%d9%88%d9%86-%d8%b3%d9%84%d8%a7%d9%85%d8%a9-%d8%a7%d9%84/. Accessed 11.01.21.

AlJaml (2008). *Al-Assad issues Law 19 related to food safety to ensure hygiene and quality of food*. https://aljaml.com/%D8%A7%D9%84%D8%A3%D8%B3%D8%AF%20%D9%8A%D8%B5%D8%AF%D8%B1%D8%A7%D9%84%D9%82%D8%A7%D9%86%D9%88%D9%86%2019%20%D8%A7%D9%84%D9%85%D8%AA%D8%B9%D9%84%D9%82%20%D8%A8%D8%B3%D9%84%D8%A7%D9%85%D8%A9%20%D8%A7%D9%84%D8%BA%D8%B0%D8%A7%D8%A1%20%D9%84%D8%B6%D9%85%D8%A7%D9%86%20%D8%B5%D8%AD%D9%8A%D8%A9%20%D9%88%D8%AC%D9%88%D8%AF%D8%A9%20%D8%A7%D9%84%D8%A3%D8%BA%D8%B0%D9%8A%D8%A9. Accessed 11.01.21.

Al-Kandari, D., & Jukes, D. J. (2009). A situation analysis of the food control systems in Arab Gulf Cooperation Council (GCC) countries. *Food Control, 20*(12), 1112–1118. Available from https://doi.org/10.1016/j.foodcont.2009.02.012.

Al-Kandari, D., & Jukes, D. J. (2011). Incorporating HACCP into national food control systems—Analyzing progress in the United Arab Emirates. *Food Control, 22*(6), 851–861. Available from https://doi.org/10.1016/j.foodcont.2010.10.013.

Al-Kandari, D., & Jukes, D. J. (2012). The food control system in Saudi Arabia – Centralizing food control activities. *Food Control, 28*(1), 33–46. Available from https://doi.org/10.1016/j.foodcont.2012.03.030.

Al-Khamees, N. A. (2007). Food safety knowledge and reported behaviour of university students in Kuwait. *International Journal of Health Promotion and Education, 45*(3), 93–99. Available from https://doi.org/10.1080/14635240.2007.10708110.

Al-Mazeedi, H. M., Abbas, A. B., Al-Jouhar, W. Y., Al-Mufty, S. A., & Al-Mendicar, Y. A. (2015). Food safety review in the State of Kuwait as a part of Arab Gulf Area. *International Journal of Food Safety, Nutrition and Public Health*, https://agris.fao.org/agris-search/search.do?recordID = United States201800173509.

Alomirah, H., Al-Zenki, S., Sawaya, W. N., Jabsheh, F., Husain, A., Al-Mazeedi, H. M., Al-Kandari, D., & Jukes, D. (2010). Assessment of the food control system in the State of Kuwait. *Food Control*, *21*(4), 496–504. Available from https://doi.org/10.1016/j.foodcont.2009.07.015.

Alrobaish, W. S., Vlerick, P., Luning, P. A., & Jacxsens, L. (2021). Food safety governance in Saudi Arabia: Challenges in control of imported food. *J Food Sci*, *86*(1), 16–30. Available from https://doi.org/10.1111/1750-3841.15552, Epub 2020 Dec 13. PMID: 33314129.

Anonymous (2015). *New alarm over "unhealthy" food in Bahrain*. TradeArabia News Service. http://www.tradearabia.com/news/HEAL_279164.html. Accessed 20.04.21.

Arab Development Portal (2020). *Trade*. Arab Development Portal. https://www.arabdevelopmentportal.com/indicator/trade. Accessed 16.02.21.

Bahrain Ministry of Health (2014). *Public health annual report*. https://www.google.com/url?sa = t&rct = j&q = &esrc = s&source = web&cd = &cad = rja&uact = 8&ved = 2ahUKEwioydv_86PwAhWLsaQKHRYHDp4QFjAAegQIAxAD&url = https%3A%2F%2Fhttp://www.moh.gov.bh%2FContent%2FFiles%2FPublications%2FX_635906124344978750.pdf&usg = AOvVaw2OSkwL3cGLaWS14afGJUVL. Accessed 20.04.21.

Baig, M. B., Al-Zahrani, K. H., Schneider, F., Straquadine, G. S., & Mourad, M. (2019). Food waste posing a serious threat to sustainability in the Kingdom of Saudi Arabia – A systematic review. *Saudi Journal of Biological Sciences*, *26*(7), 1743–1752. Available from https://doi.org/10.1016/j.sjbs.2018.06.004.

Brunel, C. (2009). Morocco-EU trade relations. In Capitalizing on the Morocco-United States Free Trade Agreement: A road map for success. Peterson Institute for International Economics. https://www.piie.com/bookstore/capitalizing-morocco-us-free-trade-agreement-road-map-success.

Busaidi, M. A. (2017). *Effective seafood safety and quality management systems: An analysis of the situation in the Sultanate of Oman*. University of Reading Department of Food and Nutritional Sciences.

CCAG (2015). *GCC guide for control on imported foods*. The Cooperation Council For The Arab States Of The Gulf Secretariat General. JFDA.

CCIB (2012). *The impact of ministerial decision 950/1 on food and beverages producers in Lebanon* (p. 96). Chamber of Commerce, Industry and Agriculture of Beirut and Mount Lebanon. http://www.ccib.org.lb/uploads/RIA%20Food%20Safety.pdf. Accessed 25.03.21.

Cooperation Council for the Arab States of Gulf (2016). *GCC guide for control on imported foods*. The Cooperation Council for the Arab States of the Gulf. https://www.gcc-sg.org/en-us/CognitiveSources/DigitalLibrary/Lists/DigitalLibrary/Agriculture%20Livestock%20and%20Fisheries/1429075065.pdf. Accessed 17.02.21.

Cortas, A. (2017). The food safety law in Lebanon: What is next? *Advanced Techniques in Clinical Microbiology*, *1*(3). Available from http://www.imedpub.com/articles/the-food-safety-law-in-lebanon-what-is-next.php?aid = 19933.

Cortas, A. (2018). A training program in food safety in Lebanon. *International Journal of Clinical Nutrition & Dietetics*, *2018*. Available from https://doi.org/10.15344/2456-8171/2018/130.

CSPI (2005). *Global & local: Food safety around the world* (p. 95). Center for Science in the Public Interest. https://www.cspinet.org/resource/global-local-food-safety-around-world. Accessed 20.03.21.

EC (2019). *Final report of an audit carried out in Egypt from 28 January 2019 to 07 February 2019 in order to evaluate the systems in place to control microbiological contamination in food of non-animal origin intended for export to the European Union (DG(SANTE) 2019-6697)*. European Commission, Directorate-general for health and food safety. https://ec.europa.eu/food/audits-analysis/act_getPDF.cfm?PDF_ID = 14389. Accessed 17.02.21.

El Haddad, G. F., Soliman, I., Mashhour, A., Gaber, M., Ait El Mekki, A., El Hindi, A., … Cagatay, S. (2011). *A review of the national and international agro-food policies and institutions in the Mediterranean Region* [MPRA Paper]. https://mpra.ub.uni-muenchen.de/66801/.

El Sheikha, A. F. (2015). Food safety issues in Saudi Arabia. *Nutrition and Food Technology: Open Access*, *1*, 1, https://www.sciforschenonline.org/journals/nutrition-food/NFTOA-1–103.php.

ElAddad, B. (2011). *Food security and food safety in Iraq*. الحوار المتمدن. http://www.ahewar.org/debat/show.art.asp?aid = 282930.

El-Jardali, F., Hammoud, R., Kamleh, R., & Jurdi, M. (2014). *K2P briefing note: Protecting consumers in Lebanon: The need for effective food safety system*. Knowledge to Policy (K2P) Center, Beirut, Lebanon. https://www.google.com/url?sa = t&rct = j&q = &esrc = s&source = web&cd = 2&ved = 2ahUKEwiundqL2bDlAhVNLpoKHS6cAisQFjABegQIABAC&url = https%3A%2F%2Fhttp://www.aub.edu.lb%2Fk2p%2FDocuments%2FK2P%2520BN%2520Food%2520Safety%2520English.pdf&usg = AOvVaw0rSe7JKiMN1T48O6FKW79N.

Eltai, N. O., El-Obeid, T., Kassem, I. I., & Yassine, H. M. (2018). *Food regulations and enforcement in Qatar. Reference module in food science*. Elsevier, https://doi.org/10.1016/B978-0-08-100596-5.22478-5.

Ercsey-Ravasz, M., Toroczkai, Z., Lakner, Z., & Baranyi, J. (2012). Complexity of the international agro-food trade network and its impact on food safety. *PLoS One*, *7*(5), e37810. Available from https://doi.org/10.1371/journal.pone.0037810.

European Commission (2016). *General food law* [Text]. Food Safety - European Commission. https://ec.europa.eu/food/safety/general_food_law_en. Accessed 16.02.21.

FAO (2004a). *Food safety and international trade in the near East region—Twenty-seventh FAO regional conference for the near East* (NERC/04/5). http://www.fao.org/3/J1653e/J1653e.htm. Accessed 17.02.21.

FAO (2004b). *The joint FAO/WHO second global forum of food safety regulators*. http://www.fao.org/3/ae018a/ae018a.htm.

FAO (2005). *Voluntary guidelines to support the progressive realization of the right to adequate food in the context of national food security*. Food and Agriculture Organization of the United Nations, Rome. http://www.fao.org/3/y7937e/y7937e00.htm. Accessed 17.02.21.

FAO (2013). *Strengthening production and marketing of Lebanese Agriculture*. http://www.fao.org/neareast/news/view/en/c/260208/. Accessed 17.02.21.

FAO (2018). *Food safety and quality: Yemen*. FAO GM Foods Platform. http://www.fao.org/food/food-safety-quality/gm-foods-platform/browse-information-by/country/country-page/en/?cty = YEM. Accessed 17.02.21.

FAO (2019a). *FAOSTAT Yemen*. Food and Agriculture Organization of the United Nations. http://www.fao.org/faostat/en/#country/249. Accessed 17.02.21.

FAO (2019b). *Food safety and quality: Risk analysis*. http://www.fao.org/food/food-safety-quality/capacity-development/risk-analysis/en/. Accessed 17.02.21.

FAO/ESCWA (2017). *Arab Horizon 2030: Prospects for enhancing food security in the Arab Region. Technical summary. Policy support and governance*. Food and Agriculture Organization of the United Nations/ Economic and Social Commission for Western Asia.

http://www.fao.org/policy-support/tools-and-publications/resources-details/en/c/1300341/. Accessed 17.02.21.

FAO/WHO (2003). *Assuring food safety and quality: Guidelines for strengthening national food control systems.* http://www.wpro.who.int/foodsafety/documents/docs/English_Guidelines_Food_control.pdf. Accessed 17.02.21.

FAOLEX (n.d.). *FAOLEX Database—Egypt*. Food and Agriculture Organization of the United Nations. Retrieved February 18, 2021, from http://www.fao.org/faolex/country-profiles/general-profile/en/?iso3 = EGY. Accessed 17.02.21.

FAOLEX (2002). *FAOLEX database—Yemen*. http://www.fao.org/faolex/results/details/en/c/LEX-FAOC046685. Accessed 17.02.21.

Faour-Klingbeil, D. (2017). *Chapter 4. The role of inequity and political incoherence as primary risk factors for food safety—A focus on the fresh produce chain. Thesis: The Microbiological Safety of Fresh Produce in Lebanon- A holistic "farm-to-fork chain" approach to evaluate food safety, compliance levels and underlying risk factors* [Thesis, University of Plymouth]. https://pearl.plymouth.ac.uk/handle/10026.1/8654.

Faour-Klingbeil, D., & Todd, E. C. D. (2018). A review on the rising prevalence of international standards: Threats or opportunities for the agri-food produce sector in developing countries, with a focus on examples from the MENA region. *Foods (Basel, Switzerland), 7*(3). Available from https://doi.org/10.3390/foods7030033.

Faour-Klingbeil, D., & Todd, E. C. D. (2019). Prevention and control of foodborne diseases in Middle-East North African countries: Review of national control systems. *International Journal of Environmental Research and Public Health, 17*(1). Available from https://doi.org/10.3390/ijerph17010070.

Farag, E., Garcell, H. G., Ganesan, N., Ahmed, S. N. N., Al-Hajri, M., Al Thani, S. M. H. J., ... Al-Romaihi, H. E. (2016). A retrospective epidemiological study on the incidence of salmonellosis in the State of Qatar during 2004–2012. *Qatar Medical Journal, 2016*(1). Available from https://doi.org/10.5339/qmj.2016.3.

GAIN (2011). *Food and agricultural import regulations and standards—Iraq* (p. 26) [FAIRS Country Report]. USDA - Global Agricultural Information Network. https://gain.fas.usda.gov/Recent%20GAIN%20Publications/Iraq%20FAIRS%20Report%202011_Baghdad_Iraq_3-24-2011.pdf. Accessed 25.03.21.

GAIN (2012). *Food and agricultural import regulations and standards—Bahrain* [FAIRS Annual Country Report]. USDA - Global Agricultural Information Network. Food and Agricultural Import Regulations and Standards - Narrative_Dubai_Bahrain_6–20-2012.pdf (apeda.gov.in). Accessed 20.04.21.

GAIN (2014). *Food and agricultural import regulations and standards -Saudi Arabia* [FAIRS Annual Country Report]. USDA - Global Agricultural Information Network. https://apps.fas.usda.gov/newgainapi/api/report/downloadreportbyfilename?filename = Food%20and%20Agricultural%20Import%20Regulations%20and%20Standards%20-%20Narrative_Riyadh_Saudi%20Arabia_9-25-2014.pdf. Accessed 19.04.21.

GAIN (2017). *Food and agricultural import regulations and standards—Narrative—Jordan* (FAIRS Annual Country Report No. JO160015). USDA - Global Agricultural Information Network. Accessed 29.04.21.

GAIN (2020). *Food and agricultural import regulations and standards country report—Egypt* (FAIRS Annual Country Report No. EG2019-0025; p. 27). USDA - Global Agricultural Information Network. https://apps.fas.usda.gov/newgainapi/api/Report/DownloadReportByFileName?fileName = Food%20and%20Agricultural%20Import%20Regulations%20and%20Standards%20Country%20Report_Cairo_Egypt_12–31-2019. Accessed 18.02.21.

GAIN (2021). *Food and agricultural import regulations and standards—Jordan* (FAIRS Annual Country Report No. JO2020-0019; p. 9). USDA - Global Agricultural Information Network. https://apps.fas.usda.gov/newgainapi/api/Report/DownloadReportByFileName?fileName = Food%20and%20Agricultural%20Import%20Regulations%20and%20Standards%20Country%20Report_Amman_Jordan_12-31-2020. Accessed 25.03.21.

GOEIC (n.d.). *General organization for export and import control.* https://www.goeic.gov.eg/en/documents/default/category/id/4/m/6-35. Accessed 18.02.21.

GSO (2018). *Conformity assessment scheme.* GCC Standardization Organization. https://www.gso.org.sa/en/conformity/gcc-conformity-assessment-scheme/ Accessed 17.02.21.

Gulf News (2003). *Unified GCC food safety laws to be discussed in Muscat.* https://gulfnews.com/uae/unified-gcc-food-safety-laws-to-be-discussed-in-muscat-1.345841. Accessed 17.02.21.

Hasan, T. K., & Gheni, N. S. (2011). *Suggested plan for national food safety policy for Iraq.* Ministry of Planning/Ministry of Health/ Minsitry of Trade/Ministry of Agriculture, https://www.slideshare.net/talal953/food-safety-policy-of-iraq.

Hufbauer, G. C., & Brunel, C. (2009). *Capitalizing on the Morocco-United States Free Trade Agreement: A road map for success. Peterson institute press: All Books.* Peterson Institute for International Economics, https://ideas.repec.org/b/iie/ppress/pa88.html.

Ibrahim, N. A., & Abdel-Haleem, A. M. H. (2016). Food regulations and enforcement in Egypt. *Reference Module in Food Sciences*, 1–6. Available from https://doi.org/10.1016/B978-0-08-100596-5.21188-8.

Irani, Z., Sharif, A. M., Lee, H., Aktas, E., Topaloğlu, Z., van't Wout, T., & Huda, S. (2018). Managing food security through food waste and loss: Small data to big data. *Computers & Operations Research*, *98*, 367–383. Available from https://doi.org/10.1016/j.cor.2017.10.007.

Jia, C., & Jukes, D. (2013). The national food safety control system of China – A systematic review. *Food Control*, *32*(1), 236–245. Available from https://doi.org/10.1016/j.foodcont.2012.11.042.

Karch, H., Denamur, E., Dobrindt, U., Finlay, B. B., Hengge, R., Johannes, L., Ron, E. Z., Tønjum, T., Sansonetti, P. J., & Vicente, M. (2012). The enemy within us: lessons from the 2011 European *Escherichia coli* O104:H4 outbreak. *EMBO Mol Med*, *4*(9), 841–848. Available from https://doi.org/10.1002/emmm.201201662, PubMed.

KUNA (2019). *The Kuwaiti National Assembly approves the draft law (the Food Authority).* https://www.kuna.net.kw/ArticleDetails.aspx?id = 2783358. Accessed 11.01.21.

Land O'Lakes, (2018). International Development awarded funds for new capacity building, food safety projects. Press releases. Washington, D.C. (October 8, 2018). https://www.landolakesinc.com/Press/News/International-Development-Awarded-Projects.

MAS (2013). *Final report round table discussion (5) Consumer Protections in Palestine in the Food Sector* (p. 8). Palestine Economic Policy Research Institute. https://www.mas.ps/download.php?id = 47f9ay294810Y47f9a. Accessed 03.04.21.

MAS (2017). *Strategic review of food and nutrition security in Palestine* (p. 108). Palestine Economic Policy Research Institute. https://www.un.org/unispal/wp-content/uploads/2018/02/WFPREV_140218.pdf. Accessed 04.04.21.

Matsuo, M. (2013). Restructuring Japanese food safety governance: Institutional changes and future challenges. *European Food and Feed Law Review*, *8*(4), 250–258, https://effl.lexxion.eu/article/EFFL/2013/4/247.

Ministry of Public Health (2021). *Public health strategy 2017 – 2022.* Ministry of Public Health in Qatar. https://www.moph.gov.qa/english/strategies/Supporting-Strategies-and-Frameworks/QatarPublicHealthStrategy/Pages/Food-Safety.aspx. Accessed 27.04.21.

MJLA (2019). *Royal Decree 24/2019 establishing the Centre for Food Safety and quality in the Ministry of Regional municipalities and water resources*. Ministry of Regional Municipalities and Water Resources. https://mjla.gov.om/eng/legislation/decrees/details.aspx?Id = 554&type = L Accessed 17.02.21.

Moore, J. C., Spink, J., & Lipp, M. (2012). Development and Application of a Database of Food Ingredient Fraud and Economically Motivated Adulteration from 1980 to 2010. *Journal of Food Science*, *77*(4), R118–R126. Available from https://doi.org/10.1111/j.1750-3841.2012.02657.x.

NFSA (2020). *NFSA's modernization of Egypt's food import control system*. The National Food Safety Authority. https://www.nfsa.gov.eg/Images/App_PP/DeskTop/App_Web/1/MyWebMedia/PDF/English%20Import%20Control%20Strategy.pdf. Accessed 16.02.21.

OHCHR (2010). *Fact sheet no. 34, The right to adequate food* (Human Rights and Fundamental Freedoms I Right to Food I Right to Health ISSN 1014-5567 No.34; p. 57). UN Office of the High Commissioner for Human Rights (OHCHR). http://www.fao.org/right-to-food/resources/resources-detail/en/c/49338/ Accessed 08.02.21.

Ragona, M., & Mazzocchi, M. (2008). Measuring the impacts of food safety regulations: A methodological review. In *2008 International congress, August 26-29, 2008, Ghent, Belgium* (No. 43864; 2008 International Congress, August 26-29, 2008, Ghent, Belgium). European Association of Agricultural Economists. https://ideas.repec.org/p/ags/eaae08/43864.html.

SAMA News (2019). *The Ministry of Economy organizes a workshop to control food safety*. سما الإخبارية. https://samanews.ps/ar/post/389461. Accessed 11.01.21.

SFDA (2015). *GRASF*. Saudi Food and Drug Authority. https://grasf.sfda.gov.sa/ Accessed 17.02.21.

STDF/YSEA (2010). *Improved capacity for ensuring the quality and safety of Yemeni seafood products- STDF 69 Final Report* (Project STDF 69 WTO-YSEA; p. 31). Standard and Trade Development Facility / Yemeni Seafood Exporters Association. https://www.standardsfacility.org/sites/default/files/STDF_PG_69_Final_Report_2009.pdf Accessed 18.02.21.

Syriandays (2021). *The Food Safety Law guarantees the quality of food produced in accordance with national and international standards*. http://syriandays.com/?page = show_det&select_page = 57&id = 17190 Accessed 11.01.21.

Tandon, S., & Vishwanath, T. (2020). The evolution of poor food access over the course of the conflict in Yemen. *World Development*, *130*, 104922. Available from https://doi.org/10.1016/j.worlddev.2020.104922.

The Official Portal of the UAE Government. (n.d.). *Food safety*. The Official Portal of the UAE Government. https://u.ae/en/information-and-services/health-and-fitness/food-safety-and-health-tips. Accessed 27.04.21.

Torayeh, N. M. (2013). The competitiveness of the Egyptian agricultural export in the EU market; should Egypt diversify its trade pattern? *Applied Econometrics and International Development*, *13*(2), 129–148. https://ideas.repec.org/a/eaa/aeinde/v13y2013i2_10.html.

UNIC (2018). *A strong representation of NFSA and SAFE in DIFSC 2018*. United Nations Information Centre in Cairo. http://www.unic-eg.org/eng/?p = 29216. Accessed 17.02.21.

UNIDO (2017). *STDF working group meeting, SPS related UNIDO project developments October 2016—March 2017*. http://www.standardsfacility.org/sites/default/files/WG_Mar17_UNIDO_Input.pdf. Accessed 17.02.21.

USP (2016). *Food fraud mitigation guidance* (p. 40) [Appendix XVII / General Tests and Assays]. The United States Pharmacopeial Convention. https://www.usp.org/sites/default/files/usp/document/our-work/Foods/food-fraud-mitigation-guidance.pdf. Accessed 02.04.21.

WFP (2018). *WFP and Egyptian government join efforts to enhance food safety in Egypt*. World Food Programme. https://www.wfp.org/news/wfp-and-egyptian-government-join-efforts-enhance-food-safety-egypt. Accessed 17.02.21.

WFP (2020). *WFP Yemen Country Brief*. World Food Programme. https://www.wfp.org/countries/yemen. Accessed 18.02.21.

WFP (2021). *Yemen Situation Report #2*. World Food Programme. https://www.wfp.org/publications/yemen-0 Accessed 27.04.21.

WHO (2001). *Report on the regional workshop on new challenges in food safety: The regional action plan*. Dubai, United Arab Emirates, 5-7 December 1999. WHO IRIS. https://apps.who.int/iris/handle/10665/254799. Accessed 11.02.21.

WHO (2015). *WHO estimates of the global burden of foodborne diseases: Foodborne disease burden epidemiology reference group 2007-2015* (ISBN 978 92 4 156516 5). https://www.who.int/foodsafety/foodborne_disease/ferg/en/ Accessed 11.02.21.

WHO (2019). *Joint statement by FAO, WHO and WTO International Forum on food safety and trade*. World Health Organization, Geneva, Switzerland. https://www.who.int/docs/default-source/resources/joint-statement.pdf?sfvrsn = 61b890c4_16 Accessed 02.02.21.

WHO (2021). *FAO and WHO mark World Food Safety Day in Iraq under the theme "Food safety, everyone's business."* http://www.emro.who.int/irq/iraq-news/fao-and-who-mark-world-food-safety-day-in-iraq-under-the-theme-qfood-safety-everyones-businessq.html Accessed 29.03.21.

WHO EMRO (2019). *FAO and WHO mark world food safety day in Iraq under the theme "Food safety, everyone's business."* WHO Regional Office for the Mediterranean. https://www.emro.who.int/irq/iraq-news/fao-and-who-mark-world-food-safety-day-in-iraq-under-the-theme-qfood-safety-everyones-businessq.html Accessed 03.04.21.

World Bank (2021). *The World Bank in Yemen* [Text/HTML]. World Bank. https://www.worldbank.org/en/country/yemen/overview Accessed 27.04.21.

WTO (2020). *High-level dialogue reviews accessions of Arab countries, marks Oman's 20th WTO anniversary*. https://www.wto.org/english/news_e/news20_e/acc_08nov20_e.htm Accessed 10.02.21.

Index

Note: Page numbers followed by "*f*" and "*t*" refer to figures and tables, respectively.

F

G

H

I

J

K

L

FSC
www.fsc.org
MIX
Papier | Fördert gute Waldnutzung
FSC® C083411

Kolibri 360 GmbH
Ferdinand-Jühlke-Straße 7
99095 Erfurt, Deutschland
produktsicherheit@kolibri360.de